Teaching and Learning with Visual Aids

A Resource Manual for Community Health Workers, Health Trainers and Family Planning Workers in Africa and the Middle East

Kathryn A. Fetter, Mari H. Clark, Catherine J. Murphy, and Jo Ella Walters

Educational Materials Unit
Program for International Training in Health (INTRAH)
School of Medicine
University of North Carolina
Chapel Hill, North Carolina

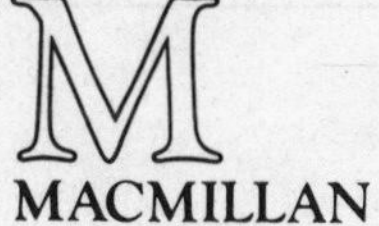

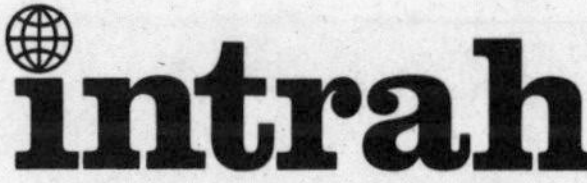

First published 1987
Reprinted 1990 (twice), 1991

Published by MACMILLAN EDUCATION LTD
London and Basingstoke
Associated companies and representatives in Accra, Auckland, Delhi, Dublin, Gaborone, Hamburg, Harare, Hong Kong, Kuala Lumpur, Lagos, Manzini, Melbourne, Mexico City, Nairobi, New York, Singapore, Tokyo

British Library Cataloguing in Publication Data
Teaching and learning with visual aids: a resource manual for family planning trainers and health workers in Africa and the Middle East.
1. Health education—Developing countries —Audio-visual aids
I. Title II. Fetter, Katherine A.
613'.07'8 RA440.55

ISBN 0–333–44815–4

Published in conjunction with Teaching Aids at Low Cost, PO Box 49, St. Albans, Hertfordshire AL1 4AX
TALC received assistance in the production of this book as a low cost edition from the Swedish International Development Authority.

Original material developd by INTRAH under USAID contract AID/DSPE–C–0058, Family Planning Training for Paramedical, Auxiliary and Community (PAC) Personnel.

Contents

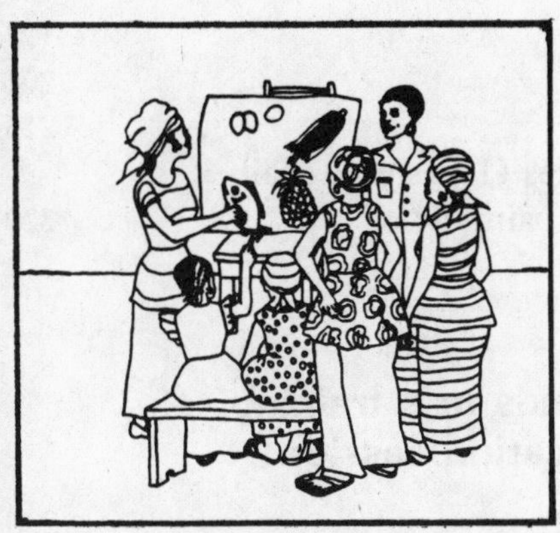

Unit 1 When to use visual aids

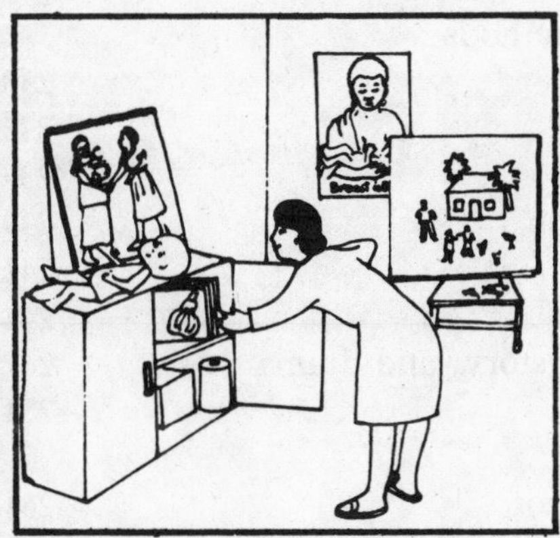

Unit 2 Deciding what kind of visual aid to use

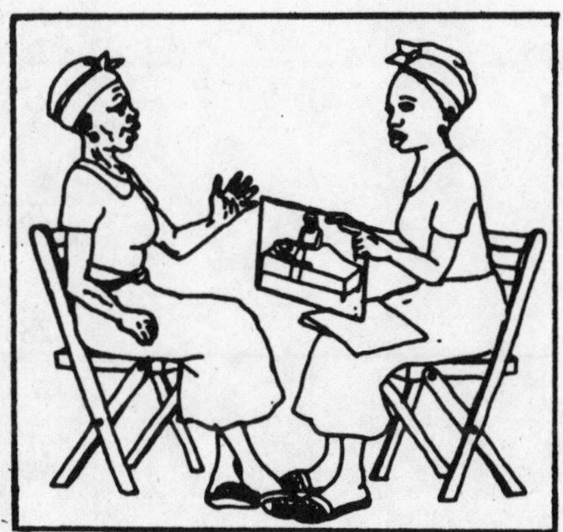

Unit 3 Planning and making your own visual aids

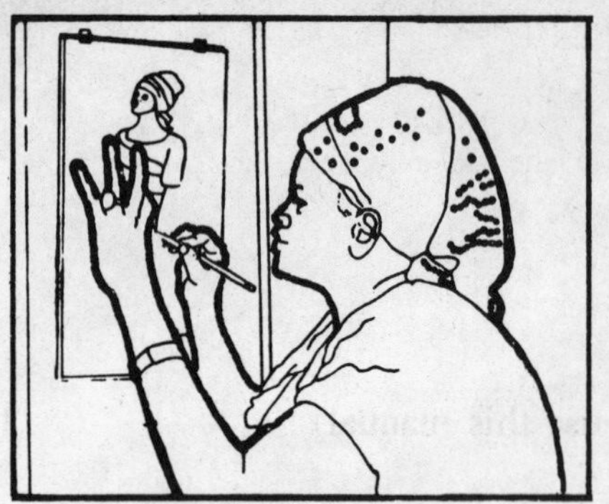

Unit 4 Production skills

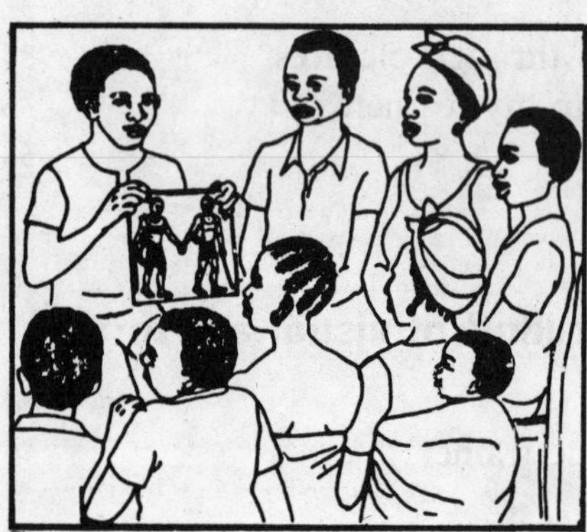

Unit 5 Using visual aids in a training or health education session

Resource pictures

To everyone using this manual

You do not require any background in art or visual aids development to use this manual.

We have designed this manual as a resource book for trainers of nurses, midwives, nutrition workers, health educators, community health workers, family planning motivators, traditional birth attendants, or other health workers in Africa and the Middle East. It can also be used for training community development workers. The trainers we have worked with are usually nurses or nurse-midwives, and many of them have helped us by field-testing parts of the manual in workshops in Kenya, Mali, Morocco, Sierra Leone, and Somalia. The manual is designed for use in pre-service or in-service training.

The manual emphasizes learning by doing and includes many suggestions for ways to actively involve your learners. We encourage you to pick and choose from the ideas and suggestions given in these units and add your own ideas. Use what you can and adapt the information and activities to your own needs and those of your particular learners. The Trainer's Guide at the beginning of the manual contains examples of ways to do this.

Although we have designed this manual for health trainers, we believe that it is basic enough to serve as a useful resource for anyone who wants to improve his or her teaching or communications skills.

Purpose of the manual

The goal of this manual is to introduce both trainers and their learners to the use of visual aids for effective teaching and learning of family health and family planning.

Objectives

A health and family planning trainer or educator who uses this manual as a resource book for his or her own teaching will learn to:

1 Decide when to use visual aids.
2 Choose the kinds of visual aids which will be most useful in a specific situation.
3 Plan and make visual aids (well designed and produced) which are part of a lesson plan.
4 Use visual aids with different teaching methods in training and health and family planning education sessions.

Acknowledgements

We would like to thank the many people who contributed to the development of this manual. We are particularly grateful to Dr Ralph Wileman, Director of the Curriculum in Educational Media and Instructional Design at the University of North Carolina at Chapel Hill. He served as our educational consultant and provided constructive criticism and constant encouragement throughout the past two years of manual development and revision. We are grateful to Dr Martha Brooke for her contributions to the initial development of some of the key ideas and activities, particularly in Units 3 and 4. We thank Elizabeth Edmands and Emily Lewis, public health nurse educators here at INTRAH, who served as consultants in developing the health and family planning content of the manual. The efforts of Pauline Muhuhu and Frank Nabwiso, INTRAH Regional Office representatives in Nairobi, Kenya, have been most valuable in providing information on specific needs of health trainers in African countries and in reviewing drafts of the manual. Participants in INTRAH workshops in Kenya, Mali, Morocco, Sierra Leone and Somalia have helped us with their suggestions for improving the activities in the manual. INTRAH staff and consultants also reviewed parts of the manuscript and contributed ideas during its development. We also thank Patricia Greenfield, Catherine Lindsey and Tony Lunde for their contributions to the artwork. We are grateful to Lynn Igoe for her assistance with the manual editing.

We would also like to recognize the valuable resource materials used to develop this manual. Specific materials are listed in the Bibliography. Particularly useful materials include *Helping Health Workers Learn* by David Werner, *From the Field* developed by World Education, and *Working with Villagers* prepared by the American Home Economics Association.

Trainer's Guide

This manual is about non-electronic, low-cost visual aids that you can make yourself. There are two reasons for making your own visual aids:

1 Visual aids that do not use equipment or electricity are more dependable and can be used in more places than visual aids which depend on electricity.

2 Visual aids that you make yourself are often more effective and interesting to your learners. This is because the symbols used in visual aids must be clear to your learners. A bed does not look the same in every country. Neither do a person's clothes, or a well, or a latrine. It is important that the symbols shown in a visual aid are clear and meaningful to your learners.

Terms used in the manual

Some users of this manual may teach in nursing schools, some may train health workers in clinics, and some may do community health education or motivation. In this book we apply the terms **teaching** and **instruction** to all of these activities. For example the seven teaching questions on which the manual is based (see Unit 2) apply equally well to health training, health education, or motivational activities.

Throughout the manual, we use the term **learner** to refer to the people you teach. These people may be nurse trainers, student nurses, nursing aides, traditional birth attendants, community health workers, villagers, or anyone whom you are teaching.

The term **visual aid** refers to anything which helps people learn through seeing. We encourage trainers to use and have their participants use such things as real objects and simple models, props for role plays and dramas, picture series, flipbooks, flannelboards, posters, chalkboards and displays.

Parts of the manual

Each of the five units in the manual begins with a page listing the objectives for the unit. These objectives tell you what your learners should be able to do by the end of that unit. The information and activities you can use to teach the objective are listed beside the objective. The evaluation section at the bottom of the page lists ways for you to tell whether your learners are meeting the objectives of that unit.

After the objectives page is a section in two columns. The column on the left of these pages is called **Information**, and the column on the right is called **Training ideas and your notes**. The column on the left contains background information which your learners will need in order to do the activities or meet the objectives of the unit. The column on the right contains ideas and suggestions on how to teach the information you have just read in the left column. It also contains ideas on how to structure the lesson and when to do which activities. This column also has some blank space where you can write your own notes on how to teach the information shown on the left.

Notice the spacing in these two columns. Begin reading whatever information is closest to the top of the page. Then, when you see some writing in the other column, be sure to read it before continuing. For example, you would read the page illustrated overleaf as indicated by the shading.

After the information and training notes section, there is a section for **activities**. The activities are very important in this manual because people learn the most and remember best when they learn by *doing*. The activities are based on the objectives. In each activity your learners practise the new ideas and skills introduced in the unit.

Sometimes an activity requires the use of certain pictures. We have included these pictures at the end of the activity. You may use them in your

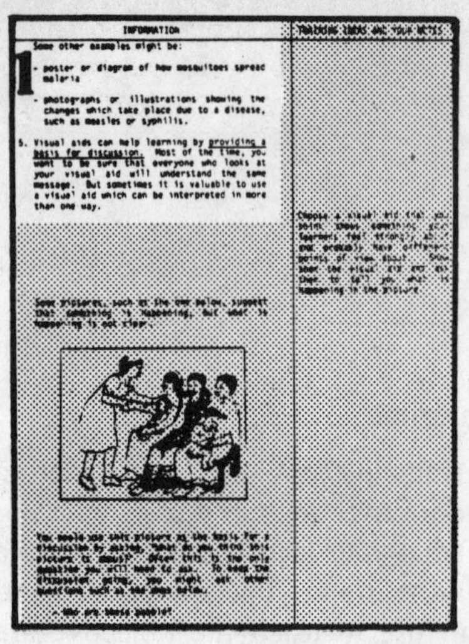

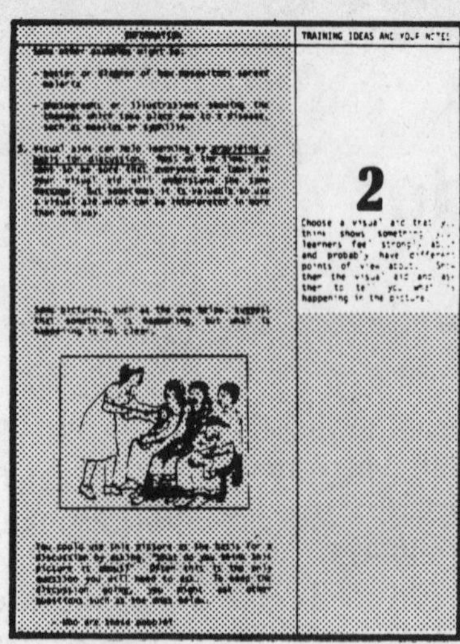

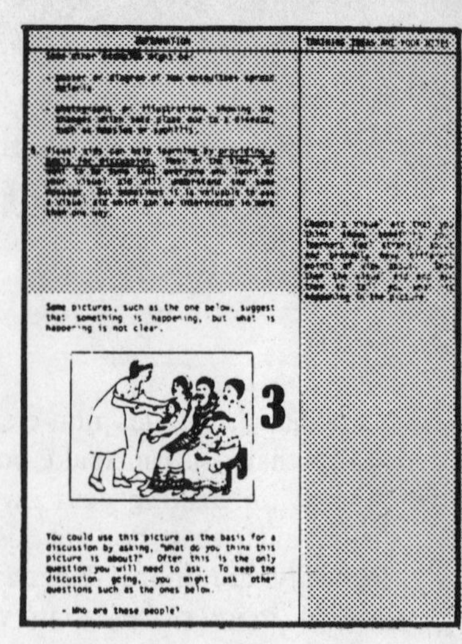

teaching by simply holding up the book to show your learners the page, but if you teach more than a few people at once, it will be difficult for everyone to see the pictures well. In this case, you can use the directions for changing the size of pictures in Unit 4 and make a larger version of the pictures to use.

Sometimes your learners will need some new information, an example, or a case study in order to do a certain activity. These things are also included with the activity. It will be helpful if you can duplicate these pages and give each person a copy to keep. If you cannot do this, then be sure to put some of the notes on the chalkboard and refer to them as you explain the example. You may find Units 4 and 5 particularly useful resources to duplicate for your learners. For example, you can use Unit 4 as a small production skills text for your learners. You will need a chalkboard or large pieces of paper to write on in all of your sessions.

We have used activities and projects for evaluation rather than tests. Activities which ask learners to apply what they have learned also contain guidelines to help you see how well your learners understand and can use their new skills. Sometimes the guidelines are in a separate section, as in Unit 4, but often they are included in the activity itself.

The Resource Pictures section at the back of the manual contains larger versions of some pictures which were used in the Information column in previous units. You can use these to teach the same information to your own learners. Use these pictures in the same way you would use pictures included with an activity.

Planning a session on visual aids (2 hours to 1 day long)

There will be situations where you would like to teach about visual aids, but you have little time. For example, in a long workshop of 5–10 days on teaching methods or health education, you may want to include a session on choosing, planning and making, or using visual aids with different teaching or health education methods. In this case you will need to relate the visual aids session to the topics and skills presented in the rest of the workshop. For example, as a part of a workshop on health education you could teach how to plan, make and use a flannelboard to help people learn the basic food groups. It is also important to demonstrate the usefulness of visual aids by using them in your own teaching. At the end of the session or day, you will want to ask your learners how useful they thought the visual aids session was, so that you can make improvements the next time you teach it.

There may be other times when you want to give a short session on visual aids which is not a part of a workshop, but must stand alone. If your learners do not know each other, it would be helpful to take a few minutes at the beginning of the session to introduce themselves and yourself. In a short session, you must make the objective very specific to fit your limited time. For example, to train traditional birth attendants to make pictures to go with a health story is too large a task for a short session, and you and your learners would be frustrated. But you may want to teach the traditional birth attendants how to use a few sets of pictures to go with health stories they are already familiar with.

The following pages contain some ideas for using this manual to plan visual aids sessions of different lengths: 2 hours and 1 day. These samples may give you some ideas for planning your own sessions on visual aids to fit the needs of your learners.

Sample Session Plan: 2 hours

Mrs Malinga is a nurse in charge of a family health clinic in a rural district. She supervises 6 traditional birth attendants (TBAs) who work and live in the communities surrounding the clinic. Every two weeks these TBAs walk to the clinic and meet Mrs Malinga to turn in their records of the mothers they have visited and the clinic referrals they have made. Mrs Malinga also uses this day for in-service training or discussion sessions with the group of TBAs. By the time the TBAs arrive at the clinic and discuss their visits and referral records with Mrs Malinga, they only have about 2 hours left for the in-service training sessions. Then they must leave if they want to reach home again before dark.

Over the past few months, the TBAs have helped Mrs Malinga make up stories and pictures to use during the home visits to teach mothers about infant nutrition, nutrition in pregnancy, and ante-natal clinic visits. Mrs Malinga pre-tested the pictures with mothers in the clinic and drew and coloured the final series of pictures on heavy cards herself. This week, Mrs Malinga is planning a session for the TBAs on how to use the picture series they have helped develop with the three health stories.

The following is Mrs Malinga's 2-hour session plan.

2-Hour Session Plan

Time	Objectives	Content	Method	Materials	Evaluation
3 minutes	The 6 TBAs will be able to use effectively the 3 sets of pictures which they helped develop as a basis for storytelling with mothers during their home visits.	What is storytelling?	Lecture-discussion (see Unit 5, Activity 1 on storytelling).	The 3 sets of pictures as examples of visual aids that can be used with storytelling: • infant nutrition • nutrition in pregnancy • ante-natal clinic visits.	
7 minutes		What is it good for?	Discussion.		
15 minutes		How do I use pictures for storytelling?	Demonstration of good use of pictures with storytelling.	One of the 3 sets of pictures.	*During session* go from pair to pair to observe their skills in practising the use of the pictures and how well they answer the mother's questions.

Continued overleaf

2-Hour Session Plan

Time	Objectives	Content	Method	Materials	Evaluation
1 hour 15 minutes			TBAs practise storytelling in pairs; each TBA practises with one set of pictures for 10–15 minutes while the other TBA acts as though she is a mother listening and asking questions.	All 3 sets of pictures.	*After session* If more mothers come to the clinic for ante-natal care.
20 minutes			Discuss questions resulting from their practice and discuss how to share the 3 sets of pictures among 6 TBAs.		If the children and pregnant mothers who come to the clinic are in better nutritional state.

Sample Session Plan: 1 day

Mrs Keino is a registered nurse who has planned a 6-week training program for 20 family health community educators. Leaders in 20 communities in Mrs Keino's region selected the family health educators to work on family health and family planning issues with people in their communities. The main tasks of the family health educators are:

1 to educate the community about good health practices,
2 to inform people about clinic services,
3 to refer people to the clinic,
4 to encourage parents to space their children.

Mrs Keino has planned workshop sessions on basic health practices such as nutrition, child spacing and prevention of diarrhoea. She has also planned sessions on how to educate individual members of the community through home visits as well as how to conduct group discussions on family health and family planning issues. As a part of her plans for teaching how to educate the community, she has planned a 1-day session on visual aids. In planning she noted that there is no electricity in most of the communities where the health educators work and few if any visual aids available. Knowing this she decided to show them only low cost visual aids that require no electricity or equipment.

To get ready for the visual aids session, Mrs Keino collected examples of different kinds of visual aids from several agencies in the capital of the province. In the Health Education Office she found a stack of old posters donated by a foreign agency. The health education officer told her that local people disliked the posters because they showed pictures of foreign people and unfamiliar objects. Mrs Keino took several of the posters so that each family health educator could adapt a poster for local people during the workshop. She also organized the visual aids that she had made herself and borrowed other visual aids made by another nurse. She collected paper, brushes, and paints from the local school for use in the workshop.

The table opposite shows Mrs Keino's 1-day session plan.

Planning a workshop on visual aids (2 or more days long)

Certain parts of any workshop lasting 2 or more days can help form a working group and keep the trainer in touch with the group. These include the opening and closing ceremonies, a 'getting acquainted' exercise, review of learners' needs and workshop objectives, 'Learning Issues,' 'Reflection and Review,' and learners' assessment of the workshop.

The purpose of the opening and closing ceremonies is to officially begin and end the workshop and to recognize the participating individuals or agencies and the contributions of the workshop. Usually officials from sponsoring or supporting agencies give short speeches. Refreshments are served.

1-Day (5-Hour) Session Plan

Time	Objectives	Content	Method	Materials	Evaluation
30 minutes	The 20 Family Health Community Educators will be able to make a simple low-cost visual aid by adapting an existing visual aid, to communicate a family health topic in their community.	Ways visual aids help learning (Unit 1)	Demonstration of visual aids. Discussion of ways they help learning.	Posters, flipbook picture series, gourd baby, photographs, real objects.	Ask them to list ways visual aids help learning.
15 minutes		Where to get visual aids and material to make them.	Open discussion sharing ideas and information encouraging using materials in new ways.	Chalkboard and chalk.	Later, follow-up and ask where they are getting visual aids.
30 minutes		Teaching questions (Unit 2) (review of topic presented earlier).	Discussion of questions to ask before teaching. Trainer gives example (Mrs Ebrahim).	Chalkboard, resource pictures, 7 teaching questions.	Later, follow-up and ask do they use the teaching questions in community work.
30 minutes		Design considerations (Unit 2).	Discussion of what makes a good visual aid.	Examples of well designed and poorly-designed visual aids.	Use of design in project. Critique of others.
15 minutes		Adapting visual aids (Unit 2).	Discussion of how to adapt. Demonstration.	Examples of adapting visual aids.	See if they apply in projects.
45 minutes		Tracing and sketching (Unit 4)	Demonstration followed by practice tracing posters. Tracing Activities 1 and 2, Sketching Activities 1, 2, and 4 (modified).	Examples of tracing, materials to trace.	Tracing in projects.
30 minutes		Using colour (Unit 4)	Demonstration followed by practice. Using colour Activity 1.	Paint, brushes, paper, examples.	Use of colour in projects.
90 minutes		Adapting a poster using tracing and colour	Individual work with help from trainer. (Unit 2, Activity 5).	Poster inappropiate for local use.	Completed project.
15 minutes		Using visual aids (Unit 5)	Demonstration of effective use.	Pictures, real objects, flipbooks, etc.	Follow-up observation of use of visual aids.

The best way to begin the work in a workshop is to have a 'getting acquainted' exercise. An example is the Visual Introduction activity in Unit 1 of this manual. This kind of activity usually allows trainers and learners to share some personal and job-related information about themselves. Usually the activity is fun and helps the learners to relax. The activity is also usually related to the skills that will be learned in the workshop. In the Visual Introduction activity, learners have fun experimenting with drawing, using the tools and skills that will be used in making and using visual aids later in the workshop.

Very early in the workshop it is a good idea to have a group discussion to find out what the participants want to gain from the workshop. You need to see how this matches with the objectives you have planned for the workshop. If necessary, you can change some parts of the workshop to meet the most important needs of your learners. It may not be possible to meet all needs of every learner, especially in a short (2–3 day) workshop.

It is also useful to set aside about 15 minutes at the beginning of each day for what we call 'Learning Issues' and at the end of the day for 'Reflection and Review.' You can use 'Learning Issues' as a time for the whole group to try to solve problems such as poor attendance, lack of transportation, or people arriving late. You can also use this time to discuss questions or ideas that learners have thought of overnight. You can use this time to give out new information based on questions or problems that arose the day before or to review the planned activities for the day. 'Reflection and Review' is a good time to review what was learned that day, what was good about the day's activities, or what could be improved. It is also a good time to give homework assignments or to give learners an idea of what you have planned for the next day or several days.

Near the end of the workshop, you will probably want to ask your participants what they thought of the workshop as a whole, so that you can make improvements for your next workshop. You can have a group discussion using specific questions about the workshop that you have thought of before the discussion. Or you can write questions on the chalkboard or on paper and ask each person to answer them.

The following pages contain some ideas on how to use this manual to schedule workshops of different lengths: 3 days, 10 days, and 12 days. These are only samples to give you ideas. You will have to plan your own workshop based on your objectives, the resources and time available to you, and the needs and backgrounds of your own learners.

Sample Workshop Plan (3 days)

Mr El Baz is a clinic nurse. He supervises nurses in his region. The nurses he supervises travel from village to village to deliver health services. At each village, he wants the travelling nurses to conduct a health education session with the villagers.

Mr El Baz decides to conduct a 3-day workshop for his travelling nurses. He wants to improve their skills in health education by teaching them different teaching methods and how they can use the visual aids available at the clinic.

Most villagers cannot read or write. Mr El Baz has observed some of the nurses' health education sessions. He sees that they need to improve their talks and demonstrations. He also wants them to be able to teach with health stories. He thinks the villagers will learn more if the nurses use visual aids within the health education sessions.

Before the workshop begins, Mr El Baz talks with the leaders of the village closest to the clinic where the workshop will be held. He arranges for the nurses to conduct health education sessions at that village. They will practise the new skills he will teach them in the workshop. Mr El Baz also gathers all the visual aids and other teaching materials he will need for the workshop.

Overall objective

By the end of the 3-day workshop, the nurses will be able to conduct health education sessions using at least 3 different teaching methods and using visual aids available from the clinic.

To fulfil the overall objective, he knew that participants needed to meet these smaller objectives:

1 Plan a health education session by answering the 7 teaching questions.
2 Demonstrate an effective use of 3 different teaching methods (talks, demonstrations, and storytelling) by following the guidelines developed for each method.
3 Demonstrate an effective use of visual aids within those methods by following the guidelines developed from the example sessions.

Following is a daily schedule for Mr El Baz's workshop.

3-Day Workshop Schedule

Time	Day 1	Day 2
8.00–9.30	Opening Remarks and Greetings. Seeing the Same Picture in Different Ways (Unit 2, Activity 3). Discuss nurses' experiences in conducting health education sessions; relate experiences to differing perceptions of words and pictures and how they affect health education. Discuss nurses' goals for workshop. Discuss workshop objectives and schedule.	Learning Issues. Demonstration as a Method (Unit 5, Activity 1: Demonstration). Use Signs of Dehydration (Unit 4, Models Activity 1, Exercises 1–3) as the sample demonstration.
9.30–10.00	BREAK	
10.00–12.00	The 7 Teaching Questions: Mrs Ebrahim's Story (Unit 2, using the Training Ideas). Parts of a Training or Health Education Session (Unit 5). Storytelling as a Method (Unit 5, Activity 1: Storytelling). Use Mrs Ebrahim's story as an example.	Making a Session Plan (Unit 5, Activity 2). • Each participant gives choice of topic and answer to Teaching Questions 1–4 (Day 1 Assignment). • Each participant answers Teaching Questions 5–7 and discusses with trainer.
12.00–12.15	BREAK	
12.15–1.45	A Talk as a Method (Unit 5, Activity 1: Lecture or talk). Use Adapting an existing visual aid (Unit 2) as a sample talk. Participants review visual aids available from the clinic. Assignment: Choose 1 topic from a list of choices to plan a health education session. (Topics will have visual aids available.) Answer Teaching Questions 1–3. Reflection and Review.	• Each participant completes a lesson plan as shown in Activity 2, Unit 5. Discuss role of learners' practice sessions (Unit 5, Activity 3). Assignment: Practice session using the visual aids. Reflection and Review.

Time	Day 3
8.00–11.30	Travel to local village. Each nurse conducts the planned health education session; others observe as previously instructed. Travel from local village.
11.30–12.00	BREAK
12.00–1.45	Sharing of observations and suggestions for improvement Each nurse writes a plan for using the new skills during the coming six months and shares the plan with other nurses and the trainer. Closing Remarks.

Sample Workshop Plan (10–12 days)

Mrs Nagali is a mid-level nurse-trainer. She provides in-service training workshops for other Ministry of Health nurses. Her workshops are usually on maternal and child health and family planning.

Many former learners have asked for further training in how to make and use visual aids for educational or training sessions. The ministry is interested in improving nurses' teaching skills. It has asked Mrs Nagali to plan and conduct a 10-day workshop on visual aids for 15–20 nurses. Her learners will be teachers in nursing schools, ward supervisors, or clinic heads. All learners provide pre-service training for nursing students, in-service training for staff they supervise, or patient education. Mrs Nagali asked most of the nurses what kind of teaching aids or supplies for making them they could get in their local areas. On the basis of their answers, she decided the workshop should be on visual aids which do not require electricity.

She decided on these objectives:

10-Day Workshop Schedule

Time	Day 1	Day 2	Day 3
9.00–10.30	Opening Ceremony. A Visual Introduction (Unit 1, Activity 1).	Learning Issues. Overview of visual aids which do not require electricity (Unit 2). Introduction to Lettering (Unit 4).	Learning Issues. Choosing a visual aid that is well designed (Unit 2). Is the Visual Aid Well Designed? (Unit 2, Activity 2).
10.30–10.45	BREAK		
10.45–12.30	Why Use Visual Aids? (Unit 1, Activity 2). Discuss participants' goals for workshop. Discuss workshop objectives and schedule.	Hand Lettering (Unit 4, Lettering Activity 1).	Tracing Skills for Making Visual Aids (Unit 4, Tracing Activities 1 and 2).
12.30–2.00	LUNCH		
2.00–3.15	Things We Have Learned Through Pictures (Unit 1, Activity 3). When to use visual aids (Unit 1). ↓	Using a Stencil to Make Letters and Words (Unit 4, Lettering Activity 2). ↓	Sketching and Tracing Skills for Adapting Pictures (Unit 4, Sketching Activities 3 and 4). ↓
3.15–3.30	BREAK		
3.30–5.00	Reflection and Review	Lettering homework assignment. Reflection and Review.	Homework assignment on Adapting Visual Aids (Unit 2, Activity 5). Reflection and Review.

Overall objective of the workshop:
By the end of the 10–day workshop, nurses will be able to conduct a maternal and child health/family planning teaching or health education session based on a visual aid which they have designed and produced.

To meet that objective, the nurses must be able to meet these smaller objectives:

1 Design maternal and child health/family planning visual aids which follow rules of good teaching and good design.
2 Produce low-cost visual aids for maternal and child health/family planning topics using locally available materials.
3 Prepare and conduct a training or health education session using a visual aid.

Below and on the next page is a daily schedule for the 10-day workshop Mrs Nagali planned for a 9.00 a.m. to 5.00 p.m. work day. A second schedule, on pages 11 and 12, shows how another trainer could adapt Mrs Nagali's plan to a 12-day workshop with daily hours from 8.00 a.m. to 1.45 p.m.

Day 4	**Day 5**	**Day 6**	**Day 7**
Learning Issues. Discuss homework and how people adapted the pictures (Unit 2, Adapting an existing visual aid). Practice in Showing an Idea in Different Ways (Unit 3, Activity 1).	Learning Issues. Need for Pre-testing Visual Aids (Unit 2, Activity 4). How to Pre-test Visual Aids: A Role Play (Unit 3, Activity 3).	Learning Issues. Summary test for week 1 (Unit 1, Activity 5 and other test questions trainers can write). Work on individual projects. Select topic and answer the 7 Teaching Questions (Unit 3, Activity 5).	Learning Issues. Parts of a Training or Health Education Session (Unit 5). Overview of Teaching Methods and Visual Aids (Unit 5, Activity 1 – choose 3 different methods).
		BREAK	
The 7 Teaching Questions (Unit 2, Choosing a visual aid which fits your training needs). Planning a Visual Aid Which Shows More Than One Idea (Unit 3, Activity 4). Divide into groups, assign topic, answer 7 Teaching Questions.	Review of group projects (Steps 10–13 of Unit 3, Activity 4).	Share and discuss individual project topics and answers to the 7 Teaching Questions.	
		LUNCH	
Review all 6 steps in planning and making a visual aid (Unit 3). Continue with Unit 3, Activity 4 up to Step 9.	Field trip to pre-test group plans for a visual aid (nursing school, MCH centre, or a community centre).	Work on individual projects with help from trainers.	Work on individual projects.
		BREAK	
Reflection and Review.	Small group discussion of pre-testing results. Assign and explain individual projects (Unit 3, Activity 5). Reflection and Review.	Reflection and Review.	Reflection and Review.

10-Day Workshop Schedule continued

Time	Day 8	Day 9	Day 10
9.00–10.00	Learning Issues. Changing Size of Pictures (Unit 4). Demonstrate square and sketching methods. Give practice assignment (Activities 2 and 3).	Learning Issues, Using Colour (Unit 4, Activities 1 and 2). Work on individual projects.	Presentations of individual projects.
10.30–10.45			
10.45–12.30	Work on individual projects.		
12.30–2.00			
2.00–3.15			Nurses' assessment of workshop. Individual conferences on projects. Display projects for closing ceremony.
3.15–3.30			
3.30–5.00	Reflection and Review.	Presentations of individual projects. Reflection and Review.	Closing Ceremony.

Including visual aids in a pre-service training program

Teaching skills and health education are often part of basic training for nursing students. Lessons on visual aids within these topics can improve student nurses' abilities to teach other health workers and to communicate with clients.

When visual aids lessons are a part of a larger training program, it is important to look at the program objectives and identify specific ways that visual aids training will contribute to them. Another consideration is the large size of most basic training classes which requires adaptation of group activities. For example, a teacher can use a large group discussion instead of a small group activity. Many small groups can work at the same time while the teacher moves among the groups. If the training program is longer than one year, it may also be necessary to develop more advanced lessons for higher-level students.

12-Day Workshop Schedule

Time	Day 1	Day 2	Day 3	Day 4	Day 5	Day 6
8.00–10.00	Opening Ceremony. A Visual Introduction (Unit 1, Activity 1). Why Use Visual Aids? (Unit 1, Activity 2).	Learning Issues. Overview of visual aids which do not require electricity (Unit 2). Introduction to Lettering (Unit 4).	Learning Issues. Choosing a visual aid that is well designed (Unit 2). Is the Visual Aid Well Designed? (Unit 2, Activity 2).	Learning Issues. Discuss homework and how people adapted the pictures (Unit 2, Adapting an Existing Visual Aid). Sketching and Tracing Skills for Adapting Pictures (Unit 4, Sketching Activity 4).	Learning Issues. Review all 6 steps in planning and making a visual aid (Unit 3). Continue with Unit 3, Activity 4 up to Step 9. Prepare for field trip.	Learning Issues. Review of group projects (Steps 10–13 of Unit 3, Activity 4).
10.00–10.30	BREAK					
10.30–12.30	Discuss participants' goals for workshop. Discuss workshop objectives and schedule. Things We Have Learned through Pictures (Unit 1, Activity 3).	Hand Lettering (Unit 4, Lettering Activity 1). Using a Stencil to Make Letters and Words (Unit 4, Lettering Activity 2).	Tracing Skills for Making Visual Aids (Unit 4, Tracing Activities 1 and 2).	Practice in Showing an Idea in Different Ways (Unit 3, (Activity 1). The 7 Teaching Questions (Unit 2, Choosing a visual aid which fits your training needs).	↓	Field trip to pre-test group plans for a visual aid (nursing school, MCH centre, or a community centre).
12.30–12.45	BREAK					
12.45–1.45	When to use visual aids (Unit 1). Reflection and Review.	↓ Lettering homework assignment. Reflection and Review.	Sketching and Tracing Skills for Adapting Pictures (Unit 4, Sketching Activity 3). Homework assignment on Adapting Visual Aids (Unit 2, Activity 5). Reflection and Review.	Planning a Visual Aid Which Shows More Than One Idea (Unit 3, Activity 4). Divide into groups, assign topic, answer The 7 Teaching Questions. Reflection and Review.	Need for Pre-testing Visual Aids (Unit 2, Activity 4). How to Pre-test Visual Aids: A Role Play (Unit 3, Activity 3). Reflection and Review.	Small group discussion of pre-testing results. Assign and explain individual projects (Unit 3, Activity 5). Reflection and Review.

12-Day Workshop Schedule Continued

Time	Day 7	Day 8	Day 9	Day 10	Day 11	Day 12
8.00–10.00	Learning Issues. Summary of test for week 1 (Unit 1, Activity 5 and other test questions trainers can write). Work on individual projects. Choose topic and answer the 7 Teaching Questions (Unit 3, Activity 5).	Learning Issues. Parts of a Training or Health Education Session (Unit 5). Overview of Teaching Methods and Visual Aids (Unit 5, Activity 1 – choose 3 different methods).	Learning Issues. Models (Unit 4). Demonstrate use of the Gourd Baby and the Birthing Box. Work on Individual projects.	Learning Issues. Changing Size of Pictures (Unit 4). Demonstrate square and sketching methods. Give practice assignments. Work on individual projects.	Learning Issues. Work on individual projects.	Participant assessment of workshop. Individual conferences on projects. Display projects for closing ceremony.
10.00–10.30	BREAK					
10.30–12.30	Share and discuss individual project topics and answers to The 7 Teaching Questions in large group.	Work on individual projects.			Presentations of individual projects.	Closing Ceremony.
12.30–12.45	BREAK					
12.45–1.45	Work on individual projects with help from trainers. Reflection and Review.	Reflection and Review.	Reflection and Review.	Using Colour (Unit 4, Activities 1 and 2). Reflection and Review.	Reflection and Review.	

Finally, textbooks on visual aids are scarce. Where duplicating facilities and paper are available, sections of the manual can be copied and used as texts. Unit 4 on 'Production Skills' and Unit 5 on 'Using Visual Aids in a Training or Health Education Session' are particularly useful for this purpose.

The following example presents some ideas for using this manual to include visual aids lessons in a basic nursing curriculum. The lesson plan assumes that the students have already learned to use several teaching methods.

Sample visual aids lessons within a basic training program

Mrs Mugambe is head tutor for a three-year program for training enrolled community nurses. The program includes teaching skills and requires that all the students prepare and give health education talks in clinics and communities. In the provincial areas where many of the student nurses will later work, the older people distrust health workers and discourage community members from attending the clinics. Many of these clients cannot read or write.

Mrs Mugambe decided that skills in making and using visual aids would help the student nurses communicate better with their clients. The other tutors in her school helped her develop a plan (see below and on the next page) to teach about visual aids during teaching skills training. Because there were no textbooks available, Mrs Mugambe applied to the Ministry of Health for funds to duplicate Unit 4 of this manual, 'Production Skills'. She and the other tutors felt that the student nurses would benefit most from visual aids lessons at the beginning of their second year of training, when they have a basic understanding of the subject and are beginning to work with clients. The tutors decided that visual aids training would fit most easily into the curriculum as a series of two-hour lessons one week apart, rather than a single block of training.

Mrs Mugambe and the other tutors developed the following general objective for the visual aids training: the student nurses will be able to conduct a community health education activity using a low-cost visual aid which they have developed. The tutors noted that the following skills would be needed to accomplish this objective:

1 selecting appropriate visual aids and teaching methods,
2 using visual aids and teaching methods effectively,
3 planning a visual aid,
4 making a visual aid.

Following these sessions on visual aids, the students will plan and conduct a health education talk and discussion in a clinic or community. The teacher will attend and evaluate as many of these sessions as possible.

Schedule for Visual Aids Training in Basic Nursing Curriculum

Duration: 10 hours (four 2-hour training sessions; one 2-hour practice session).
Additional time for health talks in clinics.

Topics	Methods and materials	Time (minutes)
Week 1		
Ways visual aids help learning	Unit 1 Activity 4 (modified); groups post solutions on the wall and teacher summarizes.	45
Types of visual aids Unit 2	Brainstorming; teacher shows visual aid types.	45
Teaching questions Unit 2	Large group discussion. Give examples.	20
Homework assignment	Unit 2, Activity 1 on Choosing Visual Aids to Fit Teaching Situations (modified as individual homework). Have students copy case study teaching questions.	10

Schedule for Visual Aids Training in Basic Nursing Curriculum (continued)

Topics	Methods and materials	Time (minutes)
Week 2		
Review of homework	Ask three students to report. Large group discussion. Teacher collects homework.	25
Design questions Unit 2, choosing a visual aid that communicates	• Lecture/large group discussion. Teacher summarizes and shows examples of each design question,	20
	• Demonstration/discussion. Teacher reviews a picture using design questions. Students review a picture as a large group (modification of Unit 2, Activity 2, Is the Visual Aid Well Designed?)	30
Adapting visual aids Unit 2, adapting an existing visual aid	Large group discussion. Reasons for adapting a visual aid. Show examples.	15
Tracing techniques	Unit 4 activities on tracing methods. Teacher demonstrates each method and assigns reading and practice for homework.	30
Homework assignment	Unit 2, Activity 5, Adapting Visual Aids, (modified, students modify MCH/FP poster).	
Week 3		
Review of homework	Teacher returns homework from week 2 with comments • Students post adaptation of posters on wall and spend 10 minutes looking at all of them and asking questions. • Large group discussion of 1 or 2 poster adaptations. Teacher collects homework.	30
Planning a visual aid Unit 3, steps in planning a visual aid	Lecture/demonstration. Teacher uses examples to show the steps in planning a visual aid.	30
Showing the same idea in different ways	Unit 3, Activity 1 (modified). • Demonstration by teacher. • Individual practice showing the same idea in different ways.	30 30
Using colour Unit 4, colouring visual aids	Demonstration by trainer. Students read colouring section in production text and practice colouring.	20
Homework assignment	Make a plan for a simple visual aid, Unit 3, Activity 2, Making a Visual Aid Which Shows Only One Idea, (modified as Unit 5, Activity 1).	10
Week 4		
Review of homework	Teacher returns week 3 homework with comments. Large group discussion. 3 volunteers report their plans, others comment. Teacher collects plans.	30
Pre-testing visual aids Unit 3	Unit 3, Activity 3, How to Pre-test Visual Aids: A Role Play. Teacher and a volunteer do a role play, (modified: only one picture tested).	45
Guidelines for using visual aids Unit 5	Unit 5, Guidelines for using visual aids with teaching methods. Teacher presents guidelines and demonstrates.	20
Homework assignment	Students make one idea visual aid using plan, test it, and be prepared to present their project next week.	10
Week 5		
Presentation of projects	Students are divided into 4 groups. Three other teachers assist in observing and give students written comments based on the guidelines for evaluating and using visual aids, Unit 3, Activity 5; Unit 5.	120

Unit 1
When to Use Visual Aids

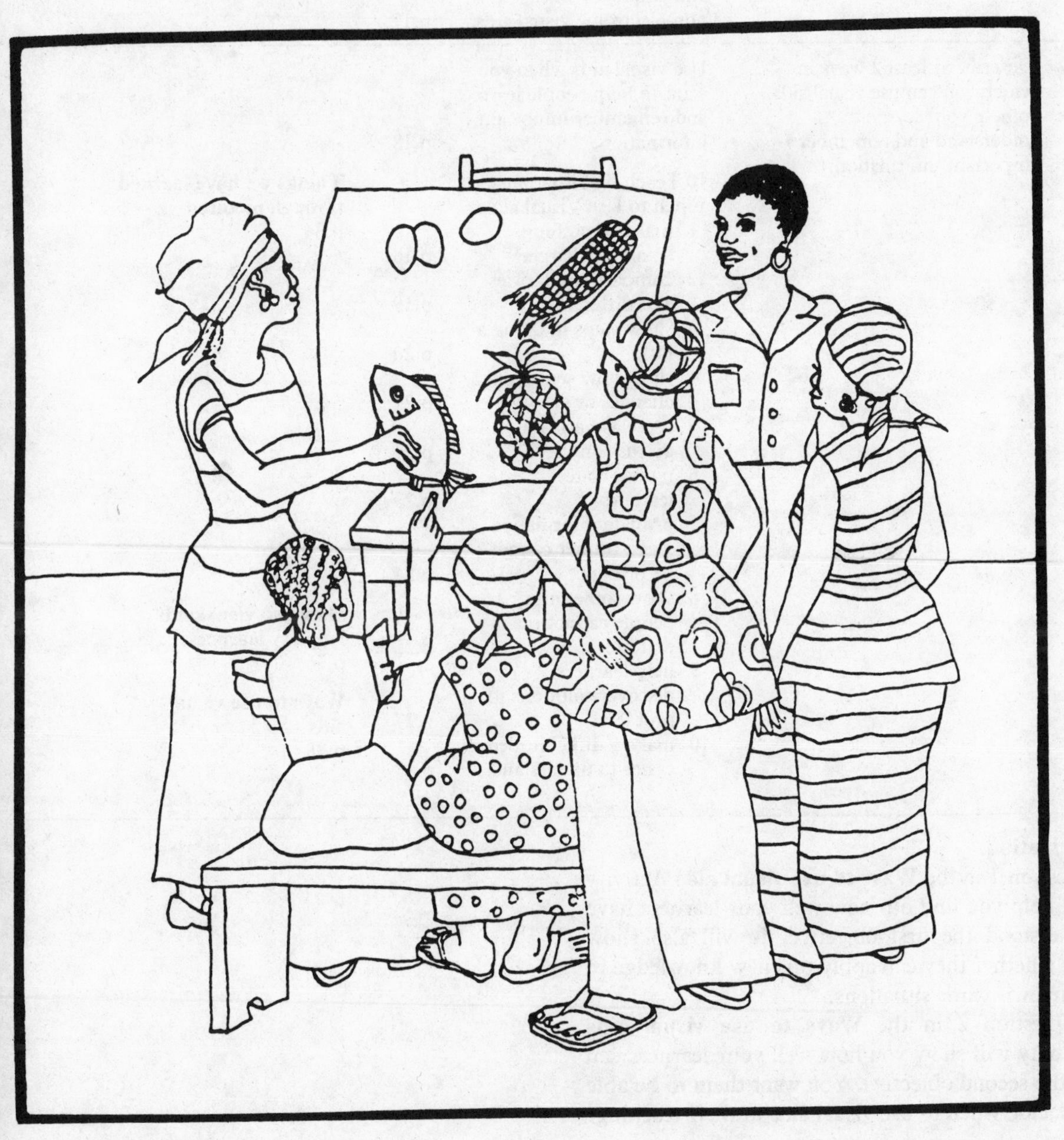

Unit 1 introduces the idea of teaching and learning with visual aids. You can use this unit to help learners explore how visual aids can make learning easier and more effective. Learners examine their own experience for things they have learned through pictures. They also look at 'Ten Teaching Situations' in which visual aids are useful. Then they discuss ways they can use visual aids in their own teaching situations.

Unit 1: When to use visual aids

Objective	Information		Activities	
1 Describe a situation which requires a visual aid.	What are visual aids? Definition of visual aids and emphasis on non-electronic visual aids.	p.17	**A visual introduction** **Why use visual aids?**	p.31 p.32
2 Describe at least 2 ways in which you can use visual aids to help your learners understand and remember important information.	Use visual aids when you want to help people learn and remember important information.	p.18		
	10 Teaching Situations. When to Use Visual aids:		**Things we have learned through pictures** p.34	
	1 make something small look larger	p.18		
	2 compare similarities and differences	p.19		
	3 show steps in doing a task	p.20		
	4 show how something changes or grows	p.21		
	5 serve as basis for discussion	p.21		
	6 review or test learners	p.23		
	7 provide information when trainer cannot be present	p.24		
	8 show something people cannot see in real life	p.25	**How can visual aids help my learners?** p.36	
	9 help learners discover solutions to problems	p.27	**Ways to use visual aids** p.38	
	10 make a difficult idea easier to understand	p.29		

Evaluation:
Question 1 in the **Ways to use visual aids** Activity will help you find out how well your learners have understood the first objective. It will also show you whether they can apply this new knowledge to their own work situations.

Question 2 in the **Ways to use visual aids** Activity will show you how well your learners can do the second objective. You want them to be able to decide when to use visual aids in their teaching.

Information | **Training ideas and your notes**

You may want to set up a display of the different kinds of visual aids before you begin. You can use these visual aids to illustrate ideas, and participants will be able to examine them to find examples of the points discussed in this unit. Try to use as many examples of the visual aids mentioned in Unit 2 as possible. Include some visual aids you have made yourself. This will encourage participants to make and use their own visual aids, too.

Begin the unit with Activity 1, in which learners draw pictures to introduce themselves to each other. Keep these drawings to use later in Unit 4, when you are evaluating the visual aid each person has made. By comparing these two projects, you can see how much progress the person has made.

Ask learners to look around the room at the different visual aids you have brought. Let them suggest their own definition of a visual aid. Write suggestions on the chalkboard as they are mentioned. Then encourage the group to agree on one definition.

What are visual aids?

Learners in the past have usually said something like this: *A visual aid is anything that helps people learn through seeing.* Visual aids can show words, pictures, or numbers. Sometimes they show only one of these things; other times they show all three.

Ask participants to name the different kinds of visual aids they see in the room. Write this list on the chalkboard. If there are questions about a particular visual aid, stop and explain briefly what it is and how it works. (See the beginning of Unit 2 for that information.)

You are already using visual aids. How often have you drawn a map on the ground, or used a symbol to describe something, or explained something by saying, 'Watch this' or 'Look at this'? We all use our eyes to help us learn and communicate with each other.

Many trainers ask, 'But are visual aids really helpful to my learners? Do they help enough that I should spend time planning and making them?'

Do Activity 2. This activity gives learners the experience of being in a situation which requires a visual aid for clear understanding.

When to use visual aids

Use visual aids whenever you want to *help people learn and remember important information.*

People in different cultures have known this for many years. This is why some cultures have developed traditions of using visual aids to explain things or help people remember things.

The Mijikenda people live along the coast of Kenya. They make wooden figures to represent relatives who have died. The wooden figures are visual aids. The carvings on each figure tell whether the person was an adult or child, male or female and whom he or she was related to. Elaborate carving means that the person had high social status in the community. Coins for eyes means that the person was wealthy.

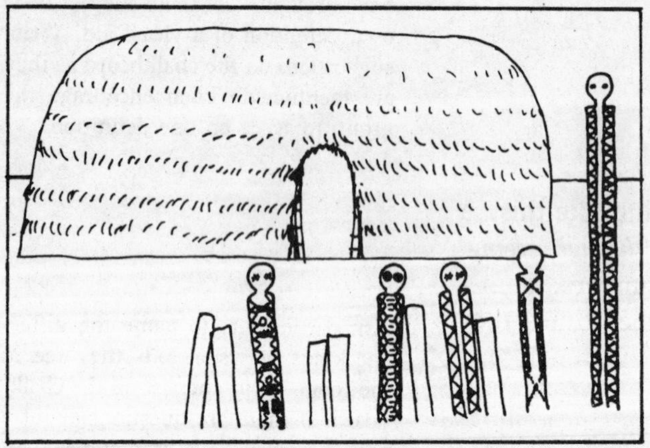

Activity 3. **Things we have learned through pictures,** asks learners to make their own list before you present any further information. The list will be a helpful reference as you discuss the following ten points. One way to teach these ten points is to present the main idea briefly, then give learners several minutes to find examples from the visual aids you have brought. Then use the examples they have found to discuss the idea more thoroughly.

1 Visual aids can **make something small look larger.** A large picture of the inner ear can help students study the small parts. A drawing or poster of an egg and sperm help learners understand what these things look like. Because the pictures are much larger than real life, learners can study them carefully.

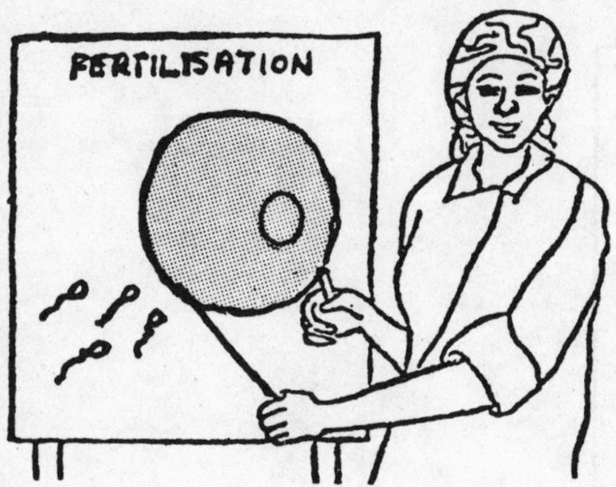

Other examples might be:

- microscopic slides of different body tissues
- a model of the inner ear
- photographs or illustrations of different kinds of cells
- photographs or illustrations of processes such as fertilization or cell division

Before going on, let learners apply what they have learned. Let them discuss whether there are any items on the list they made in Activity 3 which illustrate this point. If so write 'make something small look larger' beside that item, as explained in Activity 3. If not, move on to the next point.

If you are in a setting where your participants can take notes, ask them to write points 1–10 in their notes as you discuss them.

2 Visual aids help us **compare the similarities and differences between two things.** Show your learners pictures of two similar objects side by side, and they can look at the pictures and identify which things are the same and which are different.

The illustration below shows the drawings one nursing school instructor uses to teach her students about the differences in appearance of children with kwashiorkor and children with marasmus. She uses the pictures to help them learn the basic information, and then takes them to the clinic to see real children with these conditions.

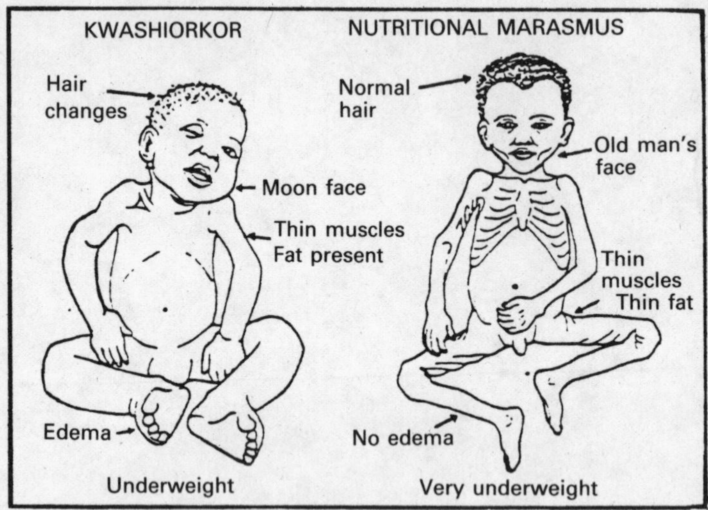

Some other examples might be:

- diagrams of a normal uterus and a tilted uterus
- different kinds of IUDs glued or taped onto a board so people can compare the sizes and shapes
- photographs or drawings of a village before and after a sanitation campaign.

Ask learners if there are any examples of this idea on the list they made in Activity 3. If so, add 'compared similarities and differences between two things' to the second list, as described in Activity 3.

3 Visual aids are an excellent way to **show the steps to follow in doing a task.** Mr Kamwengu, a nurse tutor, uses a series of pictures like the ones below to teach his students how to take temperatures.

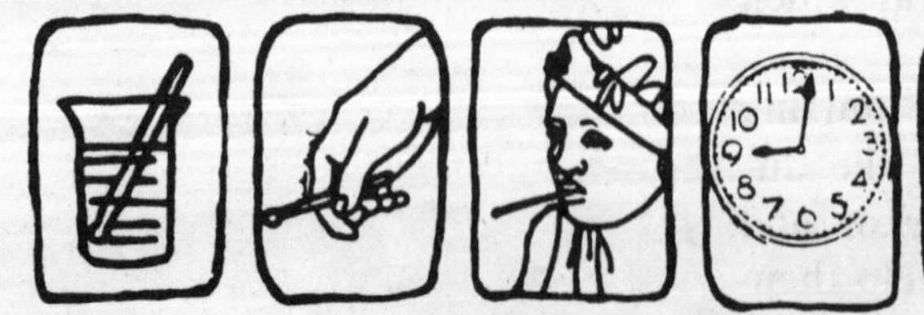

Other tasks or procedures that pictures can help show include:
- how to give an injection
- how to mix rehydration drink
- how to bathe a baby
- how to do a breast examination.

4 Pictures can **show how something changes or grows.** One picture can show all the changes which take place. These kinds of pictures are good for showing how something happens. The example below shows how blood flukes spread schistosomiasis.

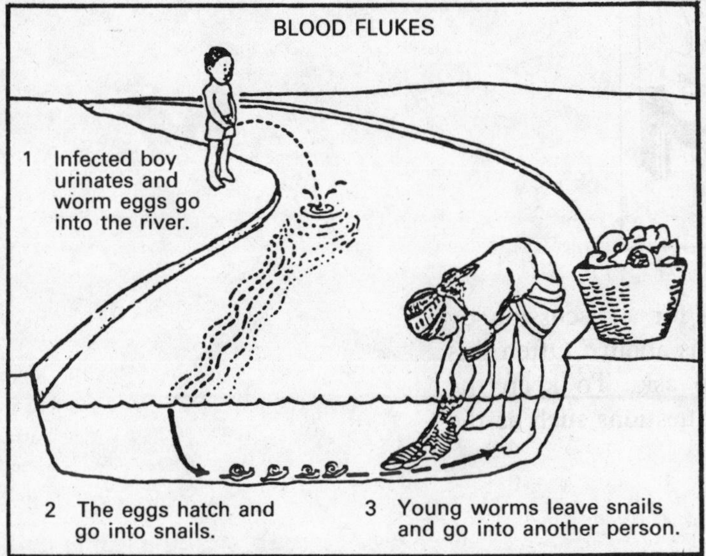

Some other examples might be:
- poster or diagram of how mosquitoes spread malaria
- photographs or illustrations showing the changes which take place due to a disease, such as measles or syphilis.

5 Visual aids can help learning by **providing a basis for discussion.** Most of the time, you want to be sure that everyone who looks at your visual aid will understand the same message. But sometimes it is valuable to use a visual aid which can be interpreted in more than one way.

Some pictures, such as the one below, suggest that something is happening, but what is happening is not clear.

Choose a visual aid that you think shows something your learners feel strongly about and probably have different points of view about. Show them the visual aid and ask them to tell you what is happening in the picture.

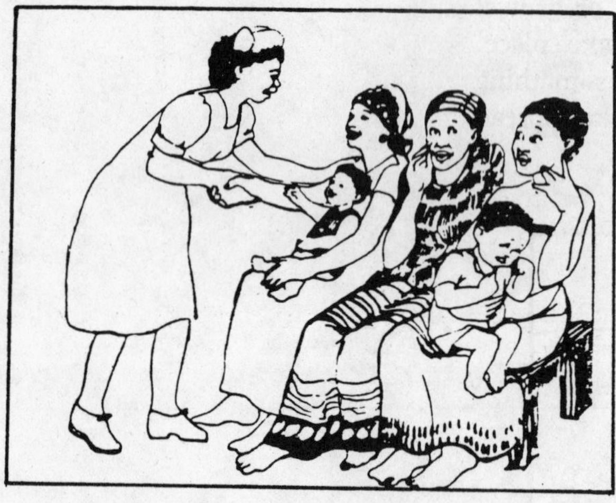

You could see this picture as the basis for a discussion by asking, 'What do you think this picture is about?' Often this is the only question you will need to ask. To keep the discussion going, you might ask other questions such as the ones below.

- Who are these people?
- What is happening in the picture?
- How do the people feel about it?

Also see the part of Activity 1 in Unit 5 on group discussion.

You can use other pictures like this one to start discussions in which the learners explore their own needs, feelings, attitudes, and expectations. For learners who will be doing any counselling, this knowledge and discussion of their prejudices and feelings is very important.

Pictures like this are also useful in community health work. A group discussion helps you learn quickly how the villagers feel about many things, and what problems need to be solved in the community.

Discussing their interpretations of pictures encourages people to observe, think and question carefully and critically.

Ask participants to suggest some other situations in which pictures like this would be useful.

Other possible examples:

- a picture of a family with many children, obviously sick and malnourished:
  You can ask, 'What is the problem presented in this picture?'
  People might respond with several answers: 'Lack of proper sanitation', or 'Lack of immunization', 'Poor nutrition', or 'Lack of family planning'.
- a picture of many women and their babies waiting in line outside a clinic:
  You can ask, 'What is going on here?'
  One person might respond, 'There has been a successful presentation on immunization.' Another person might say, 'No, there is an epidemic. The women look anxious.'

6 You can also use visual aids to **review or test your learners** to see if they really understand. After instruction, you can ask learners to identify or explain parts of a picture or other visual aid.

Flannelboards are very good for this kind of review, and learners seem to enjoy the activity. The community health worker in the picture below uses a folded blanket wrapped around a piece of wood as a flannelboard. She has been teaching the village women about nutrition, using the flannelboard as she talked about food groups. Afterwards, she asks her learners to come up and place each food in its proper group on the board.

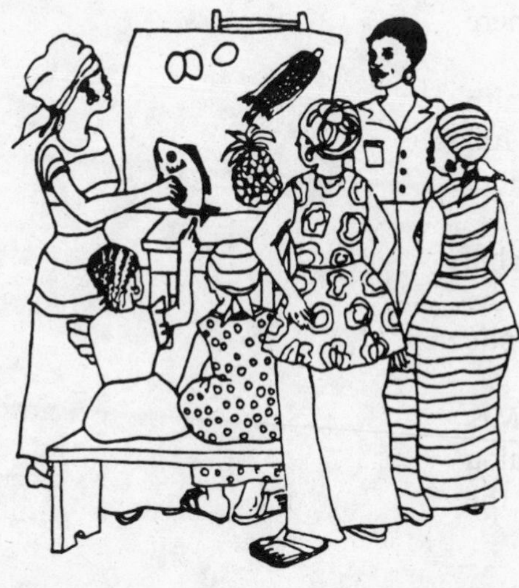

Mr Kamwengu teaches at the nursing school. He uses a series of pictures to teach the parts of the female reproductive system.

Mr Kamwengu knows that afterwards he can tell whether his students know the different parts by asking the students to draw them. He asks one student at a time to come to the front and draw a part of the complete reproductive system. If one person draws an ovary, he asks the next person to draw a fallopian tube. He asks each person to add onto the picture, until all the parts are drawn and labelled. None of his students are artists, but they all enjoy this activity. It helps them remember what they saw in the pictures.

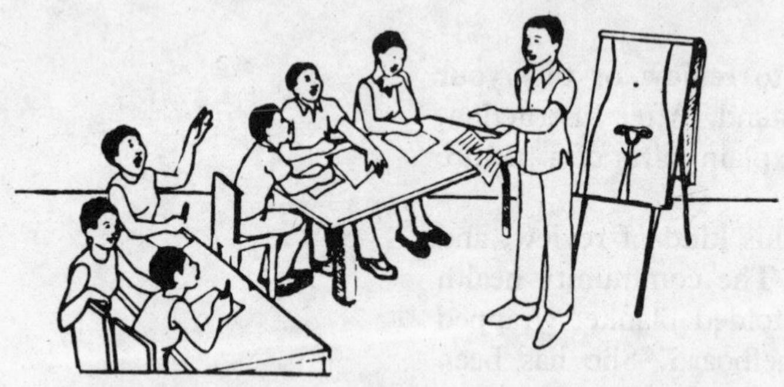

Have your learners turn to the person seated to their right. Give people two or three minutes to think of at least one way in which they could use a visual aid to test their learners. Then discuss these ideas as a large group.

7 Visual aids can **provide information when the trainer cannot be present.** You cannot always be present when someone needs to ask you about something. Sometimes you have other work you must do or you must be somewhere else.

For example, Mrs Macalou directs a community health clinic. She has one nurse's aide working for her full time. Mrs Macalou needed to make time to see more clients at the clinic.

Mrs Macalou made a poster to put over the table where clients check into the clinic. The poster shows the steps her aide should go through in taking a client's history and recording the person's complaint.

Now when her aide comes to work, she can help Mrs Macalou by seeing all of the clients first. If Mrs Macalou must be out of the clinic, the aide can still record the client's history and complaint.

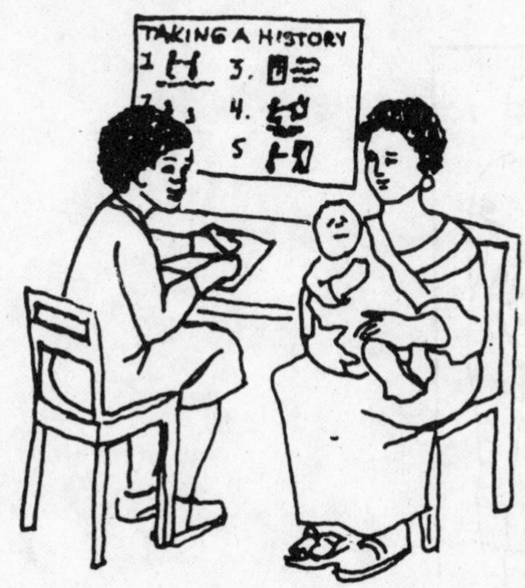

Mrs Macalou can come back to the clinic, look at the case histories, and decide quickly which patients need to be seen first.

Other examples include:

- posters, pamphlets, or displays in a clinic waiting room on ideas such as choosing a contraceptive or cooking a balanced meal
- any visual aids learners can take home with them after your presentation, such as pamphlets or hand-outs on such things as contraceptive use or pre-natal care.
- a poster or display left in the community after a health worker's visit, on topics such as 'Why space your family?' or 'Why immunize your children?'

Ask participants to think of other examples.

8 Visual aids can **show people something they can't see in real life.** The section on how visual aids can make small things look larger mentioned that visual aids help learners see things such as cells, which are impossible to see unless you use a microscope because they are too small.

Sometimes it is impossible to see things in real life for other reasons as well.

Sometimes a visual aid is useful to show something that cannot be seen because it is inside the body.

Mrs Hasan is a community health worker. She uses diagrams like the ones below to teach traditional birth attendants about the different positions the baby can have in the womb.

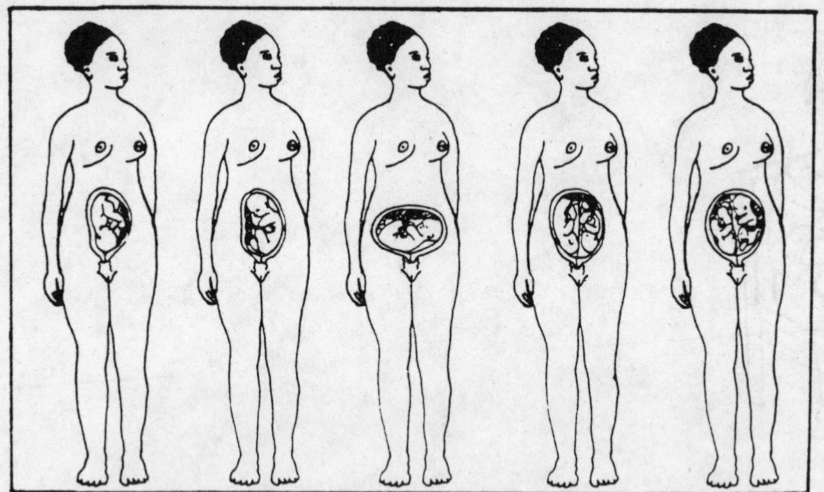

She discusses the pictures with the traditional birth attendants. Then she shows them how to feel the womb of a pregnant woman for the baby's head and buttocks.

You can also use visual aids to show your learners things which are impossible to visit in real life. You can show them pictures of an activity in a village which is too far away for them to visit. The nurse in the picture below has used drawings to make a display which she can use in clinic presentations.

You Can Have a Healthier Community
OUR Village Does
BEFORE our cleanup campaign
AFTER our cleanup campaign

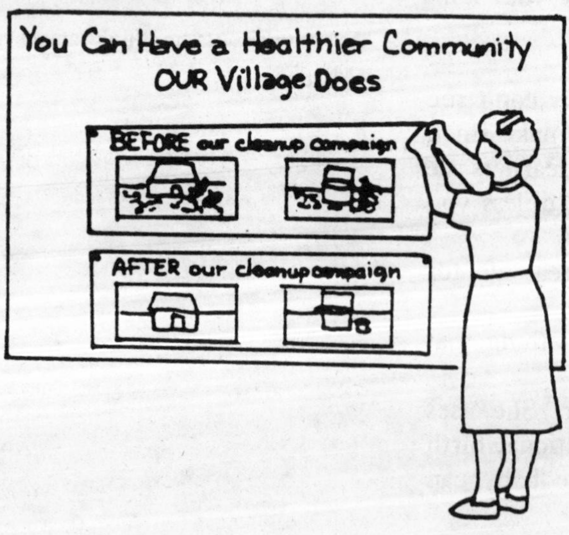

Some other examples of how visual aids can show us things that are impossible to see in real life are:

- A nursing instructor uses a series of pictures when explaining the growth of the foetus.
- A nurse/midwife uses a paper cut-out held against her body to show mothers what the womb looks like and where it is located in the body.

9 Making their own visual aids is very useful in **helping learners discover solutions to problems.** When learners make their own aids and discover the answers for themselves, learning becomes an adventure. When people are having fun learning, they remember what they learn.

Mothers and children can learn about diarrhoea and dehydration by making their own 'baby' from clay, tin cans, plastic bottles, or gourds. They can experiment with the principle of rehydration by pouring water into the 'baby' and mending the different holes with 'food'.

See Unit 4 for directions for making and using gourd 'babies'.

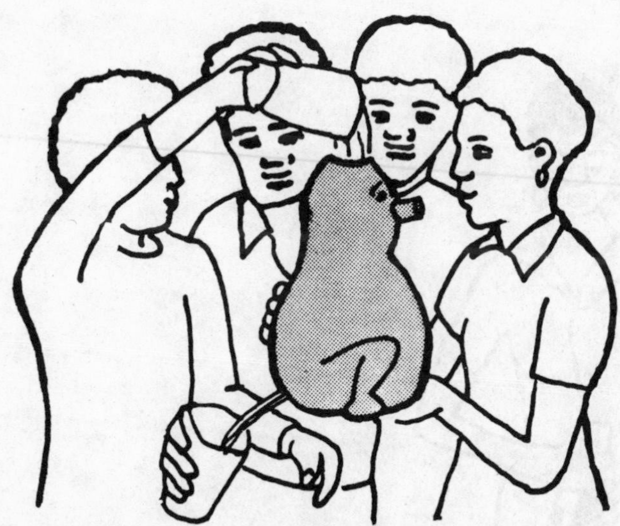

People enjoy making their own visual aids, and learn much by doing this. Mrs Keita is an example:

> Mrs Keita is a traditional birth attendant. She was in a class at the nearby clinic. There she was told that it is dangerous to ask a mother in labour to push too hard too quickly. The nurse trainer said that the opening of the

womb takes time to become large enough for the baby to pass through. The opening of the womb can tear if the birth attendant pushes on the mother's stomach or tries in other ways to make the baby go through the opening too early. The nurse trainer said that the mother's vaginal opening could tear like a cloth bag.

These were new ideas to Mrs Keita, who had always thought that trying to make the mother push was a way to help her, not hurt her.

The nurse trainer asked each person in the class to make a visual aid. She asked each person to work with an idea that was especially new or difficult.

Mrs Keita made two cloth bags and sewed two different sized elastic bands into the ends of them. She borrowed a rag doll from a friend.

When she was finished, she showed the others how the 'baby' would not pass through one of the cloth bags. The opening was too small. The opening of the second bag was large enough. Then Mrs Keita told them about the importance of not pushing on the mother's stomach.

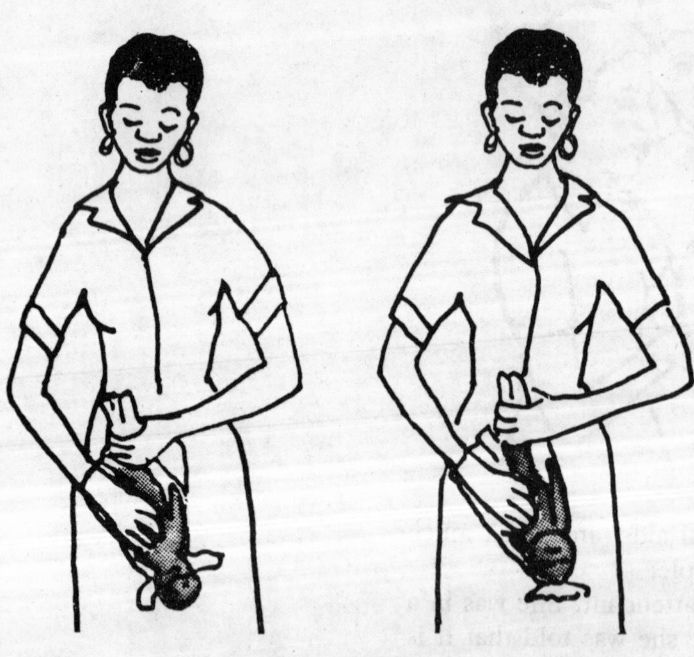

Another example:

Mrs Macalou asks clients who want to use birth control pills to draw a picture which will help them remember when to take the pills. She encourages each client to draw any kind of picture at all which will help her remember. Then Mrs Macalou asks the woman to explain the picture she has drawn. In this way, she can be sure that the woman understands and has something to take home with her to help her remember when to take her pills.

Ask learners to think of other examples.

10 Visual aids can **make a difficult idea easier to understand.** They do this by showing familiar people and things which illustrate the idea.

For example, suppose a nurse is counselling a family about the benefits of child spacing. She tells the family how child spacing means better health for the mother and for the children. But this is a new idea to the family. It is difficult to understand, because they do not know any other families who use child spacing.

So the nurse shows the family some pictures which compare child spacing to the spacing of crops. Then the family begins to understand. They know from their experience that crops grow better if they are not planted too close together.

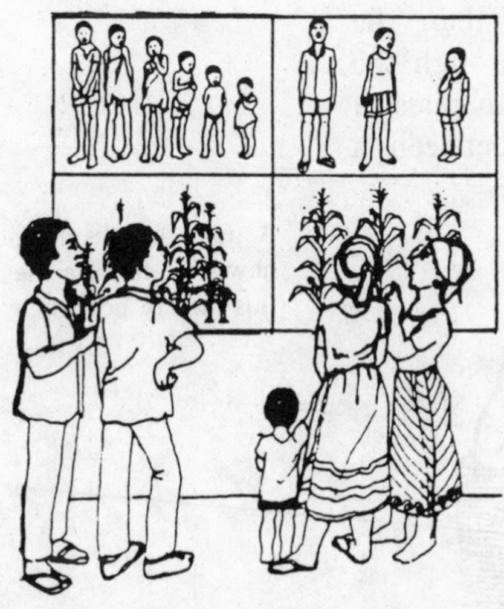

Another example is the kind of visual aid Mrs Bengaly, a nurse tutor, uses to demonstrate to her students how to tell whether a mother is losing a dangerous amount of blood during childbirth. She knows that on sheets a little blood can look like a lot.

She draws a picture on the sides of a box, showing the birth opening and the mother's legs spread and cuts a hole where the birth opening is.

Mrs Bengaly first holds up a glass container with about 500 ml of coloured water, a normal amount of 'blood'. Then she pours the 'blood' through the hole in the box onto the rags she has placed 'between the woman's legs' so the students can see what a normal amount of blood looks like.

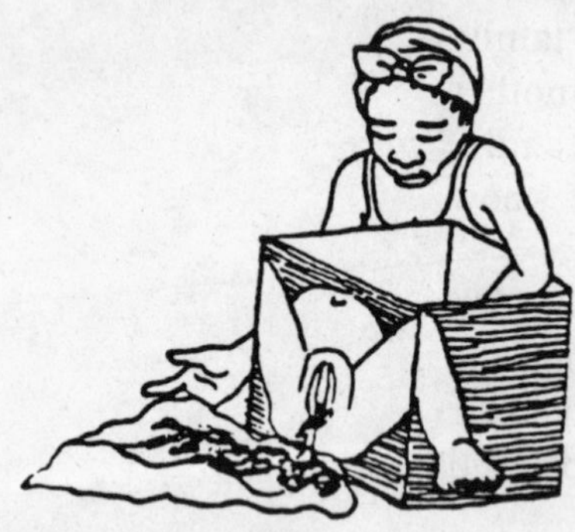

In Unit 4, Activity 2, **A birthing box,** in the section on **Making models,** shows how to make a box like the one used by Mrs Bengaly.

Then Mrs Bengaly moves the box to a place behind a clean pile of rags. Again she holds up a glass container, this time with about 800 ml, much more than the normal amount of 'blood'. She pours this through the hole again. Now her students can look at both piles of rags and see exactly what the difference between a normal and an abnormal blood loss looks like.

Activity 4 asks learners to explore how they can use the information in this unit to help their own learners.

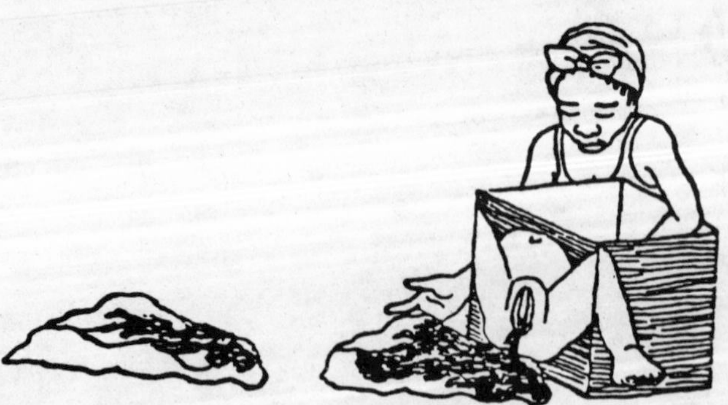

Activity 1 A visual introduction

Time 1 hour (for 15 people)

Objectives Learners will introduce themselves using pictures they have drawn themselves.
Learners will feel more comfortable working together.
Trainer will be able to evaluate learners' skill in drawing, composition, use of colour, and use of a visual aid in a presentation.

Materials needed One piece of any kind of low-cost blank paper such as newsprint or butcher's paper for each participant. 30 cm × 50 cm or larger is a good size for each piece of paper.
Coloured markers, crayons, or paint and brushes.
Pictures the trainers have prepared in advance to introduce themselves.

Instructions

1 Explain that this is an activity to help everyone to get to know each other better and to experiment with some of the drawing tools used in making visual aids. Emphasize that you do not expect people to produce great works of art. No one will be judging their drawings. This activity should be fun.
2 Explain that you will ask each person to draw on one piece of paper a few pictures showing things about themselves they would like to share with others. To demonstrate what is expected, introduce yourself using the pictures you have prepared in advance.
3 Be sure everyone has a sheet of paper and markers.
4 Ask each person to take about 5–10 minutes to draw three things which would show another person who they are and what kinds of things are important to them. Each person should print their names on their pictures. (In the past, people have drawn such things as nurses' caps, musical instruments, diplomas, children, spouses, maps, sunsets, and animals.)
5 One at a time, ask each learner to use his or her pictures to tell the group who they are and what is important to them. Allow time for questions from the group about the person's interests. Discourage criticism of the drawings and emphasize that these are not works of art, just experiments.
6 Listen very carefully during the presentations. Then you can summarize by addressing each learner by name, stating one thing you have learned about that person.
7 Post the pictures in the room so people can look at them later.

This will help them remember each other's names and interests as they are getting to know each other better.

8 Use these pictures to assess the level of skill each person is bringing to the workshop or class. Pay attention to drawing, composition, use of colour, and using visual aids in a presentation. Use this information to adapt your sessions to fit learners' needs. You can also use these pictures at the end of the workshop or series of classes to assess skills developed through your teaching.

Possible adaptations

In some areas, talking about yourself in this way is considered impolite. If this is true in your area, you can have participants do the activity in pairs. Then ask one person to introduce the other to the large group.

Activity 2

Why use visual aids?

Time

20 minutes

Objective

Learners will recognize and state that visual aids are sometimes necessary for a clear understanding of new information.

Materials needed

Pencils and paper for each participant.
Picture of the aardvark (or other animal or object to be described in activity). If you have more than 15–20 participants, you will need a larger drawing. See Unit 4 for ways to enlarge pictures.

Instructions

1 Be sure everyone has pencil and paper.
2 Explain that this activity is like a game that will lead to a discussion of teaching. Explain that you will be asking people to draw an animal based on a description from an encyclopedia which you will read to them twice. Emphasize that it doesn't matter how well they draw. Ask them to think about their reactions to the activity as they do it.
3 Read the description slowly and clearly. Do not worry if people express confusion. Ask your learners to draw whatever kind of picture the words suggest to them.

If learners want to hear the description again, read it to them again.

Tell them they have 5 minutes to complete the drawing. Let them work on the drawing for 5 minutes.

4 Ask learners how they feel about doing this activity. List some of their responses on the chalkboard to refer to later. Some of the responses you can expect are: 'not clear', 'not enough information', 'I got lost after the first sentence'.

5 Ask a few people to guess what kind of animal they have been drawing. Show participants the picture of the aardvark. Re-read the description, pointing to each part of the picture as it is described.

6 Ask people to summarize what they have learned from this activity. They should state some version of the objective for this activity. If they have difficulty, give them a hint such as: 'What has this shown you about learning new information with words and pictures?'

7 Ask learners to imagine they are nursing students and an instructor has just given them a verbal description of how an IUD is inserted, but has not shown them what the IUD or the inserter looks like! Point to the list of frustrations expressed while they tried to draw the animal. Ask them how they can apply what they have learned in this activity to their own work.

8 Summarize the activity by stating the objective ('You have stated that visual aids . . .'). Repeat their list of frustrations noting the similarity with frustrations often stated by students.

Possible adaptations

1 The aardvark seems to work well. But you may want to use another example that will be more interesting to your learners. Choose any description of an animal or object that is confusing when described only with words.

2 If time allows, in instruction 5 above, you may want to have learners post their pictures after they guess what animal it is, but before you show the aardvark picture.

3 This activity can be combined with part of Activity 3, **Things we have learned through pictures.** After instruction 7 above, have the large group do steps 1–3 of Activity 3.

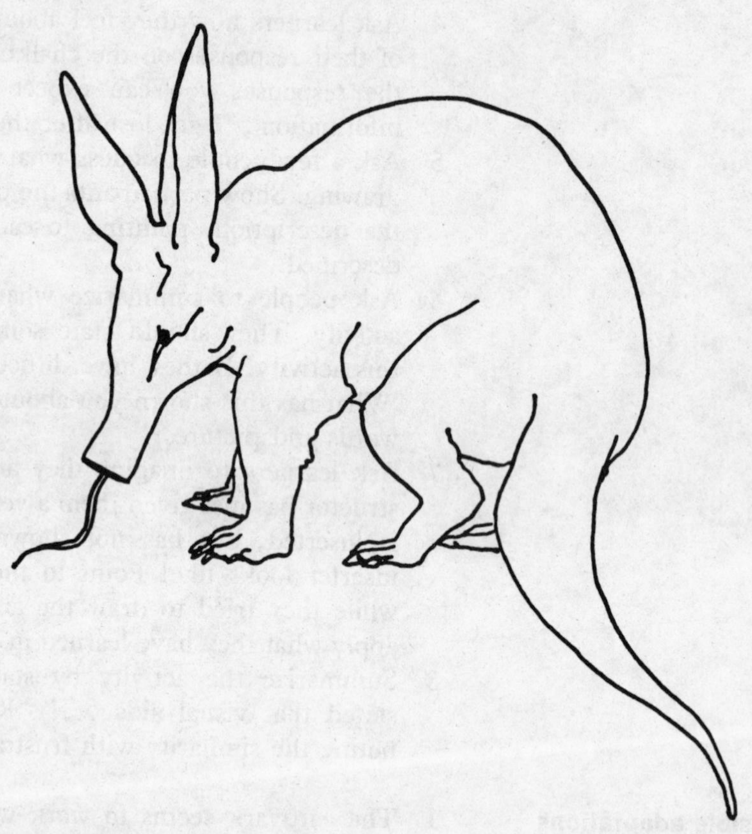

'The body is stout, with arched back; the limbs are short and stout, armed with strong, blunt claws; the ears long; the tail thick at the base and tapering gradually. The elongated head is set on a short, thick neck, and at the end of the snout is a disc in which the nostrils open. The mouth is small and tubular, furnished with a very long, thin tongue.'

Activity 3

Things we have learned through pictures

Time

45 minutes

Objectives

Learners will be able to list at least 4 things which they learned more easily because they had some kind of picture to look at.
Learners will be able to explain how the visual aid helped them learn each thing listed.

Materials needed

Several large sheets of paper, and markers or pens.

Instructions

1 Divide learners into groups of 4 or 5 people.

2 Give each group 2 sheets of paper and a marker. Ask everyone to take 3 minutes to think of at least one thing they needed to have a picture of to learn. Tell people that they may use experiences from daily life as well as classroom experiences.

Examples might be:

- what a cell looks like
- how to tie different kinds of knots
- how to sew
- what a foetus looks like
- how a foetus changes as it grows
- which road to take when travelling (Did someone draw you a map?)

3 Ask one person in each group to record the examples given by each person in their group. Ask the recorders to title the list: 'Things We Have Learned Through Pictures'. Encourage the groups to list more than 4 or 5 items if they have more that they want to add (5 minutes).

4 Have one person from each group come to the front, one at a time, and explain the items the group has listed (20 minutes). Post these lists on the chalkboard if you have one, and leave some room beside them to write another list.

5 Beside the lists, write the title, 'How the Picture Helped Me Learn'. (You can use another large sheet of paper if you do not have a chalkboard.)

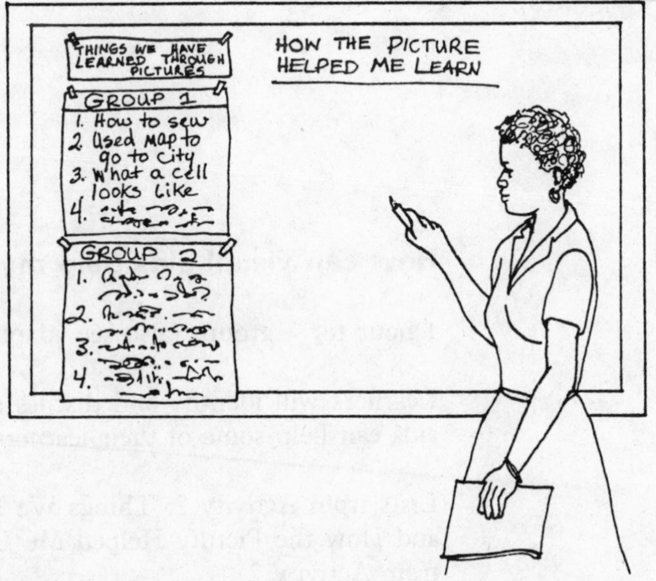

6 Explain that you will all use the lists they have made as you talk about the ways in which pictures help us learn.
7 Refer to these lists as you and your participants work your way through the 10 main ideas presented in the text. As you talk about each way in which pictures help us learn, ask learners if they see an item on the 'Things We Have Learned Through Pictures' list that is an example of that idea. Then write next to the item the way in which the picture helped the person learn.
8 By the time you are ready to do Activity 4, you will have 2 complete lists.

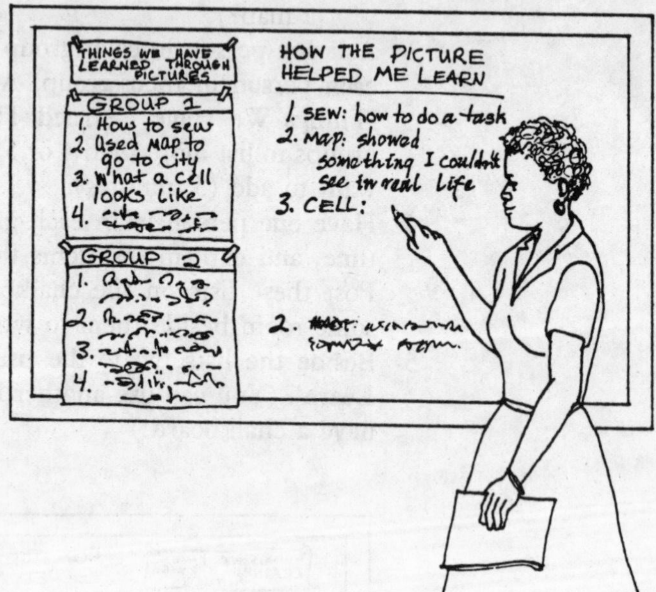

Activity 4 **How can visual aids help my learners?**

Time 1 hour for 4 groups (also see adaptation)

Objective Learners will identify and discuss at least one way in which visual aids can help some of their learners.

Materials Lists from Activity 2: Things We Have Learned Through Pictures and How the Picture Helped Me Learn. (These are already posted from Activity 2).

Class notes listing the 10 ways in which visual aids help us learn.
Paper and pencils or newsprint and markers for each small group.
A long strip of paper or a long broomstraw for each group.

Instructions

1 Ask learners to divide into small groups, with 3 or 4 people in each group.

2 Ask everyone to think of one topic his or her learners sometimes find difficult to learn (2 minutes).
Without talking, everyone writes down this topic.

3 Each group appoints one person who will act as recorder.

4 Give each group a strip of paper or a broomstraw. Ask one person to tear it into 4 unequal strips and hold the strips so they all look equal. Each of the other group members draws a strip.

5 The person with the shortest strip becomes 'the trainer'. The trainers begin the activity by sharing with the group the topic they have identified. The recorder divides the paper into 3 columns, and labels them 'Topic', 'Suggested Visual Aid', and 'How the Visual Aid Helps Learning'. The recorder writes down the topic, as in the example below (3 minutes).

6 Ask the trainer to explain to the group how he or she teaches the topic. Have other members of the group listen and try to identify the parts of the explanation learners are finding difficult (5 minutes).

7 Then ask group members to suggest visual aids which the trainer could use to help teach the topic. The recorder writes all the suggestions in the second column (5 minutes).

TOPIC	SUGGESTED VISUAL AID	HOW THE VISUAL AID HELPS LEARNING
Where the diaphragm fits	1) flash cards or series of posters 2) flipchart showing woman inserting diaphragm	

8 Beside each visual aid suggested, have the group list at least one way in which it could be *used* to help the trainer's learners (5 minutes).

Note: Groups may refer to lists if necessary. The list of the 10 ways visual aids help us learn should be especially helpful here. The recorder writes these things in the third column, beside each visual aid suggested.

TOPIC	SUGGESTED VISUAL AID	HOW THE VISUAL AID HELPS LEARNING
Where the diaphragm fits	1) flash cards or series of posters 2) flipchart showing woman inserting diaphragm	1) - shows something you can't see in real life - shows the steps involved in placing diaphragm properly

9 Meet as a large group again. Ask one person from each small group to summarize that group's activities. Post the recorder's notes (10 minutes).
Discuss the suggestions and answer any questions. (10 minutes). Draw attention to any particularly good suggestions. If some ideas do not seem to be well thought out, ask the large group to suggest other possible solutions to that trainer's problem.

Possible adaptations

If you have time, you can let the small groups consider each person's topic. Each person can become the trainer, and can take turns according to the length of the straws. Count on 15 minutes per person for the small group activities. If you have 4 groups of 4 people, the activity would take about 2 hours.

Activity 5

Ways to use visual aids

Time

1 hour if oral; 45 minutes if written

Objective

Learners will describe at least 2 ways they could use a sample visual aid to help their learners understand or remember important information.

Materials

The 3 visual aids that follow.
Pencil and paper for everyone (optional).

Instructions

1 This activity can be either written or oral. If you have a small number of learners, you can ask them to take turns answering the questions below for each picture.

2 Take off the wall the lists of 'Things We Have Learned Through Pictures' and 'How the Visual Aid Helps Learning'.

3 Post or display the 3 visual aids which follow. Be sure that everyone can see the visual aids well but that the answers beneath the visuals are not showing.

4 Explain that you are going to ask them to answer two questions. The person answering the questions may choose whichever picture he or she feels most comfortable with.

5 Have the first person come to the front. Read the first question aloud, then let the person choose which picture he or she wants to use. Ask the person to hold the picture and face the other learners as he or she answers the first question, and then the second question. If your learners are writing down their own answers to these questions, ask them to do so for all 3 pictures.

Questions: 1 Give one reason for using one of these visual aids in your own work.

2 Describe two ways you could use one of these visual aids to help your learners understand or remember important information.

6 Have the second person come to the front and choose a picture. It can be the same picture that the first person chose if the second person has different answers to the questions. Or, it can be a different picture.

7 Continue allowing learners to add their answers to the questions for all three pictures until they have run out of ideas.

8 Following the visual aids, you will find lists of possible correct answers. Learners may also suggest some things which are not on the list for that picture that seem to you to be good ideas. In this case, count that as a correct answer.

Possible adaptations

The exercises in this activity can be done with *any* visual aids. You can easily adapt the activity by choosing three other visual aids or real objects related to a topic which you know your learners are responsible for teaching. If the following 3 visual aids are not useful for your learners, do not use them — find or make your own, and make your own lists of possible answers before you begin the test activity. You can put a mark beside each item as someone mentions it. The list will also help you give people some guidance in answering the questions if they need it.

Visual Aid 1

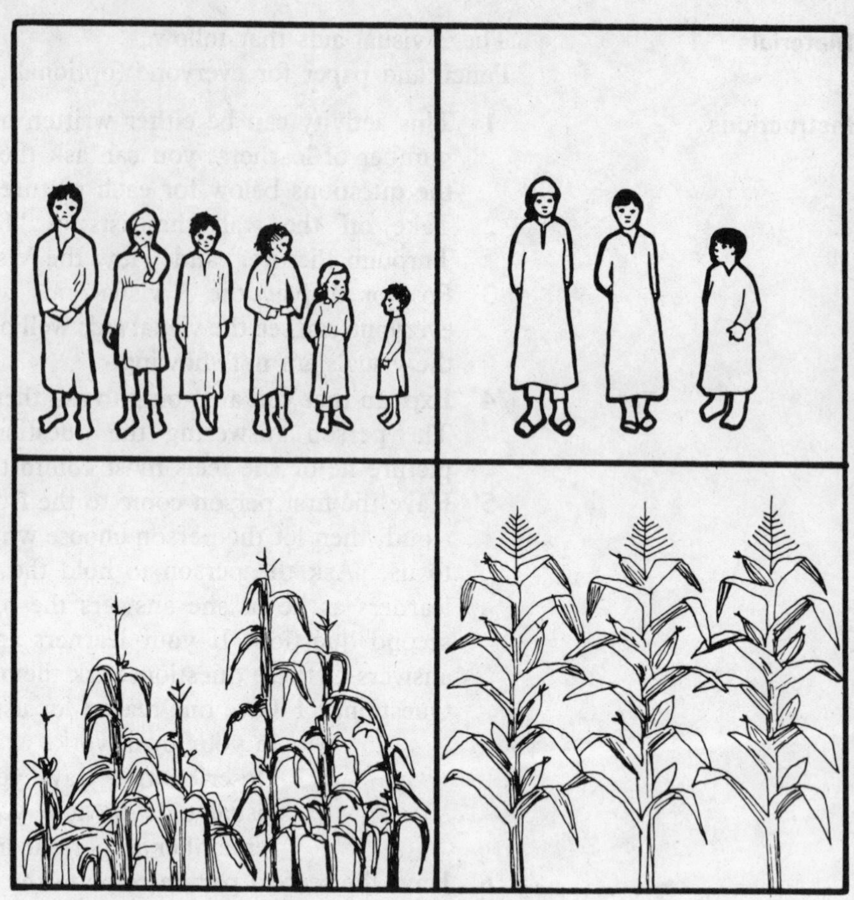

29 CHILD SPACING IS LIKE RAISING CROPS

Child spacing is like raising crops

Ways a trainer can use this visual aid:

1 *To make a difficult idea (child spacing) easier to understand* by showing how it is like planting crops.

2 *To compare the similarities and differences between two things* (crops and children).

3 *To provide information when the trainer cannot be present* (can be posted on a clinic wall).

4 *To provide the basis for discussion* of how child spacing is like planting crops. The trainer could ask, 'What do these pictures say to you?'

5 *To review or test learners*. The trainer can cover up either the top two or the bottom two pictures and have the learners sketch in the other two small pictures.

Visual Aid 2

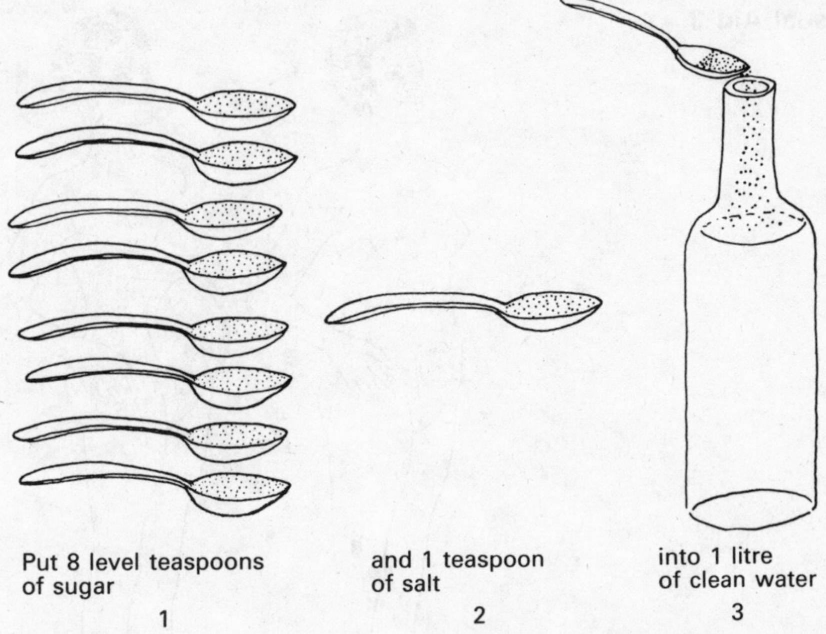

Rehydration drink to prevent and treat dehydration

Ways a trainer can use this visual aid:

1 *To show steps to follow in doing a task* (mixing rehydration drink).

2 *To review or test learners.* The trainer can cover up the labels and ask learners to explain what the pictures mean. 'What are the measurements and what are the things being measured?'

3 *To provide information when the trainer cannot be present.* The visual aid can be posted on a wall or bulletin board. It can be given to learners as a handout, or they can copy it into their notes, to use later. Mothers can copy it and take it home to hang on a wall.

4 *To make a difficult idea easier to understand.* This picture is better than reading a recipe. It shows how all the measurements relate to familiar things, such as spoons and bottles.

5 *To provide the basis for discussion.* The trainer could ask, 'Do most mothers in your area use these kinds of spoons and bottles? If not, how would you need to change this picture so that the women in your area can understand the measurements?'

Visual Aid 3

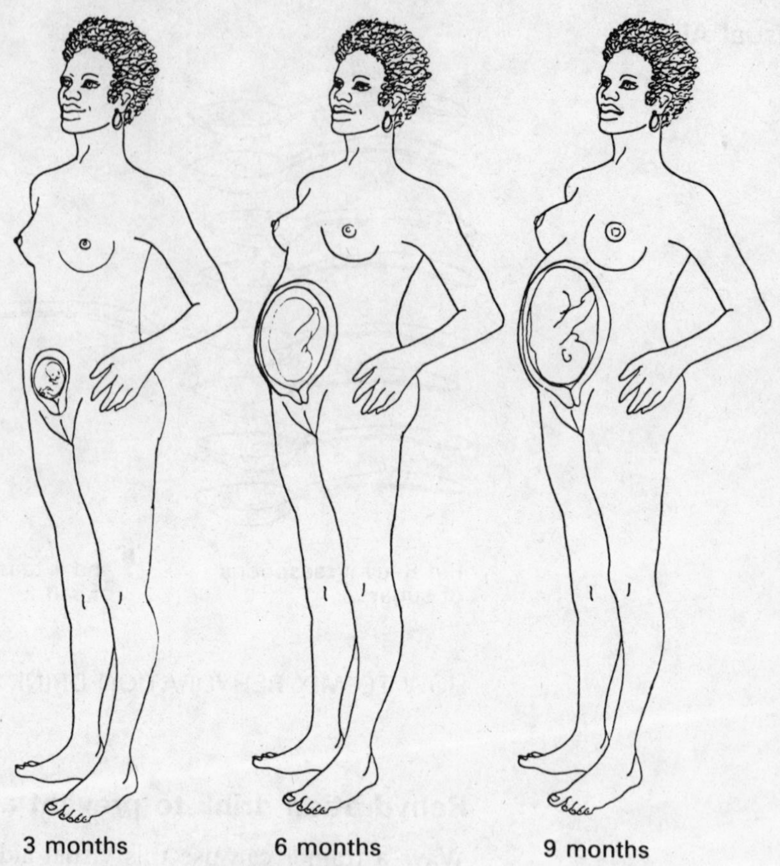

GROWTH OF THE UNBORN BABY

Growth of the baby in the mother's womb

Ways a trainer can use this visual aid:

1. *To show something people cannot see in real life* (the baby inside the mother).
2. *To show how something changes or grows* (the baby and the mother's stomach).
3. *To compare the similarities and differences* between different stages of pregnancy.
4. Perhaps *to help make a difficult idea easier to understand*. ('Where inside me does the baby grow?')
5. *To provide information when the trainer cannot be present* (can be posted on a clinic wall).
6. *To review or test the learners*. The trainer can cover up the labels and ask learners to tell how many months pregnant each of these women is.

Unit 2
Deciding What Kind of Visual Aid to Use

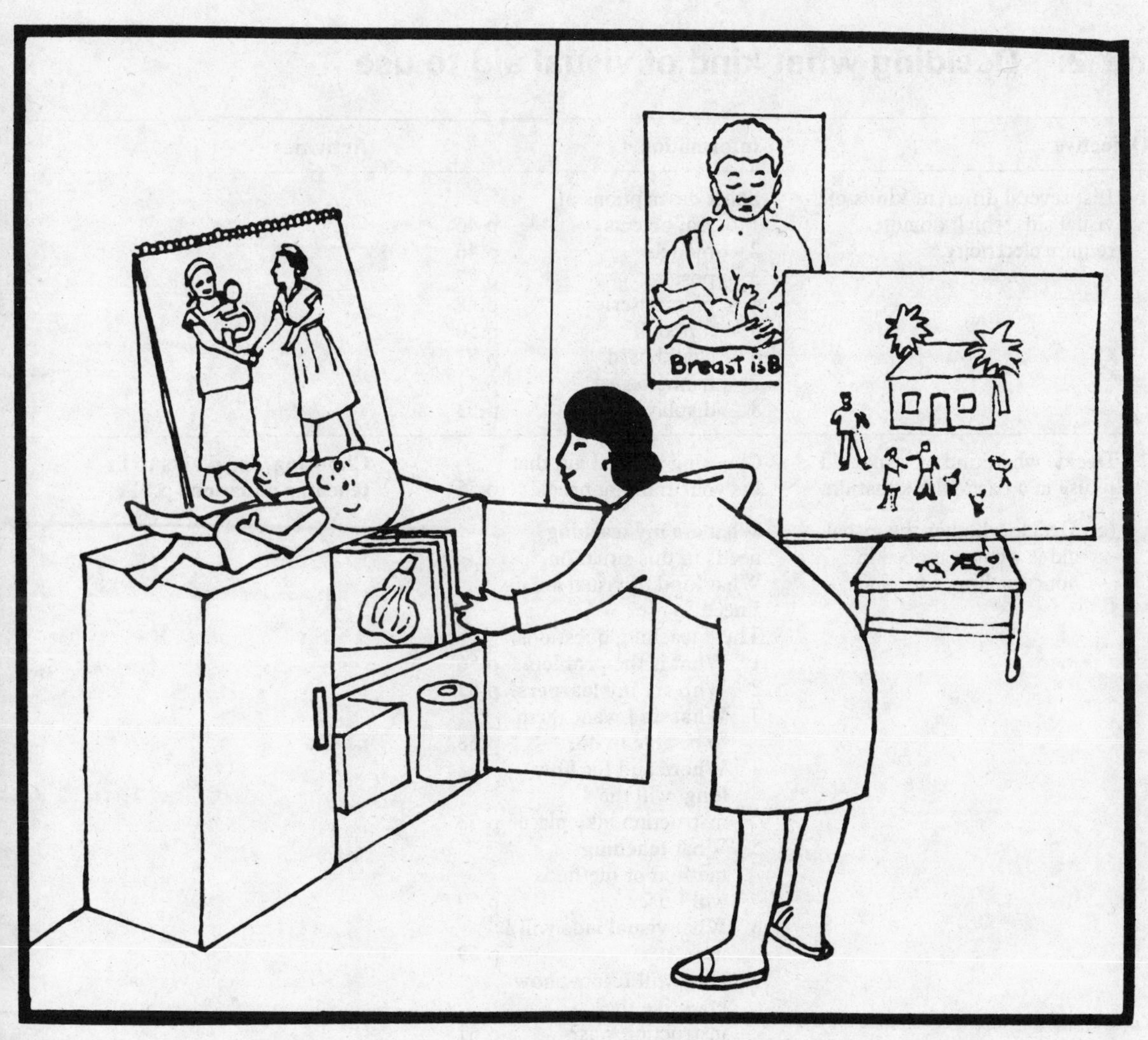

Now that your learners know when to use visual aids, Unit 2 will help them decide what kind of visual aid will be best. You can use 'The 7 Teaching Questions' in this unit to help practice choosing the best visual aid for specific teaching situations. Your learners look at different kinds of low cost visual aids. They also learn how to decide whether a visual aid is well designed. They learn how to choose visual aids for people who have little experience learning from pictures. Finally, they learn when and how to adapt a visual aid to make it more appropriate for people in their local areas.

Unit 2: Deciding what kind of visual aid to use

Objective	Information		Activities
1 List several different kinds of visual aids which do not require electricity.	Short descriptions of:		
	1 – real objects	p.46	
	2 – models	p.46	
	3 – posters	p.47	
	4 – picture series	p.48	
	5 – flipbook	p.50	
	6 – chalkboard	p.51	
	7 – flannelboard	p.51	
	8 – display	p.53	
2 Decide what kind of visual aid to use in a particular situation.	Choosing a visual aid that fits your training needs.	p.55	**Choosing visual aids to fit teaching situations** p.81
(a) Decide whether the visual aid is what you need in your teaching situation.	What are my teaching needs in this situation? What kind of visual aid do I need to use?		
	The 7 teaching questions:		
	1 **What** is the **problem**?	p.56	
	2 **Who** are my **learners?**	p.57	
	3 **What** do I want them to be able to **do**?	p.58	
	4 **Where** and for **how long** will the instruction take place?	p.58	
	5 What **teaching method** or methods will I use?	p.59	
	6 What **visual aids** will I use?	p.59	
	7 How will I know **how effective** the instruction was?	p.61	

Objective	Information		Activities
2 (b) Decide whether the visual aid is well designed.	Choosing a visual aid that is well designed.	p.62	**Is the visual aid well designed?** p.86
	The 6 design considerations:		
	1 Words and pictures should be **easy to see.**	p.62	
	2 Words and pictures should be **easy to understand.**	p.65	
	3 Information should be presented **clearly and simply.**	p.68	
	4 The visual should be **well organized.**	p.70	**Seeing the same picture in different ways** p.89
	5 The **viewer's attention** should be **directed to the important information.**	p.73	
	6 The visual should be **interesting** to the people for whom it is intended.	p.75	**Need for pre-testing visual aids** p.91
3 Adapt an existing visual aid to fit the needs of your learners.	Adapting an existing visual aid.	p.77	**Adapting visual aids** p.94
	The existing one may be:		
	1 – the wrong size	p.77	
	2 – too complicated	p.78	
	3 – offensive	p.79	
	4 – unfamiliar	p.80	

Evaluation:

Listen and watch your participants closely during the activities to be sure that they understand the new ideas.

There is an example of how to evaluate visual aids for good design in Activity 2, **Is the visual aid well designed?**

The activity, **Choosing visual aids to fit teaching situations,** contains guidelines to help you evaluate how well your learners can choose visual aids for specific teaching situations.

There are several ways for you to cover the section of this unit which introduces learners to the different kinds of visual aids. Which way you use it depends on how much time you have. See the examples of curricula in the Trainer's Guide for some ideas on how you can organize this session.

Visual aids which do not require electricity

Real objects

A real object is the real thing, not a model or a picture of it. When Mrs Kabengara teaches her nursing students about the different methods of family planning, she always shows them the real things, such as diaphragms, IUDs, and condoms.

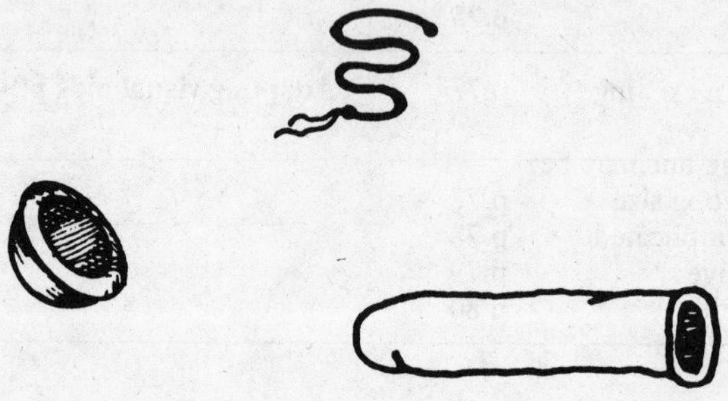

Real objects are useful when you are teaching ideas or skills which require learners to know about real things.

Models

A model is a realistic copy of something. It may be larger, smaller, or the same size as the object it represents.

Mrs Chama trains community health workers. She uses a rag doll like the one below for several different things.

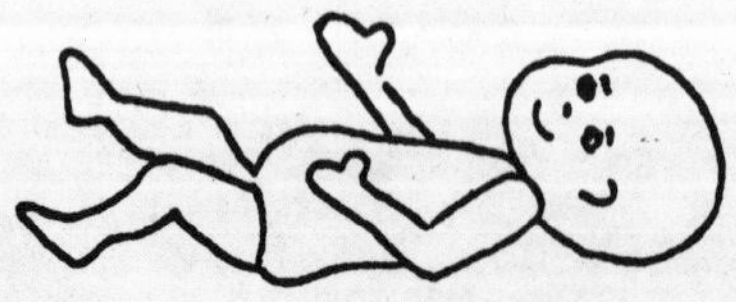

She can use it with a delivery box or a 'birthing box' to demonstrate childbearing. Her trainees can also use the doll to practise weighing a baby or holding the baby in different positions while bathing it.

See Unit 4, model making section, for instructions on how to make a 'birthing box'.

The gourd 'baby' mentioned in Unit 1 is an example of a model which helps learners discover solutions to a problem. In this case, the problem is dehydration. Learners can pull the plugs so that the water runs out, and the baby has 'diarrhoea'.

By tilting the baby backward as the water runs out, learners can see that the baby can pass urine as long as he has enough water.

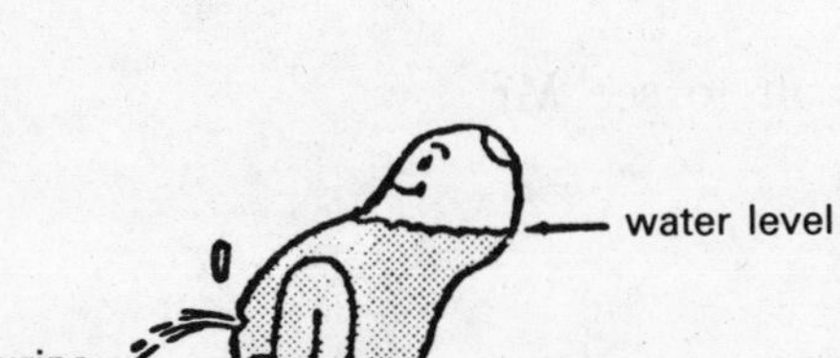

When he has lost a large amount of water, he no longer passes urine, even though the diarrhoea may continue.

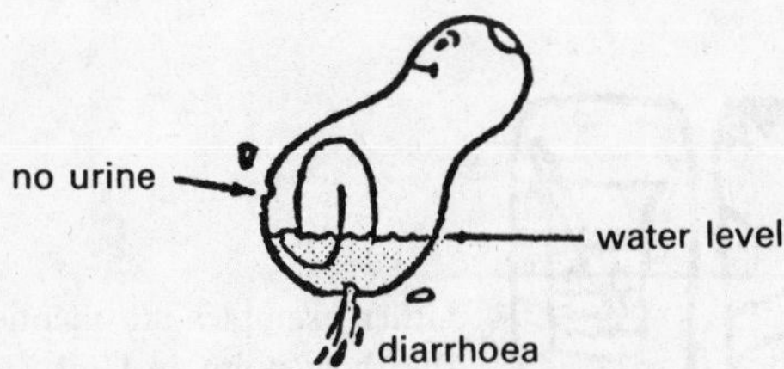

Posters

A poster is a large piece of paper or cloth which uses pictures, words, and numbers to present information. It represents only one idea or one process, and is posted for people to see. It does not need anyone to explain it.

Mr Sangare, who runs a clinic, put up a poster like the one below in the waiting room.

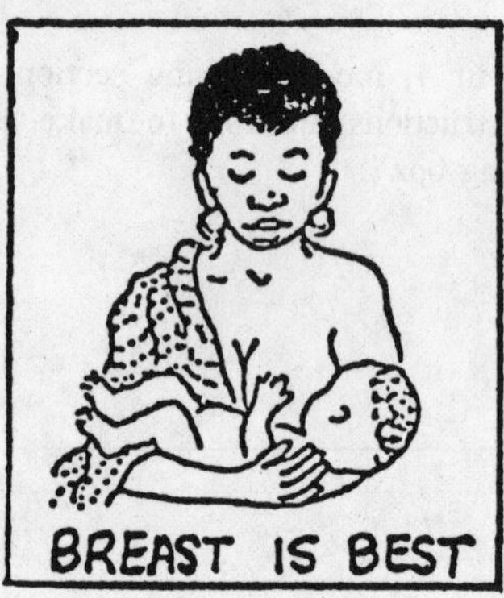

Mothers can look at the poster while they wait to see Mr Sangare.

Picture series

A picture series is a set of drawings or pictures which can be used in several different ways.

Mr Kamwengu, the nurse tutor, used this set of pictures to help his students learn how to take temperatures.

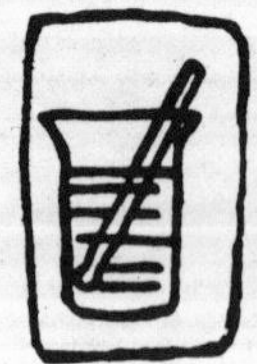
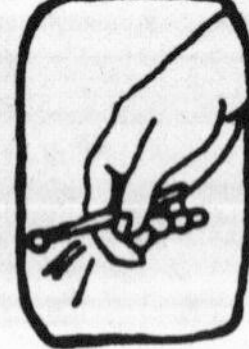
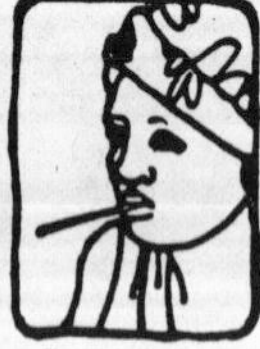
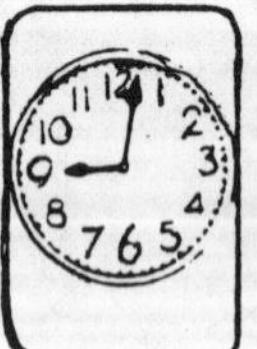
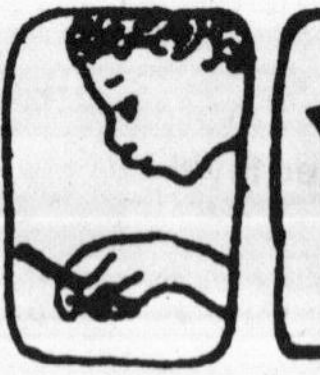

Other examples are mentioned under the third point in Unit 1 — *the steps to follow in doing a task*.

A set of pictures can show the steps to follow in doing a task, such as taking a temperature, but a series of pictures can also be used to show how something changes or grows. The series of pictures below shows how a fertilized egg begins to grow.

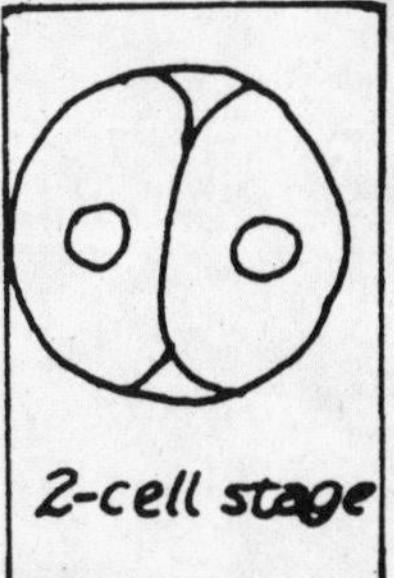

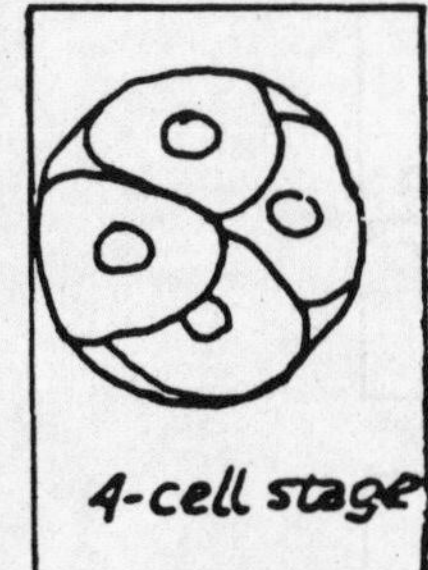

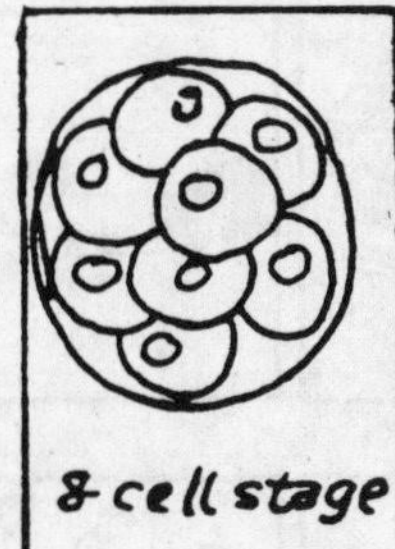

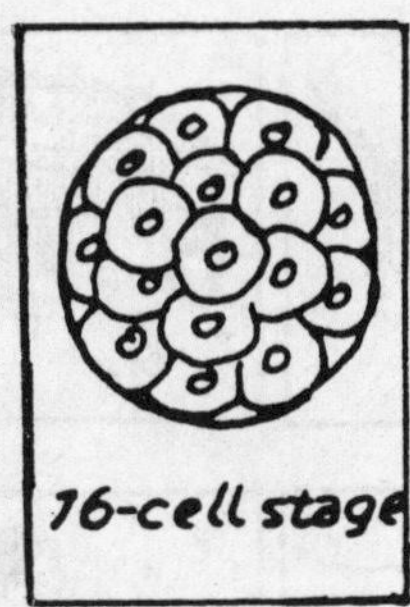

A picture series can show several things of the same kind that belong together or are used together. Mrs Dissa talks with the village women about nutrition, using a set of pictures for each different food group. Then she mixes pictures from the sets. Then she asks the women to pick out the picture which does not belong in the series.

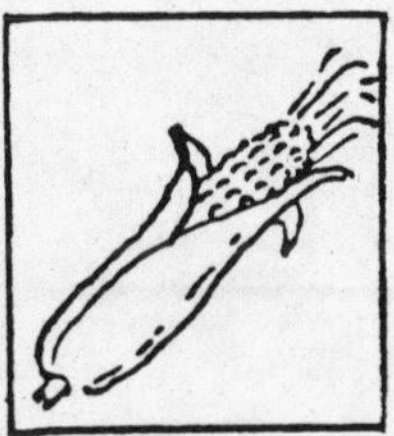

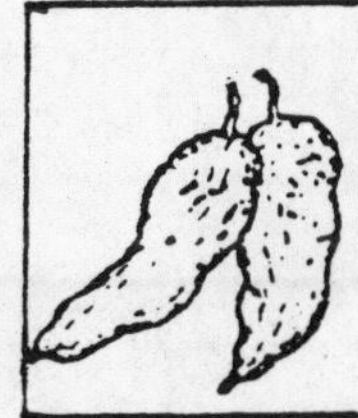

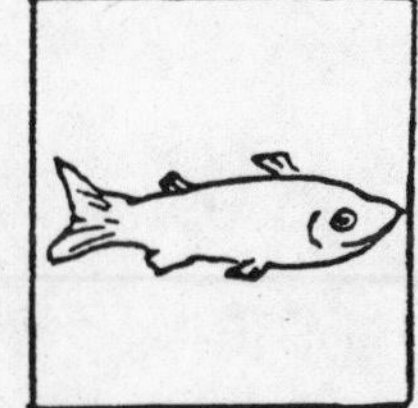

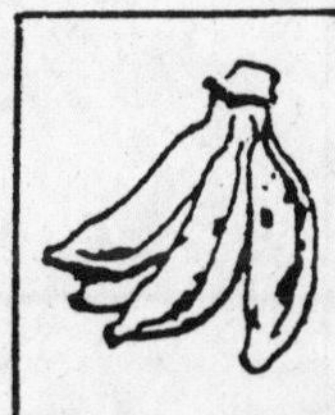

The maize, cassava, and bananas belong together because they are all starches.

The fish does not belong in the series because it is a protein.

A picture series is excellent for telling a story. Mrs Dissa also uses the set of pictures below to tell villagers a story about how a man with diarrhoea or worms spreads the disease to his whole family.

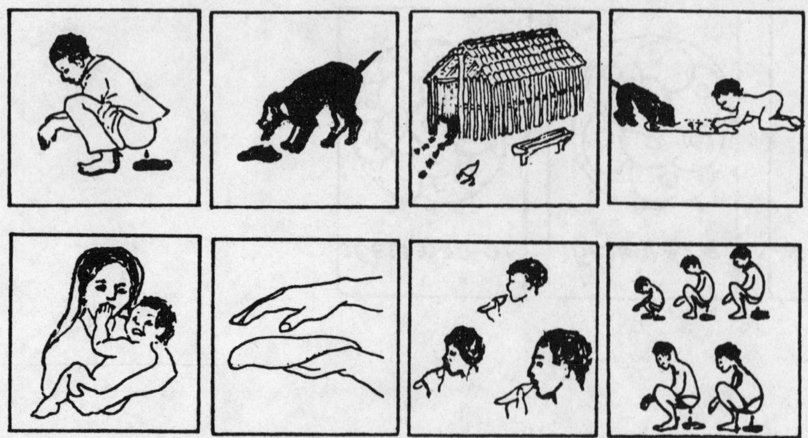

Flipbook

A flipbook is a series of pictures bound together in a particular order. They usually tell a story or show steps in a process.

Mr Kyara has a flipbook on interviewing which he uses with his nursing students.

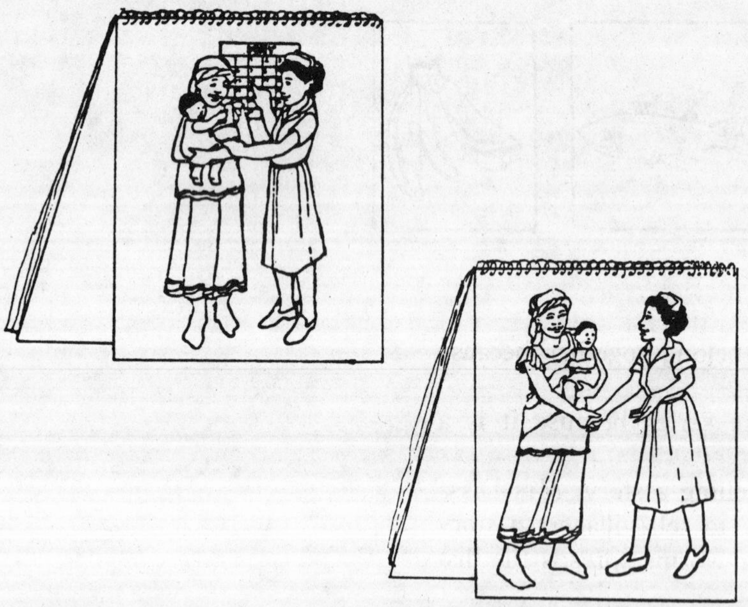

He shows his students one picture and then leads discussion about the picture. Then he 'flips' the book to the next picture.

Chalkboard

A chalkboard can be any dark coloured, flat surface on which you can write with chalk. Chalkboards can be used for drawing or stencilling pictures as well as writing words. Mrs Fatma draws a picture like the one below on her chalkboard. Then she shows her nursing students where the pituitary gland is and where the ovaries and uterus are.

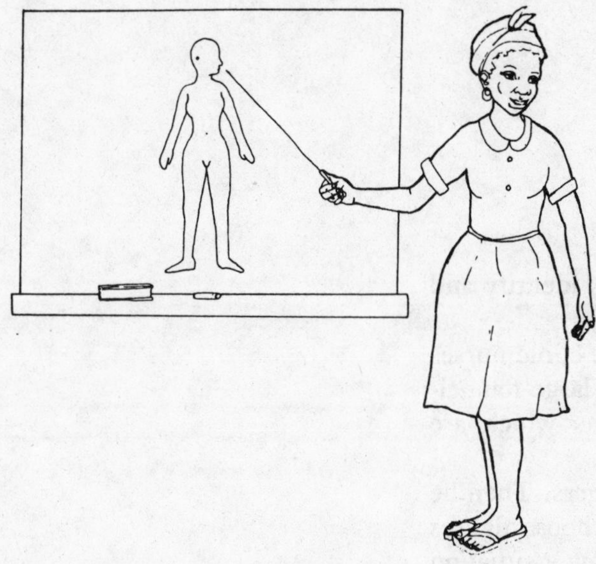

Flannelboard

A flannelboard is a board made of flannel, felt, or other rough cloth. Pieces of the same cloth are cut into shapes of objects. These objects will stick to the board, because of the rough surfaces. Sand or wheat chaff can also be glued onto the backs of the cloth pieces to help them stay on. The flannelboard should be tilted slightly backward to help the pieces stay on.

Flannelboards are useful for presentations because you can add or move around objects as you speak. This is what the community health worker in Unit 1 was doing when she presented information on the food groups to the village women. Then she checked to see what the women had learned by asking them to come up and place the different 'foods' in the correct group on the flannelboard.

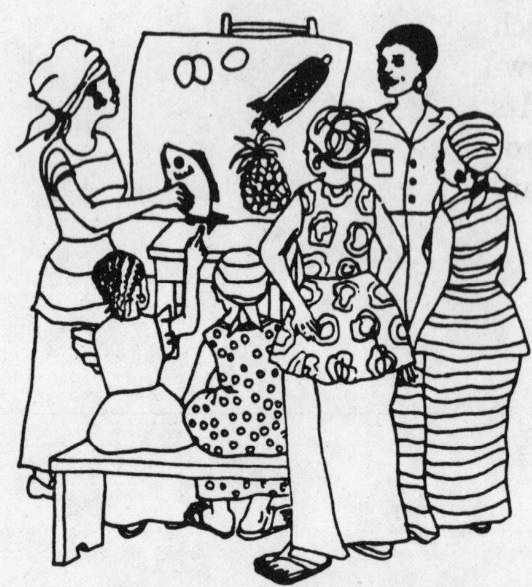

Flannelboards can also be used to help learners identify and solve problems.

Many of Mr Soulama's workshop learners are clinic nurses or community health workers. He has made a large flannelboard, and many different figures and objects which are common to communities in that region.

He asks his learners to pretend they are villagers. Then he asks a few learners to come to the front and choose figures and objects and place them on the board to show a situation which is a problem in their 'community'. Then they explain the situation they have shown, and everyone discusses possible ways to solve the problem.

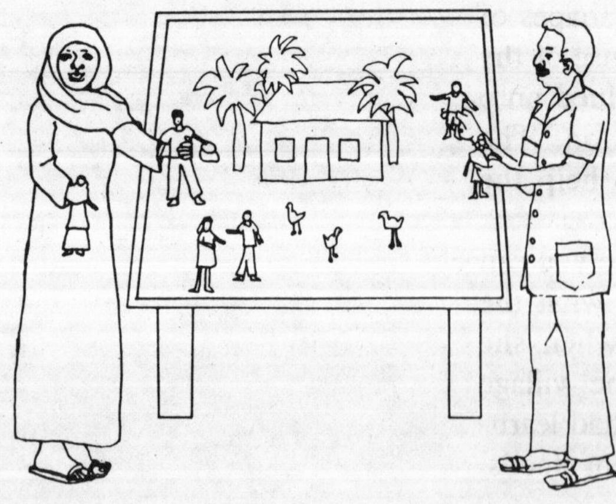

In this way, Mr Soulama's learners see how they may use a flannelboard to help villagers identify and talk about their problems.

Display

A display is an exhibit, organized around one idea or theme. It usually includes different kinds of visual aids, such as real objects, models, and posters. The main purpose of a display or exhibit is to attract attention and give information. It is sometimes useful to have someone present with the display to answer questions, but this is not always necessary.

Two effective kinds of displays can be made very simply: a rope display and a pole display. Both are easy to make and easy to move from place to place.

See Unit 4 for instructions on making rope displays and pole displays.

Mrs Goko had an idea for a display using live plants.

She planted two plots of ground in front of the clinic. In one plot, she planted very many yams close together. In the other plot, she left space between the plants as in a normal garden.

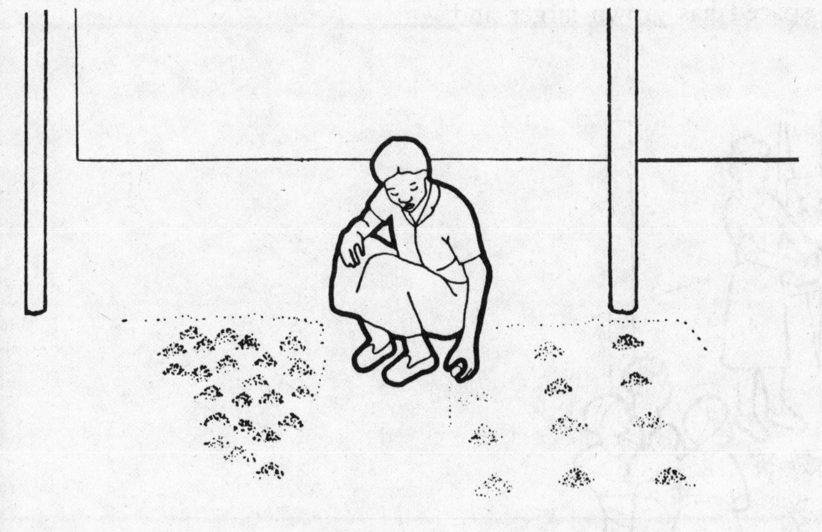

When the plants were large, she hung a rope display from the clinic roof to the ground behind the plants. She made posters and tied them to the ropes with pieces of string.

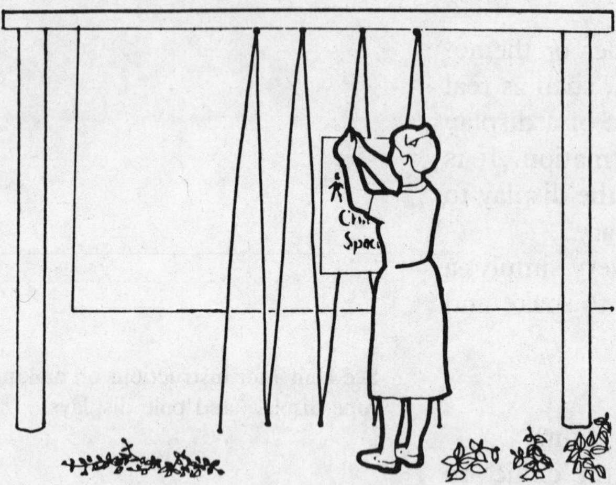

Now people coming to the clinic can see the posters and look at the plants to see that the healthier ones are the ones which had more space to grow.

Mrs Goko also gives talks using the display. To show how children spaced at least two years apart are usually larger and stronger, she pulls up one yam from each of the plots, and shows that the one which was spaced has grown larger and healthier.

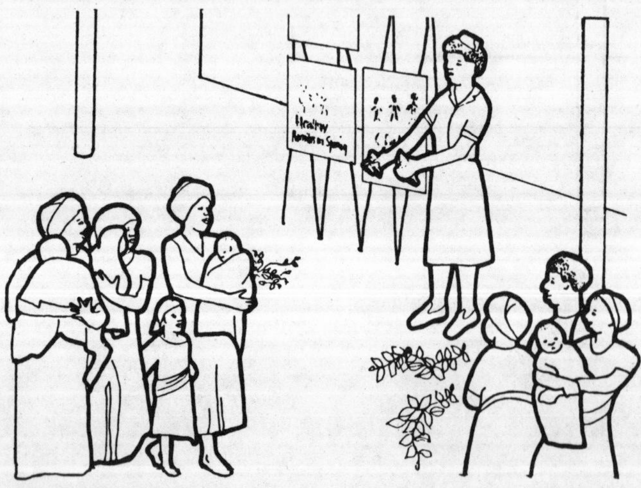

Choosing a visual aid that fits your training needs

'What kind of visual aid do I need to use?'

Choosing a visual aid which will be effective for your learners is only part of planning a training session. Trainers must identify specific training needs before they can know what kind of visual aid is best to use.

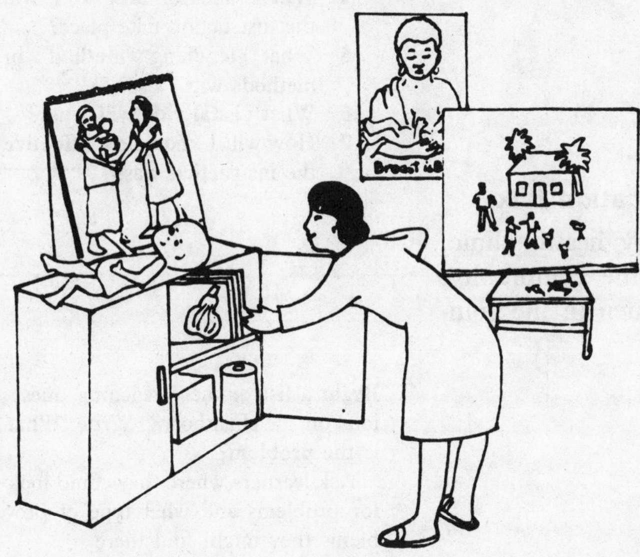

Series of images adapted from *Why Family Planning*?
© Collier Macmillan Limited 1982

The following story tells about Mrs Ebrahim's plans for using visual aids in a health talk. It illustrates the 7 teaching questions that anyone must ask to decide what visual aid to use.

There are larger versions of the pictures in the Resource Pictures section at the end of the manual. (See the Trainer's Guide for how to use that section.)

One way to teach this section is first to present the story and pictures which follow. Display or post the pictures one at a time as you tell the story of Mrs Ebrahim.

Then go back through the pictures and have the learners identify the teaching questions and suggest important things to consider under each.

The 7 teaching questions are:

1 **What** is the **problem**?
2 **Who** are my **learners**?
3 **What** do I want them to be able to **do**?
4 **Where** and for **how long** will the instruction take place?
5 What **teaching method** or methods will I use?
6 What **visual aids** will I use?
7 How will I know **how effective** the instruction was?

Story: Mrs Ebrahim plans a health education talk

Mrs Ebrahim is in charge of a community health clinic. Kwashiorkor is a widespread problem in the community. Mrs Ebrahim wants to talk with more women in the community about nutrition.

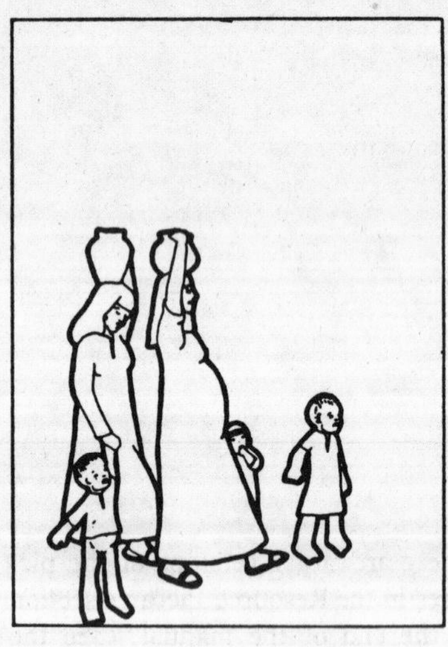

Series of images adapted from *Why Family Planning*?

Begin a list of the 7 teaching questions on the chalkboard. Write '**What** is the **problem**?'

Ask learners where they could look for problems and what type of problems they might find there.

They might suggest:

1 in the community
- health and illness
- community health education

2 in the agency
- staff skills
- clinic management
- client education and follow-up.

Ask learners how they could find out problems. They might suggest:

- Ask the people involved, such as members of the community, clients, or clinic staff or manager.
- Observe for themselves what goes on in the clinic or community.
- Check the clinic or the community records.

Ask learners what are some other important things to consider when deciding on problems to solve.

Information	Training ideas and your notes

They might mention:

- Sometimes there are too many problems and you have to decide which are the most important to solve, so rate the problems according to how common they are and how serious they are.
- Some problems can't be solved by training or education.
- Sometimes a high level official tells you what problem to solve.

Ask learners what problem Mrs Ebrahim identified.

She wants to talk with women who are not regular clients at the clinic. Many of the women do not come to the clinic because they do not know about the services it provides. Many of the women in the community are not literate.

Write the second teaching question on the chalkboard, '**Who** are my **learners**?'

Have learners suggest a list of important things for a trainer to know about his or her learners if the training is to be most effective. Write these things under the question '**Who** are my **learners**?'

Be sure the following ideas are mentioned:

- How many people will be in the session?
- What are the backgrounds and life-styles of these people?
- What things are important to them?
- What do they want from the training?
- What do they know already?
- Will they be required to attend or will they choose to attend?
- What might keep them from attending?

Ask learners to copy these questions into their notes as you discuss Mrs Ebrahim's situation.

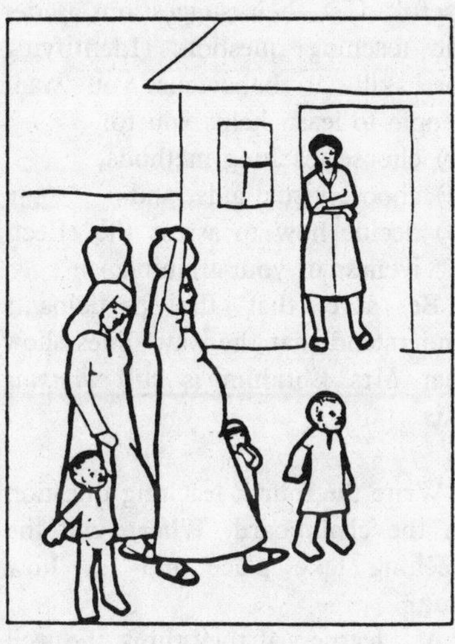

Series of images adapted from *Why Family Planning*?

Mrs Ebrahim wants the women to know that kwashiorkor is caused by not enough protein in the child's diet. She wants the women to be able to name at least 3 high protein foods they can feed their children.

Information	Training ideas and your notes

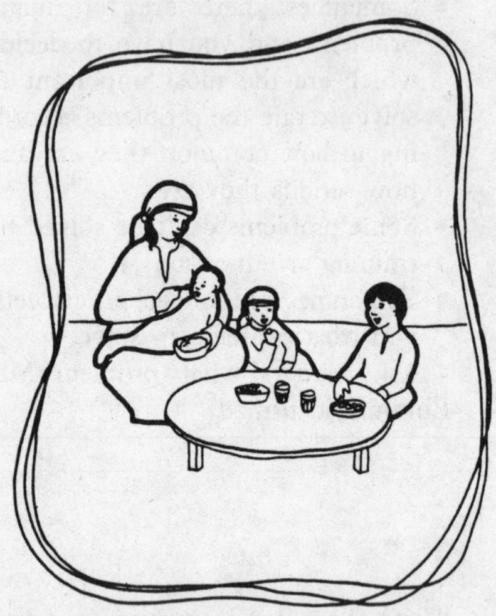

Series of images adapted from *Why Family Planning*?

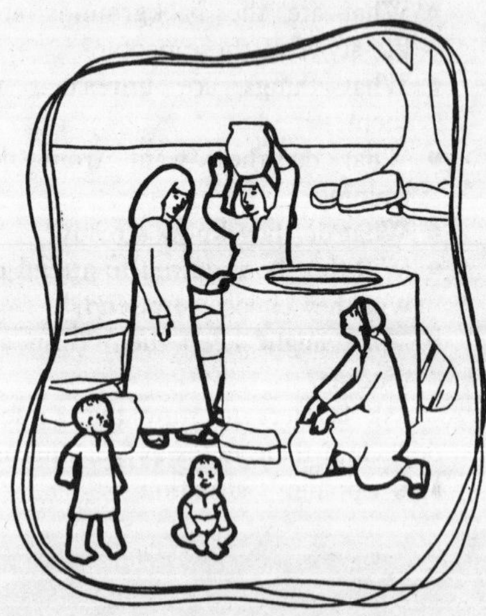

Series of images adapted from *Why Family Planning*?

Explain that the wavy lines around some of the pictures are meant to show that this is what Mrs Ebrahim is *thinking*.

Ask participants if they recognize what Mrs Ebrahim is doing (deciding on her objective).

Write the third teaching question on the chalkboard:
'**What** do I want them to be able to **do**?'

Lead a discussion of the learners' understanding of what an objective is. (Learning objectives are statements of exactly what the learners will be able to do as a result of the teaching or training.)

Ask learners why objectives are useful. List their suggestions under the teaching question. (Identifying the skill or behaviour you want people to learn helps you to:
(1) choose teaching methods,
(2) choose visual aids, and
(3) decide how to assess the effectiveness of your training.)

Be sure that the participants understand that the wavy lines show that Mrs Ebrahim is still *thinking* this.

Write the fourth teaching question on the chalkboard: **Where** will the teaching take place and for **how long**?

Ask learners if they think the well is a good choice. Why or why not?

Have learners suggest important things to think about concerning the setting for the instruction. List these under the teaching question.

Some things they may mention are:

- Will the session be indoors or outdoors?
- Is there electricity? Lights?
- Will there be chairs or tables?
- Are there chalkboards?
- Will it be noisy or will there be other distractions?

Information	Training ideas and your notes

- How comfortable can I make the place for my learners?
- How much time do my learners have to spare?
- How much time do I have to spare?

Mrs Ebrahim decides that the well is a good place to meet with the women, while they are drawing water. The women will be busy and will not be expecting her. So she must have something with her which will get and hold their attention and interest them. They have little time to listen to her, so she decides to spend ten minutes talking with them.

Write the fifth teaching question on the chalkboard: 'What **teaching method** or methods will I use?'

Have learners list under this question the important things in choosing a teaching method. Be sure that the following ideas are mentioned:

- What do my answers to the **who** and **what** questions tell me about what teaching method or methods to use?
- How can I best help my learners to learn what I want them to?
- Can I use more than one method to make the sessions more interesting?

Mrs Ebrahim has noticed that the women often tell stories to each other when they are at the well. She thinks the women would be interested in hearing a health story. She plans to tell a story about a mother whose child gets kwashiorkor.

See Unit 5 for more on using different teaching methods.

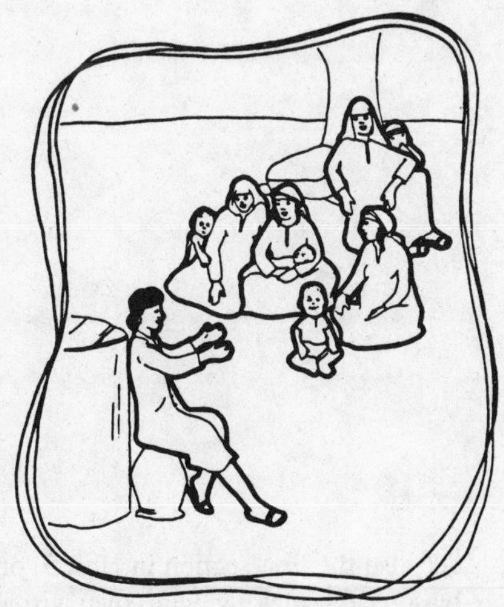

Series of images adapted from *Why Family Planning*?

Write the sixth teaching question on the chalkboard: 'What **visual aids** will I use?'

Have learners suggest things they would consider in choosing a visual aid for Mrs Ebrahim to use. They may suggest:

- must be easy to carry
- must be suitable for using with storytelling method
- must be interesting enough to get and hold the women's attention.

Ask them to suggest the general things they think are important when choosing a visual aid. Write these under the teaching question.

They may suggest:
- What visual aids are *available* to me? What can I find that is already made?
- What visual aids can I *make*?
- How much *time* and what *materials* do I have to make my own? Is it practical to make my own?

Mrs Ebrahim wonders what kind of visual aid she can use.

Mrs Ebrahim then wonders if she has any flipbooks or pictures in the clinic which would be useful for this meeting. She looks through her cabinet to see what she has. She does not find anything.

Ask learners to suggest all the sources they can think of which are available to them for visual aids. Include agencies and shops at the national and local levels. Ask participants to copy these into their notes for future use in their jobs.

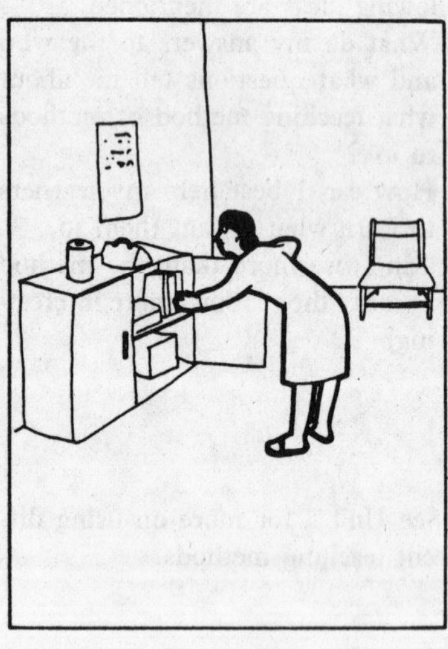

Series of images adapted from *Why Family Planning*?

Mrs Ebrahim knows that she can use a series of pictures of kwashiorkor again and again in her work. She decides to take the time to make her own picture series on kwashiorkor.

She also decides to take real food examples to show the mothers during her talk.

See also the first section in Unit 3, on reasons for making your own visual aids.

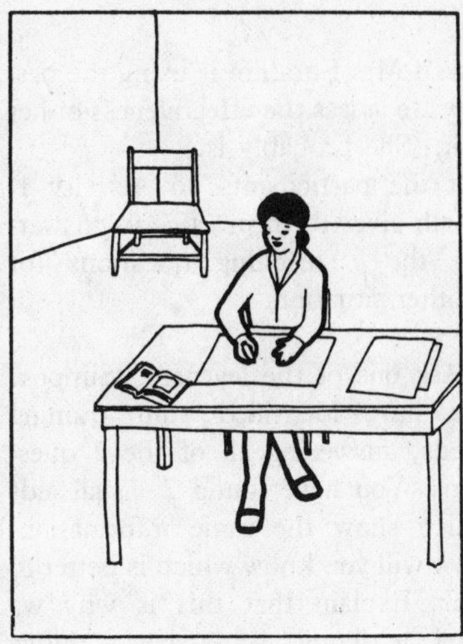

Series of images adapted from *Why Family Planning*?

Mrs Ebrahim notices the reactions of the women during her talk with them. The women seem interested. They ask questions. Mrs Ebrahim can tell from their questions that they understand the information in the story. Afterwards, when Mrs Ebrahim shows them pictures or examples of high protein foods, the mothers can name at least three.

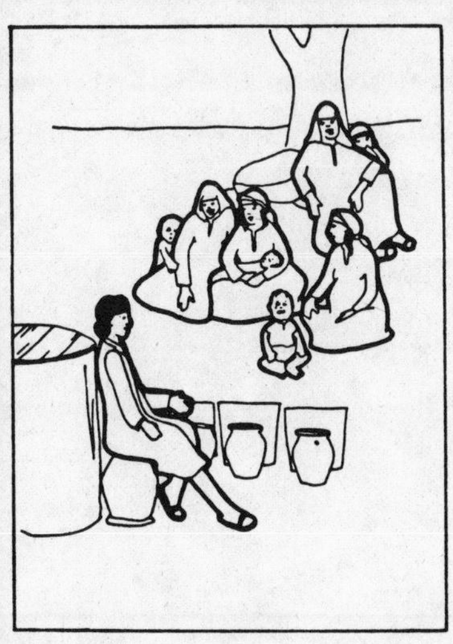

Series of images adapted from *Why Family Planning*?

Write the seventh teaching question on the chalkboard: 'How will I know **how effective** the training was?'

Ask participants to suggest some reasons why assessment is valuable. Write these under the teaching question.

They may say:

- It helps us find out if the training worked.
- It helps us know what to change to make the training more effective.

Mrs Ebrahim can also tell that the talk was effective if she sees more women coming to the nutrition sessions at the clinic.

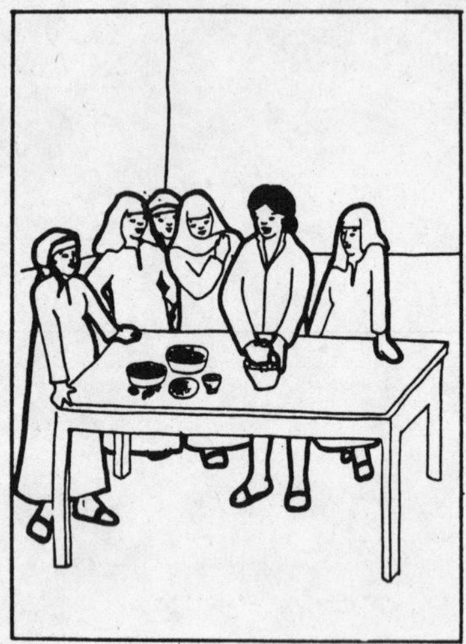

Series of images adapted from *Why Family Planning*?
© Collier Macmillan Limited 1982

Ask if Mrs Ebrahim is using the best ways to assess the effectiveness of her talk. (She probably is.)
Let the participants do Activity 1, which gives them practice in answering the 7 teaching questions for another situation.

Ask one of the learners, 'Suppose you have identified your training needs, answering all of the 7 questions. You have found 2 visual aids which show the same information. How will you know which is better to use?' Explain that this is why we need to know some basic things about design.

The 6 design considerations are to help us tell a good design from a bad one.

You can enlarge the pictures in the text and use them to teach this session. Or you can find your own examples and use them.

Choosing a visual aid that is well designed

Answering the 7 teaching questions will tell you what *kind* of visual aid you need. It will also tell you what *information* needs to be included in the visual aid, as when Mrs Ebrahim decided on the story she wanted to tell.

The following 6 design considerations help you decide how well the visual aid communicates the message. The considerations encompass 15 questions: ask these questions as you review visuals that you may use to teach. Also keep these questions in mind as you plan and make your own visual aids.

1 Words and pictures should be **easy to see.**

a) Are the words large enough to see?
If there is lettering, it should be large and thick enough to read easily. Compare these two examples of good and bad lettering.

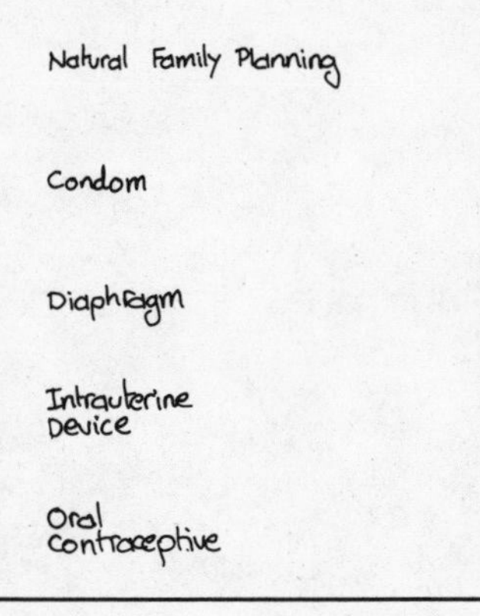

Natural Family Planning
Condom
Diaphragm
Intrauterine Device
Oral Contraceptive

Hold examples up for everyone to see. Newspapers, advertisements, posters, and books are good sources for examples of lettering. See also Unit 4, **Lettering** for more details.

b) Are the pictures large enough to see?

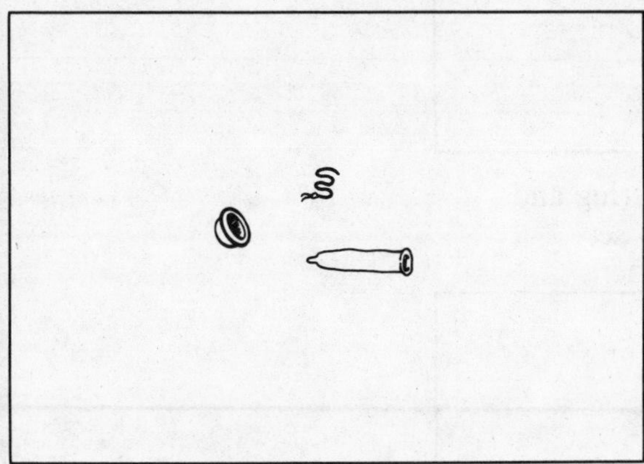

These drawings are too small–people can't read them.

Hold up this picture or another example like it and ask learners what is wrong with it. (The pictures are small and hard to read.)

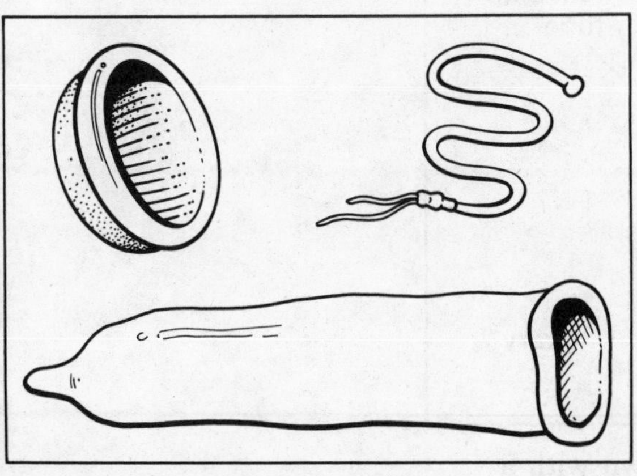

These drawings are large and people can read them.

Hold up this picture also and ask learners whether they find it easier to read and understand.

If you cannot enlarge these pictures, you can easily draw them on the chalkboard as you discuss this point.

c) Are the words and pictures bold enough to see?

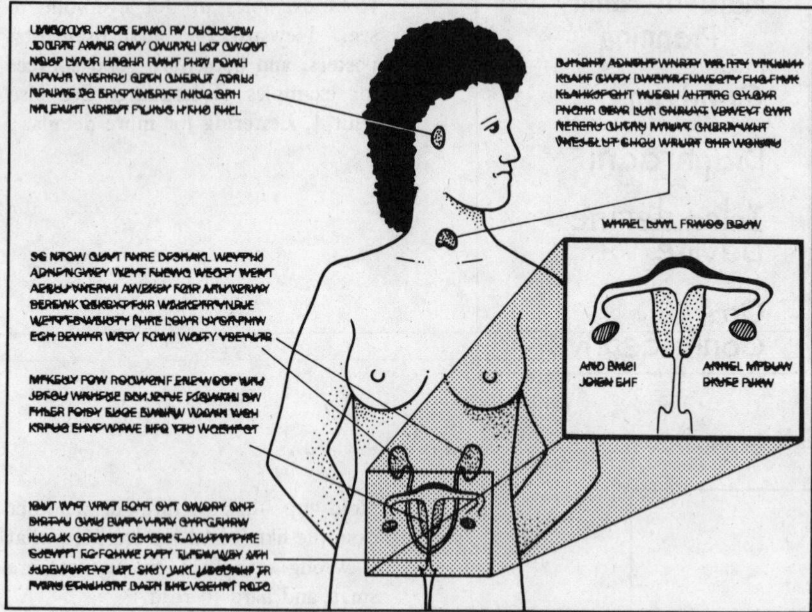

This drawing is large enough to see but the lettering and pictures are too small and detailed for people to see.

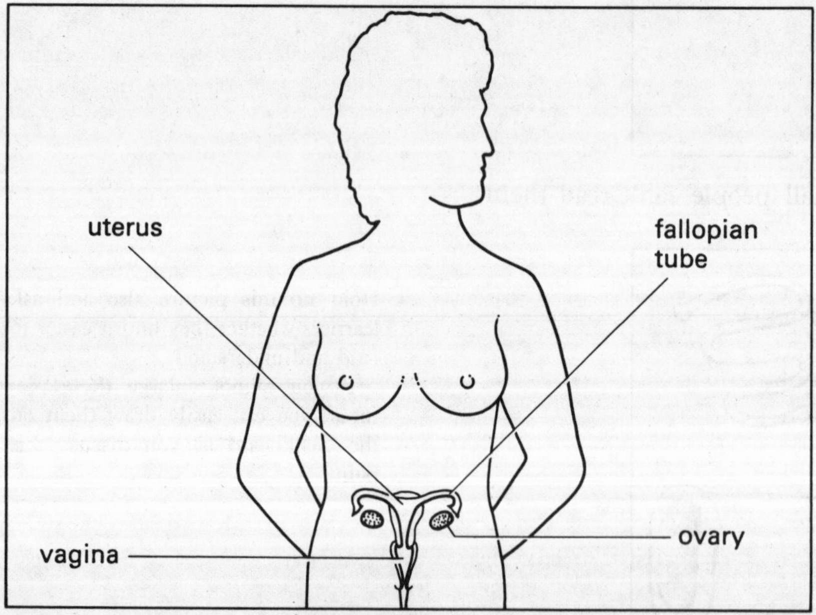

This drawing is large enough to see and is drawn with a bold line so that people can see it.

2 Words and pictures should be **easy to understand.**

a) Are unfamiliar words or pictures used? Using an illustration style showing people, actions, objects and words which are familiar to your learners will make the visual aid easier to understand.

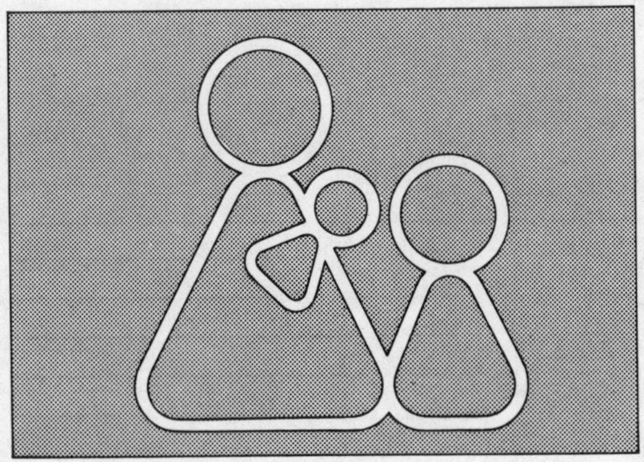

This stylized visual of a mother and children would be unfamiliar to many people.

Hold up the picture. Ask learners to recall other examples of unfamiliar styles which they have seen. These may include cartoons of dancing food or very sophisticated graphics which only use abstract shapes.

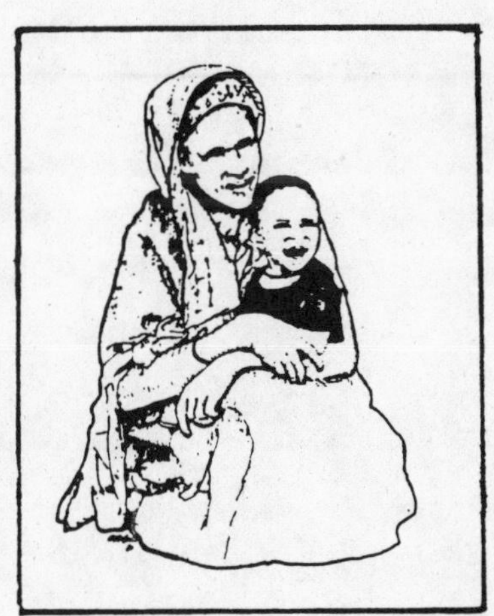

This picture of a mother and child would be more familiar to people in East Africa.

If possible, use other examples more appropriate for your learners. Ask participants to describe other examples from their experience.

b) Are all figures or objects on the same scale? Notice in the picture on the left that the pineapple appears to be as tall as the man. But have you ever seen a pineapple that big? Of course not. Showing the pineapple and the man on two different scales is confusing.

On the right, the man is holding a pineapple. The man and pineapple are on the same scale and are easy to understand.

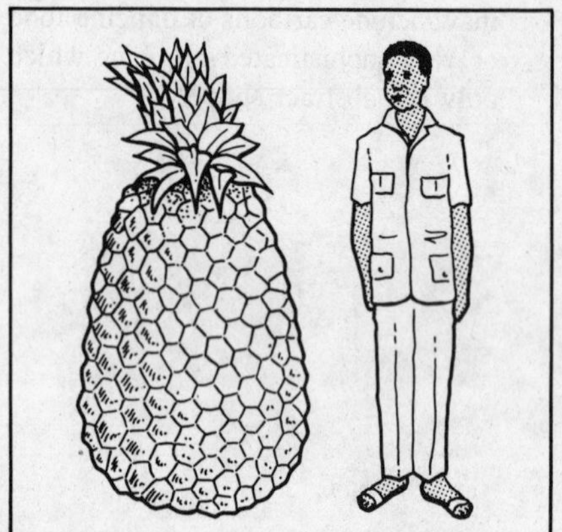

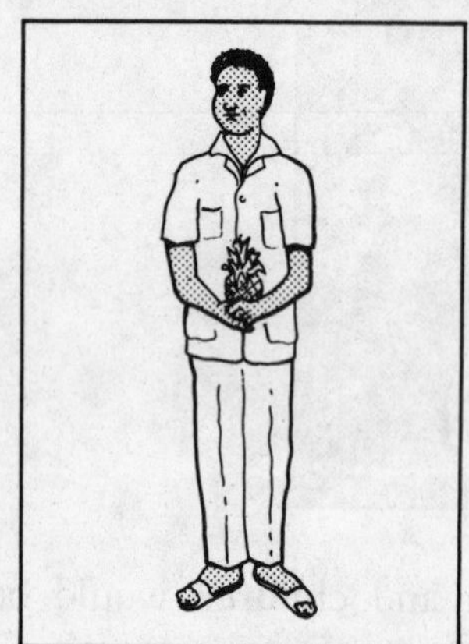

c) Are full figures shown, rather than parts of figures? A whole figure is more like what we see in daily life.

It is easy to recognize the picture below that shows a mother nursing a baby.

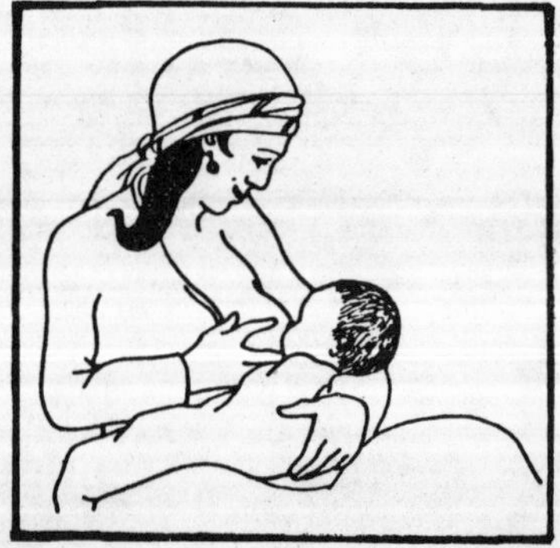

Adapted from *Prenatal Nutrition and Breastfeeding*

It is not easy to recognize the following picture which shows only the baby at the mother's breast.

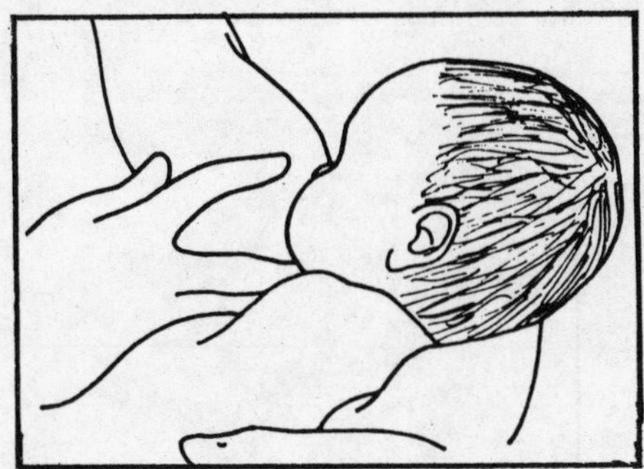

Adapted from *Prenatal Nutrition and Breastfeeding*

When it is necessary to look at only a part of something, use the whole figure drawing as a starting point to show where the part fits into the whole. Then show a picture of the part you want to discuss. You can leave the whole figure picture as a reference while you talk about the part.

You can explain where an IUD is placed in a woman's body by first showing where the womb is located on a picture of the woman's whole body.

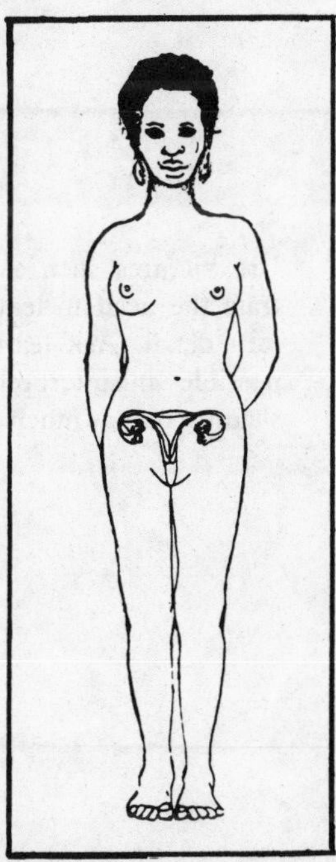

Then you can show a picture of the part of the body where the IUD will be placed, and show how the IUD fits.

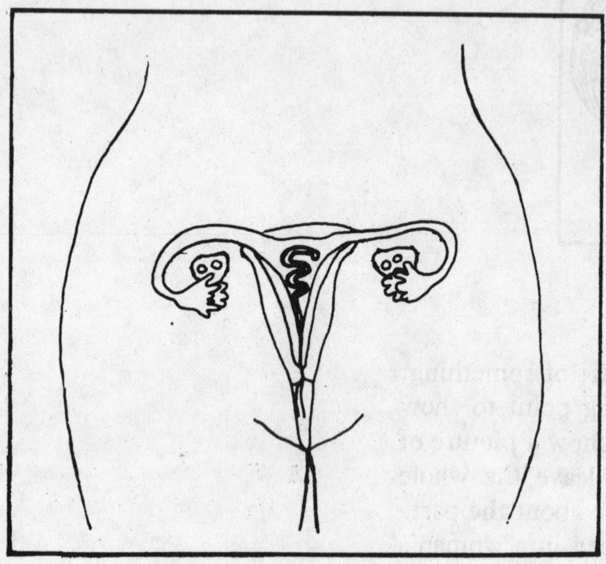

3 Information should be presented **clearly and simply.**

a) Are there unnecessary details? Show only what is necessary to the main idea. Details in clothing or background, or artistic shading may draw people's attention away from the main idea. Too many figures, objects, or actions may distract or confuse learners.

Use pictures such as these to illustrate the need to leave out unnecessary detail. Ask learners to suggest possible misinterpretations due to shading or too much detail.

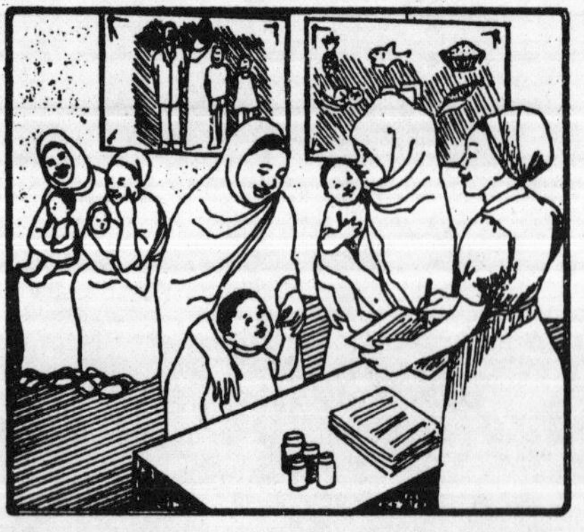

The posters which the artist put in the background are very distracting. The people in the poster can be seen as a family watching through a window, or as people standing in a doorway, or trapped in a box. The 'floating' food in the other poster is also confusing, and the shading is distracting.

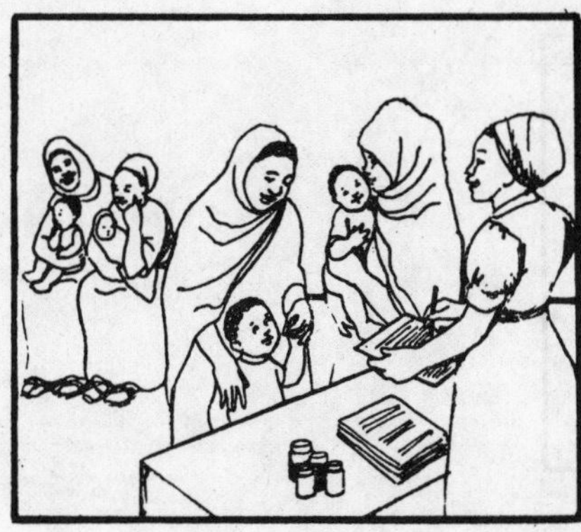

Point out that it is easy to trace pictures and use only the necessary information.

Activities for learning and practising these skills are in Unit 4, **Tracing.**

The picture above is much easier to look at. The mothers making their appointments is all that is shown in this picture.

b) Is there one main idea for each picture? Too much information at once is confusing.

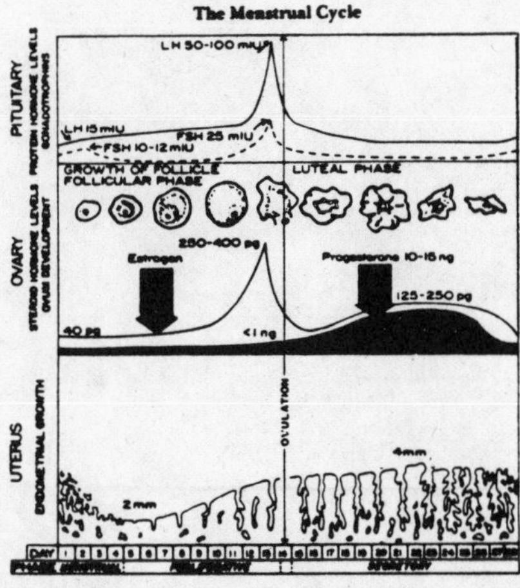

Possible sources for other examples of this idea are books on how to build or make things and technical textbooks.

The picture above shows too many aspects of the menstrual cycle at the same time.

A good picture shows only one idea and gives only the necessary information. You need more than one picture to show something like the menstrual cycle which involves several ideas. The pictures below show aspects of the cycle more simply.

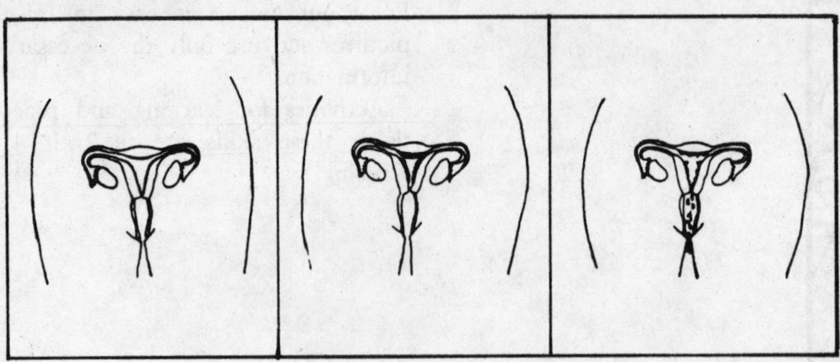

4 The visual should be **well organized.**

a) Is there a margin of blank space around the outside? Keep important pictures and words away from the edge of your poster or display. This will help the people looking at the visual to focus on what is important.

KEEP YOUR HOME CLEAN
AND
A CLEAN HOME IS A HEALTHY HOME

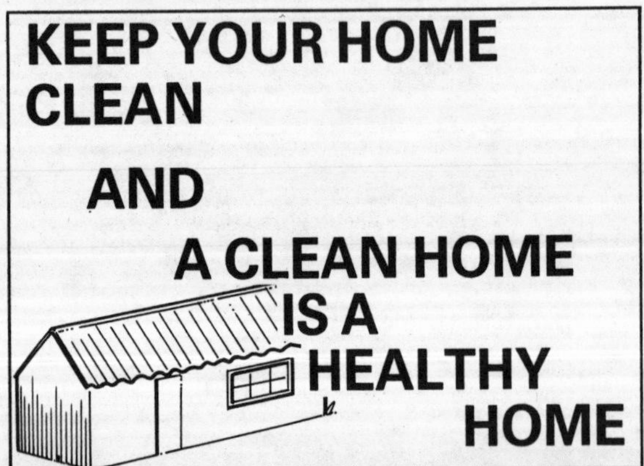

In this visual there is no margin and the words and picture are too spread apart.

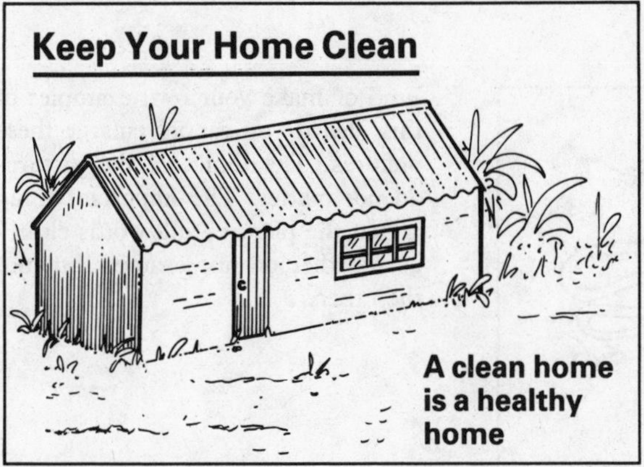

Here, a margin around the edge of the picture helps define the area that should be looked at.

b) Does the picture fill the space?

Show learners larger versions of these two pictures or another example of this idea. You can easily show the idea by sketching 2 simple posters like this on the chalkboard. Choose objects which are simple to draw, such as medicine vials or diaphragms.

Ask learners which is a better poster. Then make this point about pictures and words filling the poster.

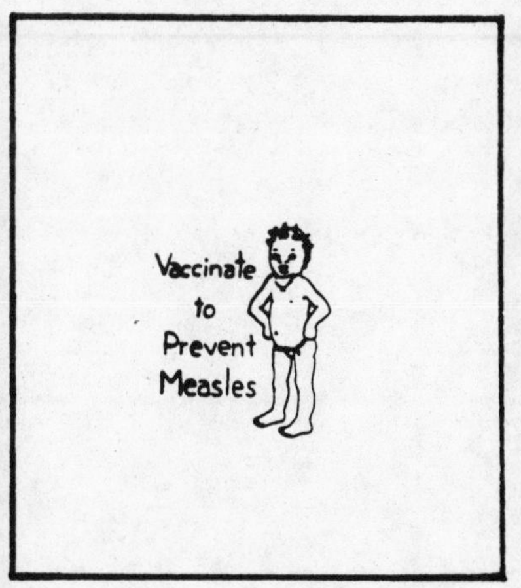

The picture and words are too small for the space.

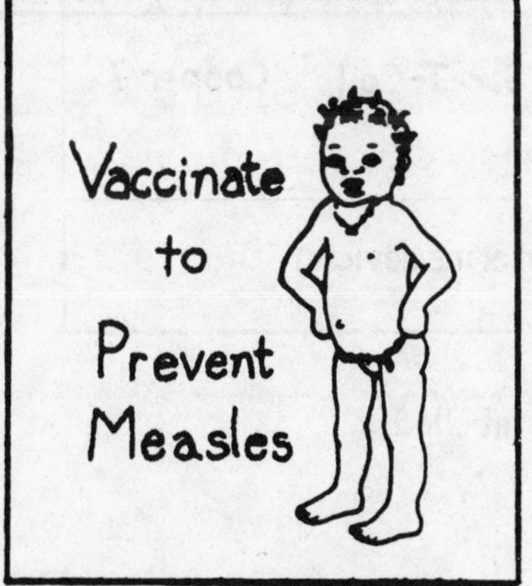

The picture and words fill the space.

c) If words are used is it clear what words go with what picture?

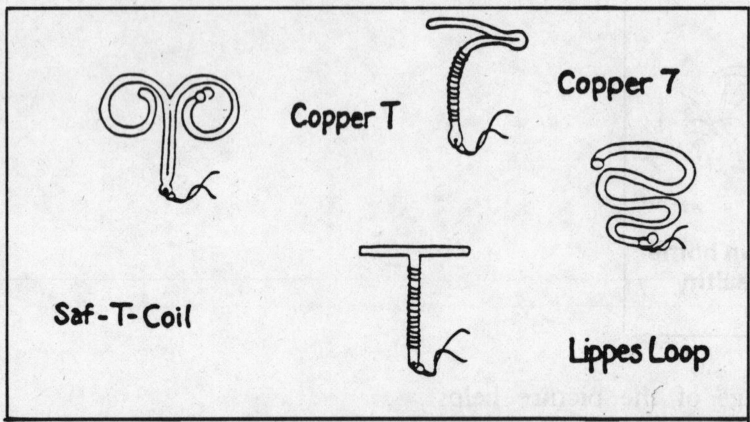

It is difficult here to tell what word goes with what picture.

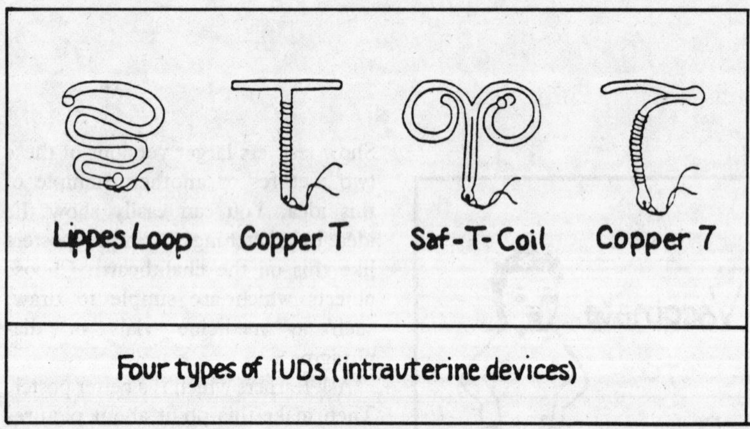

Four types of IUDs (intrauterine devices)

Here, the pictures are clearly labelled.

Find or make your own examples of this idea if you cannot enlarge these pictures. The topics of the pictures do not matter. The important thing is that the pictures and words clearly go together on one example but not the other.

5 The **viewer's attention** should be **directed to the important information.**

a) Are the important things the centre of attention?

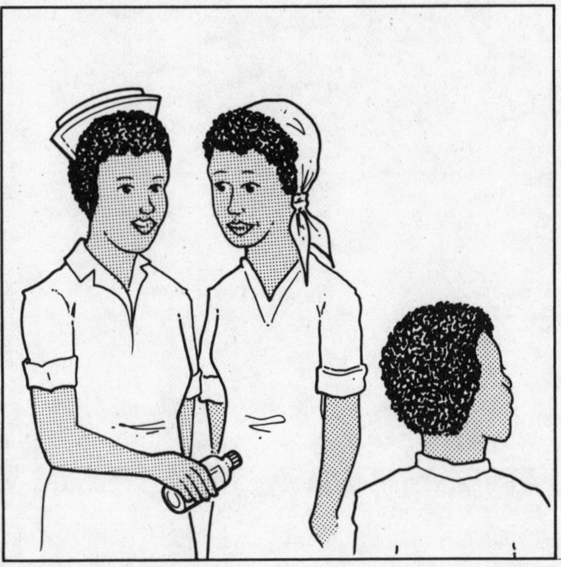

There are three people in this picture. They are all talking about something. The centre of attention is not clear.

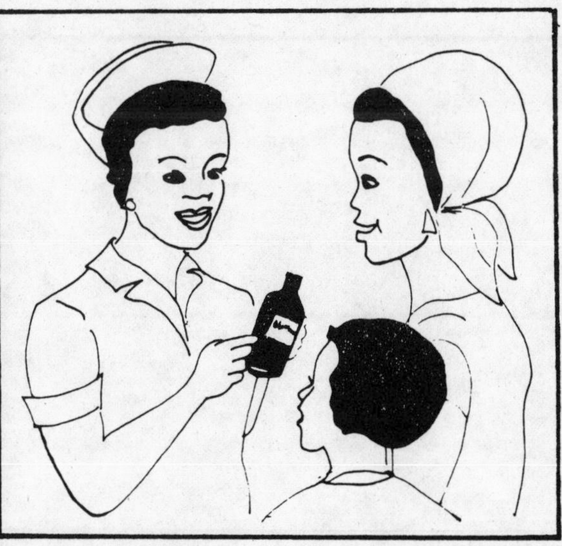

The bottle is the centre of attention. The people are all facing the bottle. The nurse is pointing to the bottle.

b) Would colour or some other visual technique help guide the viewer's attention?

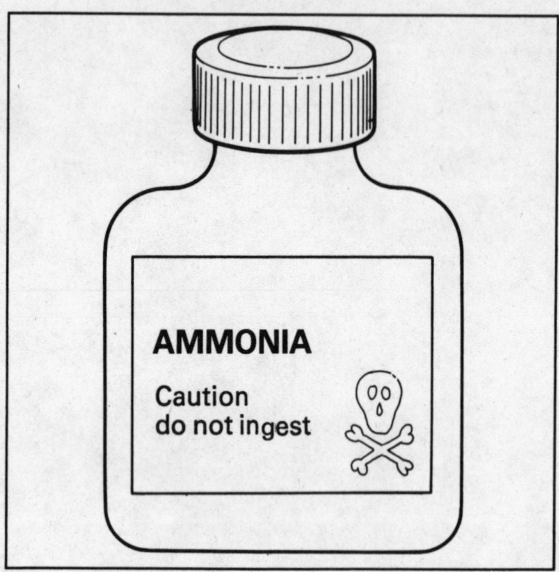

This drawing is of a substance that is poisonous.

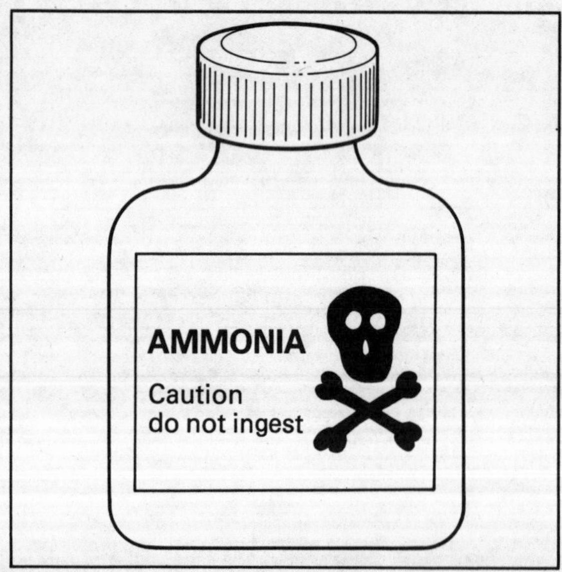

This drawing is of a substance that is poisonous; the skull and crossbones are grey. They could be printed in red or some other 'danger' colour.

6 The visual should be **interesting** to the people for whom it is intended.

a) Are the objects and figures in the visual based on the experience of the learner?

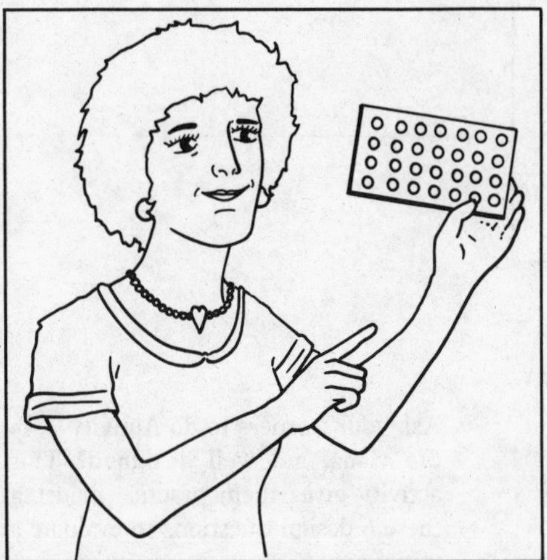

This picture of an American woman is not appropriate if you are expecting people in Africa to identify with her.

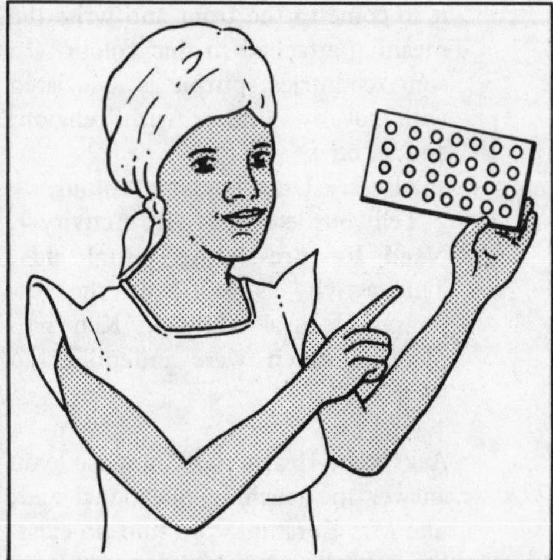

People shown in visuals should be chosen with the audiences in mind. Visuals designed for people in developing countries should include figures they are familiar with.

Ask learners to suggest some questions they can ask themselves to determine what visual aids might be interesting to their learners. List these on the chalkboard. If the questions below are not mentioned, you can suggest them.

- What do my learners seem most interested and eager about?
- What things do they respond positively to?
- What do they like to look at?
- What local crafts, artwork, or events do they find interesting?

b) Does the design and style fit local ideas about what is attractive?

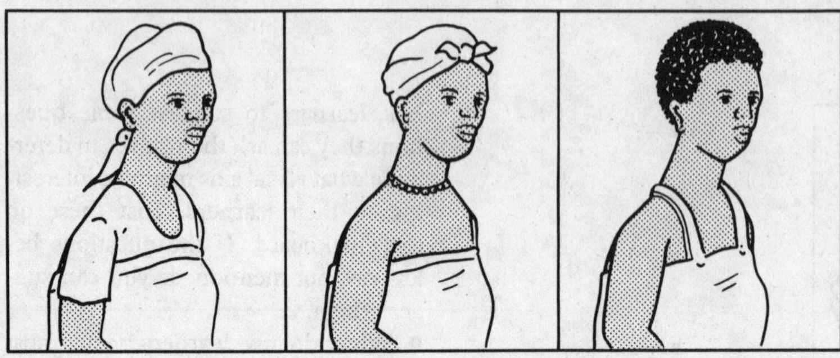

There are many ways to draw people. You should draw them in a style that will both attract and hold your viewer's attention.

Ask your learners to do Activity 2, **Is the visual aid well designed?** This activity gives them practice in using these 6 design questions to evaluate a visual aid.

Have your learners discuss what meanings they associate with what colours. Ask them to name colours common in their areas. List these on the chalkboard. Then, beside each colour, ask the person who suggested it to come to the front and write the meaning attached to that colour. (In some countries, purple is associated with royalty, orange with religion, and so on.)

Also see Unit 4, **Using colour.**

Tell your learners to do Activity 4, **Need for pre-testing visual aids.** This activity is based on the responses of rural adults in Kenya to pictures which were unfamiliar to them.

Ask your learners, 'Suppose you answer the teaching questions, and, like Mrs Ebrahim, you find no existing visual aid which meets your needs? And suppose you do not have much time to make one? What else can you do?' (You can modify or *adapt* an existing visual aid.)

Adapting an existing visual aid

You can enlarge some of these pictures in the text or find your own examples to teach this session.

You may think of more than the following 4 reasons for adapting visual aids in your area. If so, just be sure that you have examples of each reason for your learners to compare.

1 Sometimes it is necessary to adapt a visual aid because it is the **wrong size** for your needs.

Example: Mr Kamba has seen a picture in a book which he feels would be useful, but there are 40 students in his class. What can he do?

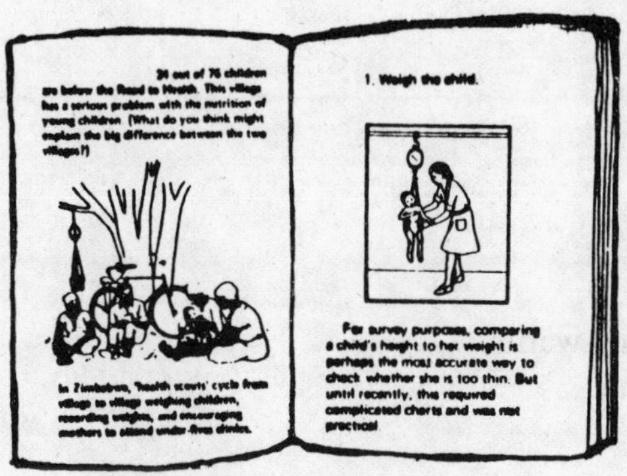

Ask learners why this picture would not be useful in the example situation. (Wrong size.) Ask how they would modify the picture.

Tape the picture up on the chalkboard or wall.

Mr Kamba uses one of the techniques for changing the size of pictures described in Unit 4 to make a poster from the picture.

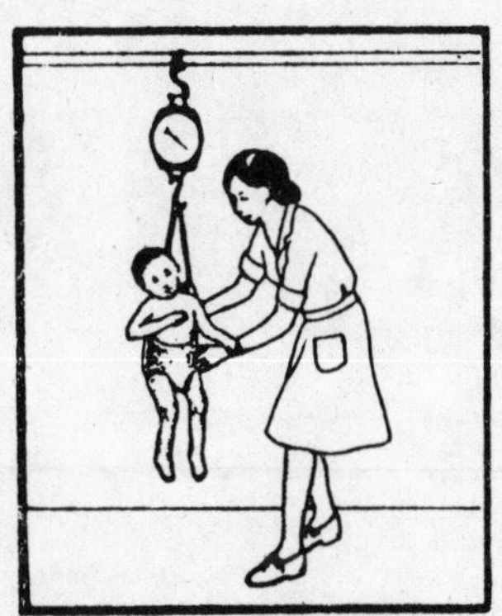

Hold up this picture also, and tape it next to the other picture.

You may also find your own examples. Choose them to suit your learners and your region.

2 Sometimes a visual aid is **too complicated** for your learners or your purpose.

Example: Mr Makambera found this picture of the glands which affect fertility. He wants to use it with his first-year students in community health nursing.

Present this pair of pictures in the same way you presented the first pair.

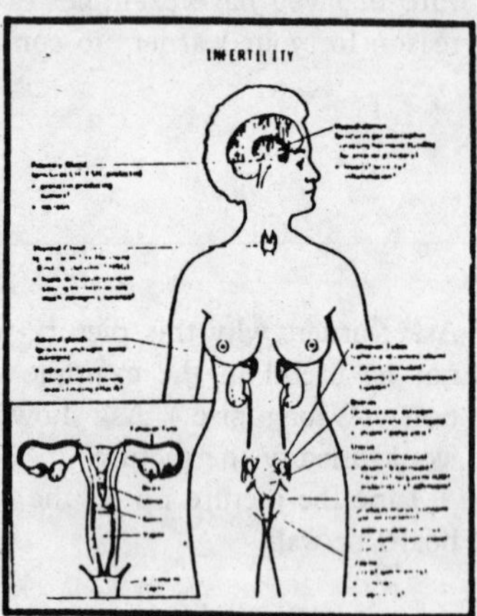

He traces the picture, putting in the parts he wants shown, and leaving out unnecessary information.

See Unit 4, **Tracing,** for an explanation of how to trace like this.

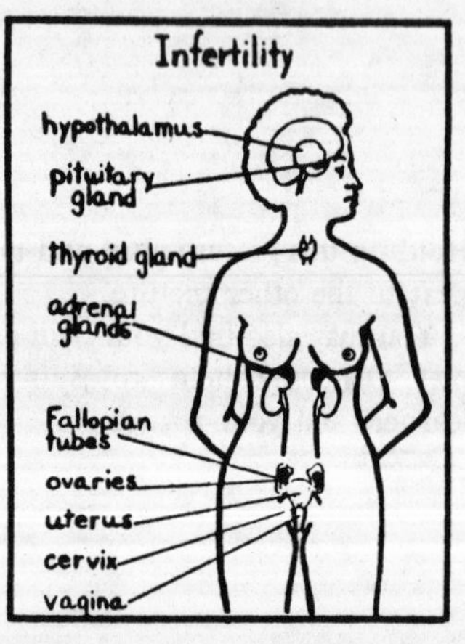

3 A visual aid which is quite acceptable to some people may be **offensive** to others.

Example: Mr Mwikale wants pictures to use for a community talk on adolescent sexuality. This picture is one of a series he has found. He believes that the naked figures will be offensive, because both men and women will be attending the talk.

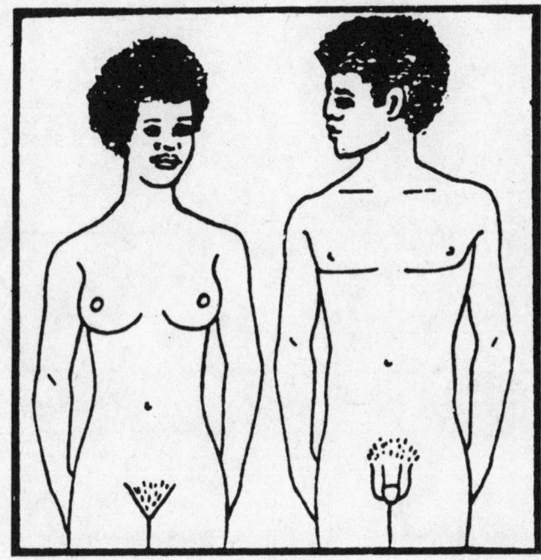

He traces and sketches to add clothing to the figures.

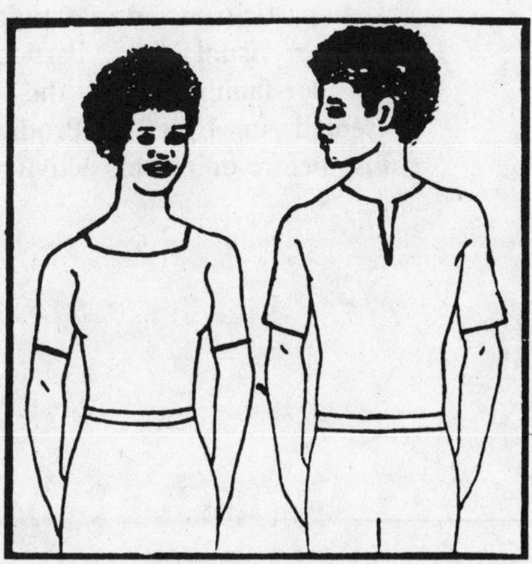

4 A visual aid may show **unfamiliar** people, objects, or words.

Example: Mrs Addo likes to use as many pictures as possible because many of her rural clients are not literate. The only picture she can find on oral contraceptives is foreign.

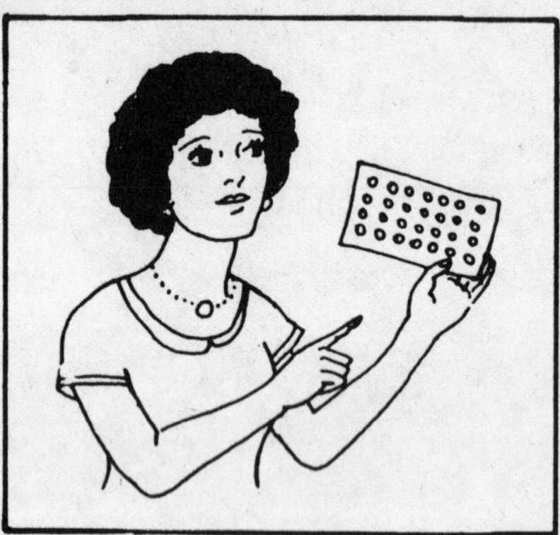

She sketches and traces to change the woman's clothes and face, so that the picture looks more like the women she talks with in the villages.

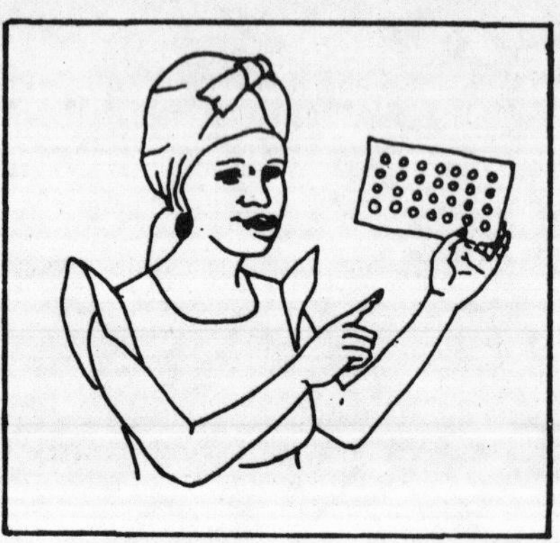

Lead a short discussion on the ways a visual aid can be modified or adapted. (You can adapt by adding, removing, or changing details or ideas.)

Let participants do Activity 5, **Adapting visual aids.** Participants must be familiar with the skills presented in Unit 4, **Production skills**, before doing this activity.

Activity 1 Choosing visual aids to fit teaching situations

Time 45 minutes

Objective Learners will use the 7 teaching questions to choose visual aids and plan a teaching lesson.

Materials Copies of the attached case studies or others you have written.
A list of the 7 teaching questions. These will be on the chalkboard if you have presented them as suggested. You can also leave the pictures on display for people to refer to.
Pencil and paper for the learners.

Instructions

1 Write the 7 teaching questions on the chalkboard if you have not already done so. Ask learners to copy these questions into their notes. Learners can use the questions later in planning their own teaching or training sessions.
2 Divide your learners into small groups of about 4–5 people.
3 If possible, give each small group a copy of all the case studies. If you have enough copies, give each person a copy of the case studies.

Otherwise, write the case studies on different sheets of paper and give one to each group.

Be sure you only give participants the case study description, *not* the list of possible answers to the 7 teaching questions.

4 Assign a different case to each small group. Explain that groups will have 15 minutes to discuss the case. The group must answer the 7 teaching questions for planning the teaching session required in the case.
5 Have a member of each group present their case study and answers to the 7 teaching questions to the large group (5 minutes). Allow time for discussion.
6 When all presentations are finished, ask the participants if this has been helpful practice for them. Why or why not?

Possible adaptations

1 Write your own case studies to show situations familiar to your participants.
2 If you have more time, ask each small group to answer the 7 teaching questions for more than one case study. It does not matter if more than one group works on the same case study.
3 If time is limited, have each small group do the same case study. Then one group can report their answers to the 7 teaching questions. The other groups can add their suggestions during

the following discussion (30 minutes).

Learners can use remaining case studies for practice in their own time.

Evaluation

Have your learners answer the 7 teaching questions and choose visual aids for their own teaching problem which they may be working on during the workshop.

Case 1: Encouraging mothers to bring their children to the clinic for immunizations

The health worker in a small rural clinic is concerned because many babies in the area are dying from diseases that could be prevented by immunizations. She is concerned because mothers in the area do not bring their babies to the clinic for these immunizations. Her assistant, who lives in the village, told her that the women fear that the immunizations will poison their babies. They have heard rumours of babies dying after such immunizations and they prefer to use their own herbal remedies for illnesses. The health worker observes that the women gather every week under a tree in the village to pound their grain, talk, and sing. The women are busy with many tasks and only stay under the tree about one hour or less.

What can she do to encourage the women to bring their babies to the clinic for immunizations? She has some paper and paint that she brought from the regional capital. The village has no electricity.

The following are *possible* answers to the 7 teaching questions for this case study.

1 **What problem:** many babies in the area are dying from diseases that could be prevented by immunizations
2 **Who:** women with babies
3 **What:** bring their babies to the clinic for immunizations
4 **Where and how long:** under the village tree where women gather to pound their grain; 15 minutes
5 **Teaching methods:** songs, stories, or a talk about immunizations for babies
6 **Visual aids:**
   (a) existing materials: paper and paint, the mothers' children who are sick with a childhood disease
   (b) materials she can make:
      (1) pictures to illustrate her songs or stories about immunizations
      (2) drawing of children showing symptoms of each of the diseases that could be prevented by immunizations
7 **Effectiveness:**
   (a) Observe whether the women pay attention to her presentation

and ask questions or offer their own stories about diseases or immunizations.

(b) Count the number of women who bring babies to the clinic for immunizations *before* and *after* the session.

Case 2: Teaching a community how to build a latrine

The local health committee has asked the health worker in the regional clinic to visit their community and teach local volunteers how to build a latrine. The village is in a remote area accessible only by foot, donkey, or boat. Most of the villagers have never seen a latrine. The newly appointed health committee heard from a visiting health worker that many of the stomach pains and diarrhoea problems in the community could be reduced by building and using latrines. Wood is available locally. The villagers have digging tools. In one day a health worker can usually demonstrate how to build a latrine.

What is the best way for the health worker to teach the volunteers how to build a strong effective latrine?

The following are *possible* answers to the 7 teaching questions for this case study.

1 **What problem:** stomach pains and diarrhoea problems in the community

2 **Who:** village volunteers

3 **What:** build a latrine in an acceptable location

4 **Where and how long:** in the community; 1–day demonstration activity

5 **Teaching methods:**

(a) lecture/demonstration (lecture about materials needed to build latrines, where to build them, and the steps in building a latrine)

(b) help the villagers build a latrine in an acceptable location

6 **Visual aids:**

(a) existing materials: wood, digging and carpentry tools, paper, crayons

(b) materials to make:

(1) drawings of people building a latrine, showing the different steps in locating and building the latrine

(2) wooden model of the best type of latrine for this village

7 **Effectiveness:**

(a) During construction:

(1) to see how effective your explanation was, count the number and kind of requests villagers make for re-explanation of steps in building a latrine;

(2) count the number and kind of mistakes made during the construction.

(b) After building the first latrine, return to the village at regular intervals to see if new latrines are being built; also check to see if they are building them correctly and placing them in acceptable locations.

Case 3: How to inform mothers of young infants about nutrition

The health worker is in a small clinic in a poor area at the edge of a large urban centre. She is concerned about the large number of cases of infant malnutrition that she sees in her community. She talks with some of the mothers. They have little money for food. They feed their babies bread and macaroni with broth from the stews that the adults eat. Most of the mothers cannot read. They are not aware of the dried milk and soybean meal distributed free in a nearby clinic. The mothers who have heard of this free food have not bothered to go to the clinic to get it. They have never prepared such food. They do not know how to cook it. Some think that it is animal food not fit for humans.

The health worker has paper and drawing materials. How can she inform these mothers about nutrition to help them improve the health of their children?

The following are *possible* answers to the 7 teaching questions for this case study.

1 What problem: large number of cases of infant malnutrition

2 Who: mothers in a poor community at the edge of a large urban centre

3 What: improve their babies' nutrition through use of dried milk and soybean meal

4 Where and how long: in the community; in the clinic; 15-minute demonstrations

5 Teaching methods: community displays or exhibits; food preparation and tasting demonstrations at the clinic

6 Visual aids:

(a) existing materials: paper and drawing materials, dried milk and soybean meal samples

(b) materials to make:

(1) a display with drawings to illustrate that (a) free food is distributed at the clinic, (b) cooking demonstrations are given at the clinic, and (c) humans can eat the dried milk and soybean meal cooked in the clinic demonstration

(2) a cooking fire, foods made at the clinic demonstrations

7 Effectiveness:

(a) Count the number of mothers who come to the clinic for the food demonstrations.

(b) Count how many mothers come to the clinic for free food.

Case 4: Teaching nurses about breast-feeding

A nursing instructor is sitting at home after the evening meal. She watches her 5-year-old daughter play with her dolls. She is thinking about a unit on breast-feeding which she must teach. She has about 3 weeks to prepare for a 2-hour session on breast-feeding for her 20 community health nursing students. She wants her students to be able to explain the advantages and possible problems in breast-feeding. She also wants them to be able to teach good breast-feeding practices to pregnant women. She has already found large photographs of abnormal breast nipples. She also has some posters which show a smiling mother breast-feeding her baby with words saying, 'Mother's Breast is Best'. She knows that the school has chalkboards and a supply of paper, pencils, and coloured crayons.

Answer the 7 teaching questions to explain how this instructor might prepare for her class session.

The following are *possible* answers to the 7 teaching questions for this case study.

1 **What problem:** nursing students need to know more about breast-feeding
2 **Who:** 20 community health nursing students
3 **What:** explain the advantages and possible problems in breast-feeding; teach good breast-feeding practices to pregnant women
4 **Where and how long:** classroom; for 2 hours
5 **Teaching methods:** lecture, discussion, demonstration, role play
6 **Visual aids:**
   (a) existing materials: large photographs showing abnormal breast nipples, 'Mother's Breast is Best' posters, chalk and chalkboard, paper, pencils, crayons, her daughter's dolls
   (b) materials to make:
      (1) a set of drawings showing the advantages and possible problems in breast-feeding
      (2) role descriptions for a role play of a nurse explaining breast-feeding to pregnant women; guidelines for role play; guidelines to assess the nurse's role
7 **Effectiveness:**
   Divide students into 5 groups of 4 students each. Have each group act out the role play at the same time. Have students use guidelines to assess each other's performance in the role of the nurse.

Case 5: Teaching adolescents how pregnancy occurs

A community health nurse in a large town is concerned about the increasing numbers of teenage pregnancies. There is no sex education in the school and tradition discourages parents from talking to their own children about sex. She wants the adolescents in the area of her clinic to understand how pregnancy occurs and to be able to explain accurately to their friends. She has arranged to give a 20-minute health education talk in a classroom in the local school to 20 schoolgirls, age 12–14. She has a large flipbook with pages showing phases of the menstrual cycle and how fertilization takes place. She also has a flannelboard with pieces showing the male and female reproductive organs. She has a chart showing the growth of a foetus from 3 months to 9 months.

The following are *possible* answers to the 7 teaching questions for this case study.

1 **What problem:** increasing numbers of teenage pregnancies in a large town
2 **Who:** 20 schoolgirls, age 12–14
3 **What:** explain how pregnancy occurs
4 **Where and how long:** in the classroom for 20 minutes
5 **Teaching methods:** group discussion, lecture, role play
6 **Visual aids:**
(a) existing materials: flipchart, flannelboard, chart
(b) materials to make: role descriptions for a role play explaining to another girlfriend how pregnancy occurs; props for role play
7 **Effectiveness:**
Ask girls to explain how pregnancy occurs using the reproductive organ pieces on the flannelboard. Observe role play explanations of pregnancy.

Activity 2

Is the visual aid well designed?

Time

45 minutes

Objective

Learners will evaluate sample visual aids using the design considerations.

Materials

A copy of the 6 design considerations for each person.
One poster or picture for each group. (Choose sample visual aids carefully to include some good and bad examples of design.) Describe the people for whom each picture is intended.
Paper and pencils and markers for each small group.
Picture of the hookworm included with this activity.

Instructions

1 You may want to present the example of the hookworm picture before you begin this activity. Show this picture to your learners and lead a group discussion on how the 6 design considerations apply to the picture. Then your learners will be more ready to apply the design considerations to other pictures.

2 Ask learners to divide into small groups with 3 or 4 people in each group.

3 Give each group one of the posters or pictures and a piece of paper and pencil or a sheet of paper and marker. Describe the people for whom each picture is intended.

4 Ask each group to look carefully at their poster or picture and apply the 6 design considerations.

5 Also ask them:

(a) If the visual aid is in colour, has colour been used for a purpose? If yes, what purpose or purposes?

(b) How would you change this visual aid to improve the design? How would you change it to make it communicate better?

6 Ask learners to sketch how the poster or picture should be changed.

7 Ask one person from each group to show the sample poster or picture to the large group. Ask this person also to explain how the small group applied the considerations and changes made in the revised sketch.

8 Encourage other people to offer comments on the sample poster or picture and the sketch prepared by the small group.

9 Summarize the important ideas mentioned during the activity, emphasizing the use of the design considerations.

Possible adaptations

If time is limited, you can do this activity in a large group, by holding up the pictures and asking learners to answer the design considerations (approximately 20 minutes).

Answers to the 6 design considerations

These are answers that learners in other workshops gave when looking at the picture of the hookworm on the next page. The picture is intended for rural people.

When you use this example, try to colour the picture, so that you can discuss the use of colour with your learners. Use one very bright colour for the worms (perhaps orange or red) and another colour that is darker for the rim of the magnifying glass (such as dark blue).

1 **Easy to see?** Yes. The word and pictures are large and bold.

2 **Easy to understand?** Difficult to understand.

The magnifying glass will be confusing because most people have never seen one. They will not understand that the magnifying glass makes things larger. They will probably think that the worms are snakes because they are so large on the page.

3 **Clear and simple?** Not clear, fairly simple.
The dots between the worms are confusing. The small worms on the outside of the picture are unnecessary.

4 **Well organized?** Yes.
The arrangement of words and pictures on the page is good. There is a white border around the outside of the picture and words. There is only one picture, and it is clear that the words describe that picture.

5 **Directs the eye of the viewer?** Yes.
Uses colour contrast, light and dark contrast and a circle to direct our attention to the hookworms.

6 **Interesting?** No
Probably the rural people would see the picture as snakes flying in the air or in a pool of water. It could be frightening or unbelievable. The worms appear to be talking to each other. This could also be unbelievable and uninteresting to the rural people.

Suggestions to improve the picture

Write the title larger.
Eliminate the magnifying glass, the small worms outside, the dots inside, and the faces on the worms.

Visual Aid

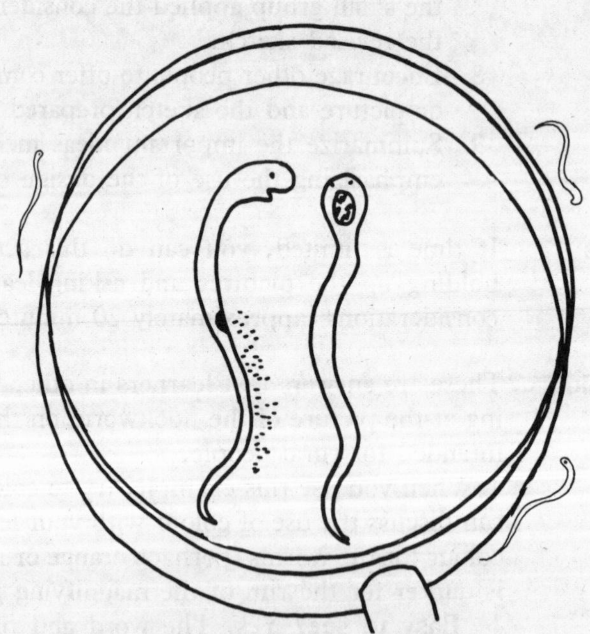

hookworms

Activity 3

Seeing the same picture in different ways

Time

30 minutes

Objectives

This activity will enable learners to:
(a) explain how people can see different things in the same picture but be equally 'right';
(b) explain how students' and clients' interpretations of pictures will affect their work as health and family planning educators and community workers;
(c) state the importance of trying to understand and respect the viewpoints of their clients.

Materials

Copies of the first picture on the next page (if possible one for each participant), or one copy large enough for everyone to see. Blackboard and chalk, paper and felt pens.

Instructions

1 Give each person a copy of the picture or show them a large version. Ask learners to look at it for 5 minutes and be prepared to say what they see in the picture.
2 Ask for the descriptions. List the descriptions and the number of people who gave each.
3 Point out which descriptions were given by the most people.
4 Write the following questions on the chalkboard:
(a) Why did we see different things in the same picture?
(b) What comparisons can we draw from our own experiences?
Lead a discussion of those questions.
5 Summarize the discussion. Emphasize that as trainers we must respect people's perceptions in any situation, and recognize that a person's background and environment affect the understanding of pictures. Emphasize that health educators and community workers must use pictures and teaching methods appropriate to the experiences of the people with whom they work.

Possible adaptations

The lower drawings on the next page outline two of several possible figures that can be seen in the upper picture adapted from W. H. Hill. Both the 'young woman' and 'old woman' can be seen in the picture. Other figures are possible. You may wish to use these or similar drawings to show how people 'fill in' information in a picture to understand it. The drawings also show how people ignore parts of a picture that do not make sense.

SEEING THE SAME PICTURE IN DIFFERENT WAYS

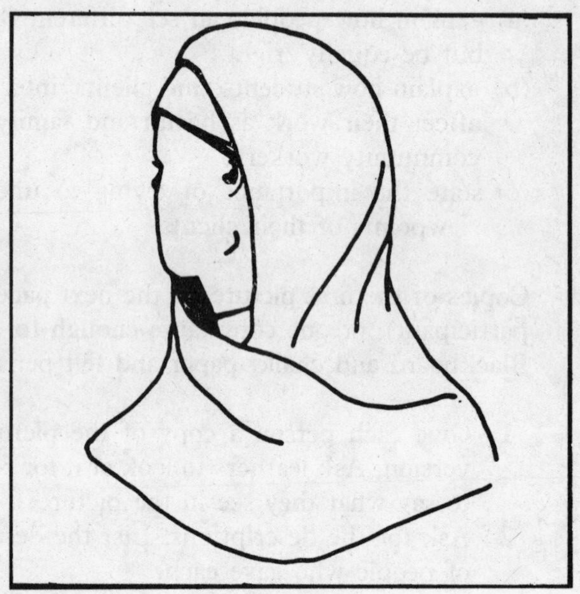

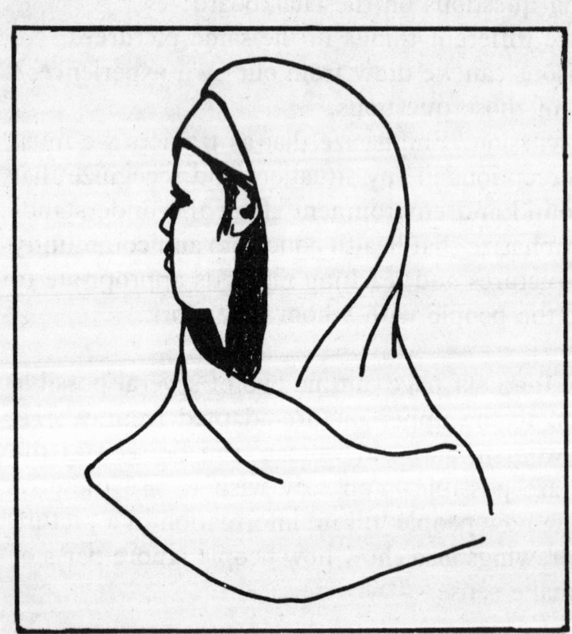

The 'young woman' in the picture

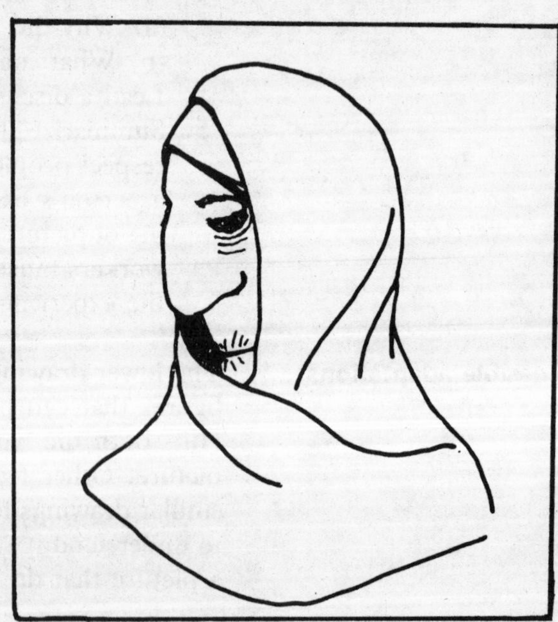

The 'old woman' in the picture

Activity 4

Need for pre-testing visual aids

Time 30 minutes

Objective Learners will identify and discuss the need for pre-testing pictures with the people for whom they are intended.

Materials Larger copies of the following pictures. You may also find your own pictures that have been pre-tested. See 2 under 'Possible adaptations'.
Pencil and paper for each participant.
If possible, for each participant make a copy of the page which summarizes how people in Kenya reacted to the drawings.

Instructions

1 Tell the learners that you are going to play a visual game. Explain that you will hold up several pictures, one at a time. Each person is to write down what the picture is about, without talking to each other. This is not a test!

2 Hold up each picture and ask, 'What do you think this picture is about?' Make sure everyone can see each picture. You may use the pictures in any order. Be sure everyone has time to write an answer to the question before you hold up the next picture.

3 When you have finished, hold up the pictures again. Show them one at a time, in the same order as before. Ask the learners to say what they have written for each picture. Encourage discussion of the different things participants 'saw' in the pictures.

4 Explain that these pictures were designed to be used with illiterate people in Kenya. Before they were used, they were tried out with groups of illiterates to see if they understood what the pictures were about. Explain the results of the pre-testing, as summarized on the following page. Distribute the handouts if you have them. If you use other pictures, give information about the results of pre-testing them.

5 Ask the learners what they think this game demonstrated. The game is meant to show that it is important to *try out* or pre-test pictures, *with people like the people you want to reach, before you use the pictures*.

6 Have learners suggest reasons for trying out pictures in this way. List their reasons on a chalkboard or large sheet of paper if possible. Be sure the following ideas are covered:

(a) Pre-testing helps us find out whether the pictures are appropriate and meaningful to our intended learners.

(b) Pre-testing enables us to discover any unexpected reactions or interpretations.
(c) Pre-testing shows us what things need to be changed and in what way.

Possible adaptations

1 If time is limited, you may want to choose only a few pictures for the game. Choose some pictures which are hard to understand, some which are easy to understand, and some which are understandable but demand careful attention.

2 If you have a few extra minutes, your learners may even comment on the way you encouraged honest responses from them:
(a) emphasis on having fun, not testing them, so that their anxiety was minimized
(b) using the open question, 'What do you think this picture is about?'
(c) allowing them plenty of time to answer
(d) being careful not to be critical of their responses
These are all ways to get reliable reactions from the people who are looking at your pictures.

PICTURES FOR RECOGNITION IN PRE-TESTING SITUATION

Percentages refer to correct responses of illiterate rural adults in field-tests with groups ranging from 162 to 793 people.

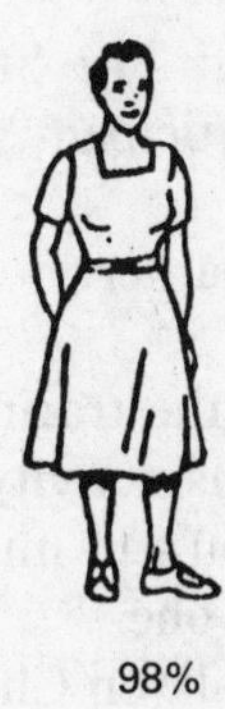

98%

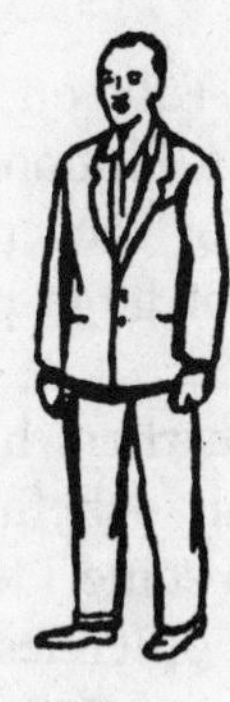

98%

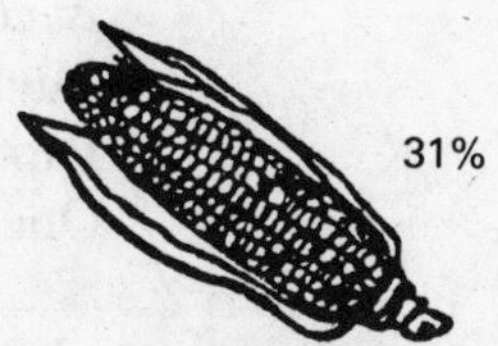

31%

Misconceptions: tortoise, crocodile, pineapple, bird, fish, mosquito, man

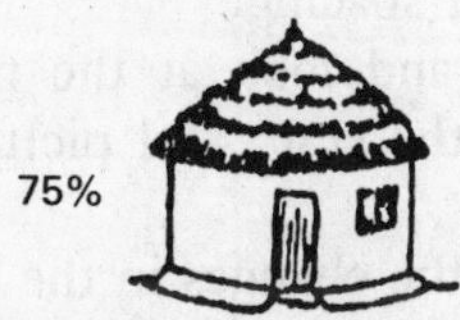

75%

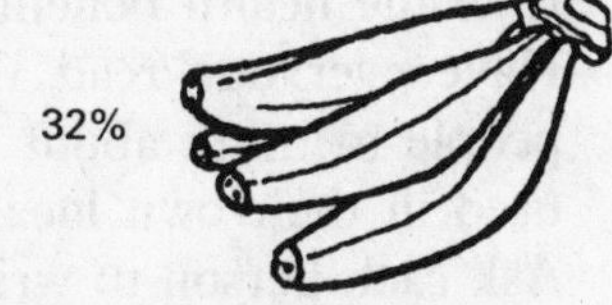

32%

Misconceptions: fingers, palm, bird, flowers, tree, man

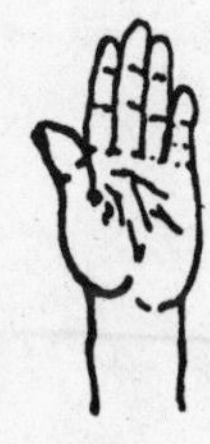

69%

11%

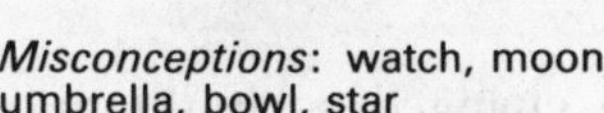

Misconceptions: watch, moon, umbrella, bowl, star

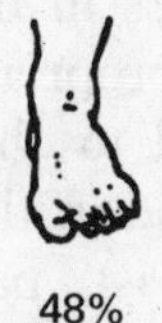

48%

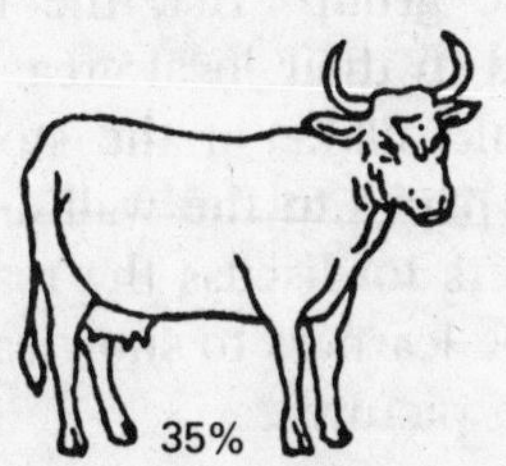

35%

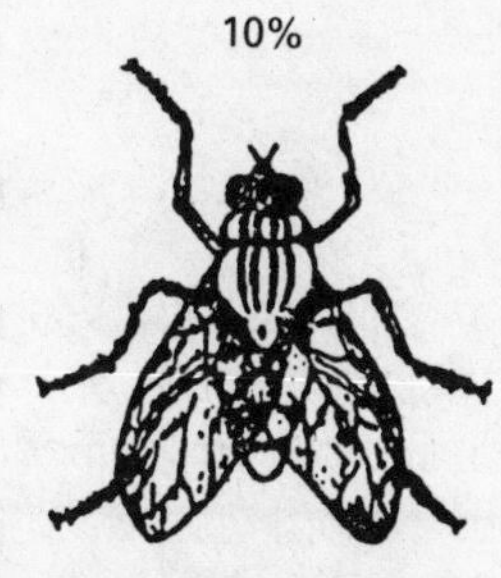

10%

Misconceptions: butterfly, bee, locust, spider, mosquito, grasshopper, cockroach, crab

Activity 5

Adapting visual aids

Time

1 hour

Objective

Learners will make changes in the pictures and story of a flipbook in order to make it more appropriate for use in their own local area.

Materials

A copy of 'Health Talk on Child Spacing: The Story of Fatu and Musu' made up as a flipbook for each participant.
Paper and pencils for each participant.
One or two sheets of large paper and a marker.

Instructions

1 Be sure your learners have practised the tracing and sketching skills from Unit 4 before they do this activity. The Trainer's Guide contains some ideas on how you can mix the skills from Unit 4 in with other lessons like this one.

2 Give each learner a copy of 'Health Talk on Child Spacing: The Story of Fatu and Musu'. Explain that this story can be used with individuals or small groups of mothers or couples to illustrate the health benefits of child spacing.

3 Have everyone read the story and look at the pictures. Ask people to think about whether the story and pictures could be used in their own local area.

4 Ask each person to write down the changes in the story, if any, to make it more acceptable to people in their local area.
In the past, learners have suggested changing names, phrases, or even the actual events in the story.

5 Ask learners to choose one of the pictures in the story to change. Their task is to use their tracing and sketching skills to change the figures in the picture. Participants are to make the figures more appropriate for the people in their local area. They may also need to change the pictures to fit more with the changes they made in the story.
In the past, participants have changed such things as faces, gestures, or the style of dress.

6 Meet again as a large group. Ask the learners whether the flipbook could be used in their local area. Ask them to explain the changes they would make in the story and the pictures. Tape a large sheet of paper to the wall and write the suggestions. Encourage learners to discuss the reasons for the changes they suggest. Allow the learners to show each other the changes they have made in the pictures.

Possible adaptations

1 If time is limited, you can ask the learners to adapt only one figure in one picture, rather than the whole picture. You can use a poster instead of the flipbook and ask your learners to change the words and pictures.
2 You can assign this activity for homework and have the group discussion as the next day's opening session. This gives learners more time to think about how they could use the flipbook and the changes they would make.
3 You can do this activity with several small groups. Give each group a different visual aid to review and adapt to be more suitable to their local situation. Then each small group shares their suggestions with the large group.
4 You can hand out a different picture series or flipbook.

Health talk on child spacing 'The Story of Fatu and Musu'

Produced by Family Planning International Assistance Project with
Preventive Medical Services Project
Family Health Division
Ministry of Health and Social Welfare
Monrovia, Liberia

Objective

To show people the importance of spacing their children two to three years apart, so that both mothers and children will live long, healthy lives. People in Liberia like to have plenty of children. This is a good thing, but if the children are born too close together, the children will not live long, and the mothers will not be healthy. People need to know that if they take time and space their children, they can have large, healthy families.

This health talk does not show all about the different methods of child spacing available to people in Liberia. If people in your clinic want to know more about how to space their children, take time and explain the different methods they can use.

Take time when giving this health talk. Learn the story yourself. Use your own town's name, name the people in the story with names from your own tribe, and name the health worker and the clinic she works in. Show each picture one at a time, and make sure all the people listening to the talk can see the picture.

Note to the trainer

You can enlarge the following pictures in this manual to make a flipbook to use as you tell 'The Story of Fatu and Musu' to your learners. Read the story that goes with each picture as you hold up the enlarged versions.

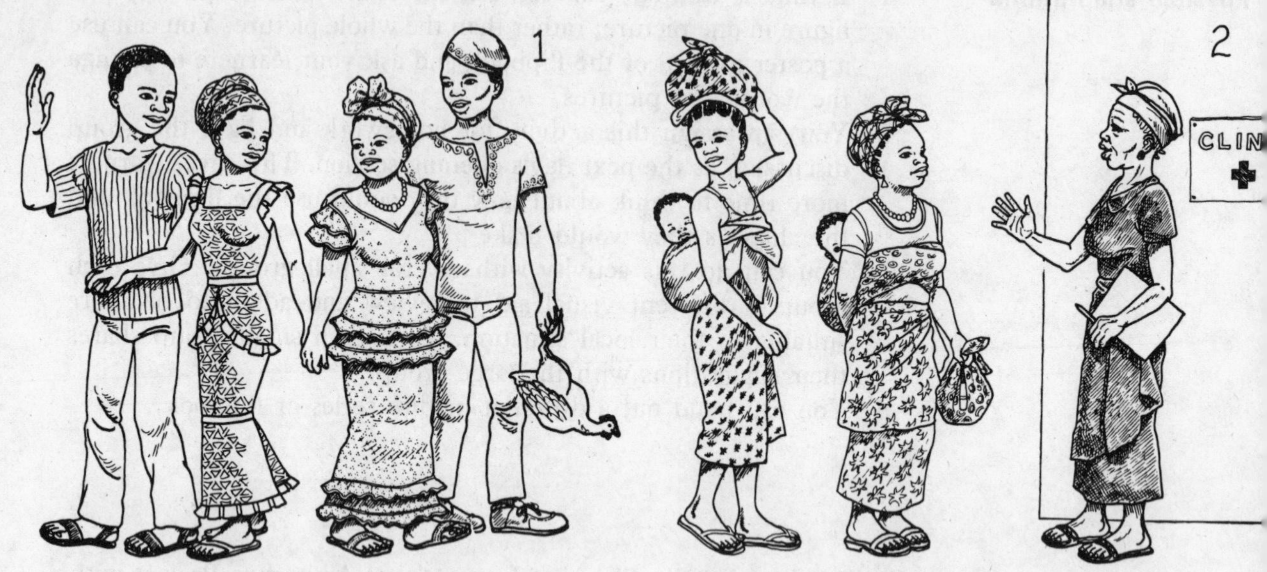

PICTURE 1: Fatu and Musu are good friends. They grew up in the village together. Both of the girls grew up to be fine, fat and healthy. When they became older, they found men who really loved them. When they were both 16, they got married to different men at the same time. Fatu married Flomo, and Musu married Kerkula.

PICTURE 2: Soon both of the women got pregnant. When the time came, both mothers delivered fine sons. After the babies were born, both women carried their sons to the clinic. They learned different things about keeping their babies healthy and about staying strong themselves. One thing they learned about was child spacing. Each woman went home and advised her husband about what she learned.

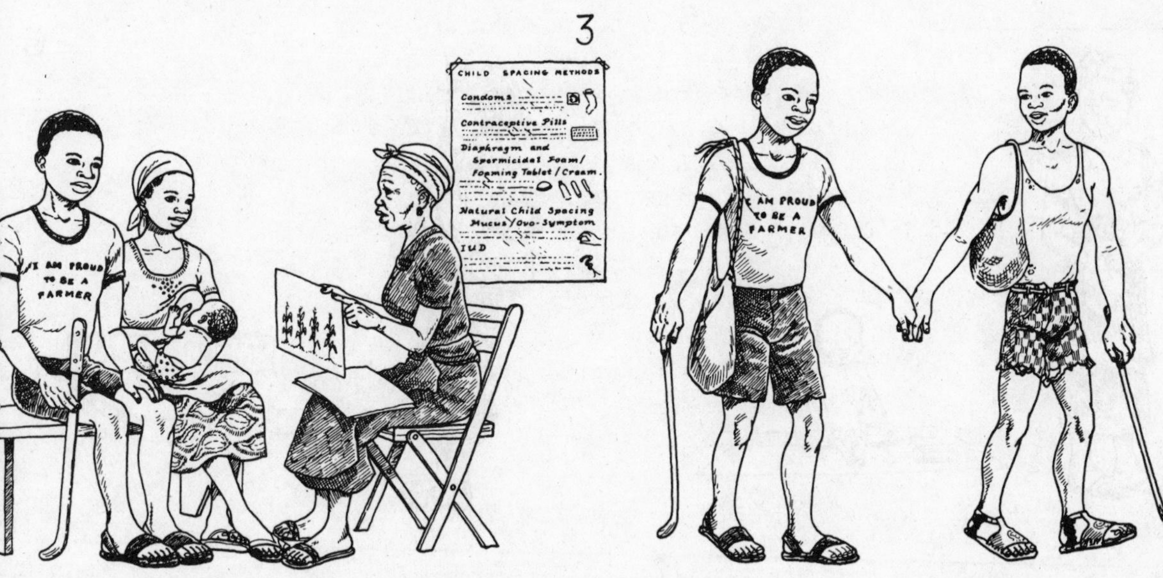

PICTURE 3: When Fatu went home to Flomo, he found what she had to say interesting. He was convinced that it was good to use child spacing medicine so that his wife could rest before their next baby was born. They went to the clinic and listened to the nurse. She explained that children cannot be born too close together, or they will be weak. Just like farmers know corn cannot be planted too close together, or the plants will not grow big. She explained the different child spacing methods, and Fatu and Flomo agreed on a method to use together.

When Musu went home to her husband, Kerkula, she found that the man was against the idea of child spacing. He wanted to have many children as quickly as possible.

PICTURE 4: One day the two men met out on a farm. Flomo greeted his friend Kerkula and said, 'My friend, you are looking happy today! What news?' Kerkula said, 'Ah, yes Flomo, today I have good news. Of course you know that two months ago my wife Musu bore me my first son and made me a proud man. Well, I just learned that the woman has belly again! Soon I will have plenty of children to work on my rice farm, and I will be a rich man!'

When Flomo heard this he laughed to himself. He said, 'Kerkula, I too want a large family so that I will one day be a rich man myself. But I am a young man now and I will take time with having more children. My own wife, Fatu, bore me a fine boy the same time your child was born. He is strong and healthy. Because we want him to remain healthy, my wife and I are practising child spacing for two or three years. When that time has passed, we will have another child. I know it is better to wait two or three years between each baby. That way the children and the mother will stay strong. Of course, it will take some time, but one day I will have a family bigger than your own! It is foolish to have children so close together. The children will not be healthy. You will see that my way is best!'

The men parted and went their separate ways. Each thought the other was foolish. Each man thought that his way was the best way to have a large family.

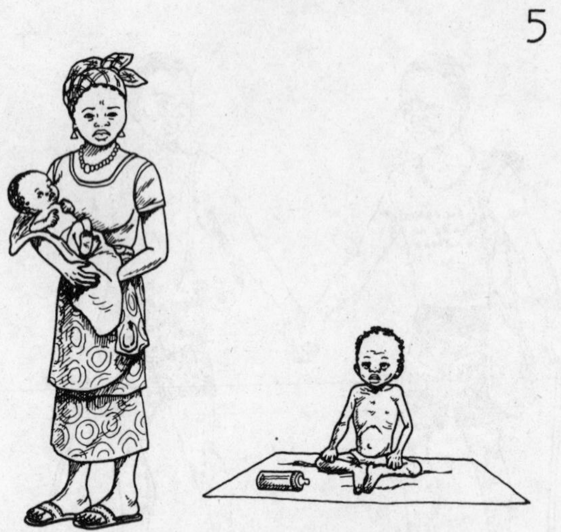

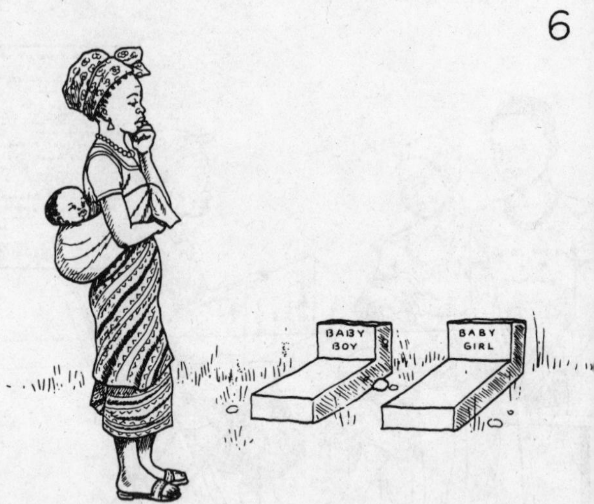

PICTURE 5: Before Musu's baby could walk, her second baby was born. Two months after Musu delivered her second baby, her first child became very sick. Since Musu did not have enough milk for two babies, the first baby was taken off the breast. He became very weak and dry. It was not long before the poor, sick child died.

Musu was very sad her first baby died. She also felt afraid that the new baby would go back too. Even the new baby was looking very dry and small. And those were not the only things troubling Musu. She knew that she had belly again, and she was feeling too weak and tired.

PICTURE 6: It was not long after Musu's third baby was born that her second child died. Musu was very troubled. She knew that she must do her best to keep her third baby healthy. She was afraid that she might even have belly again, for the fourth time. She herself was no longer fat and fine. She looked very tired and dry.

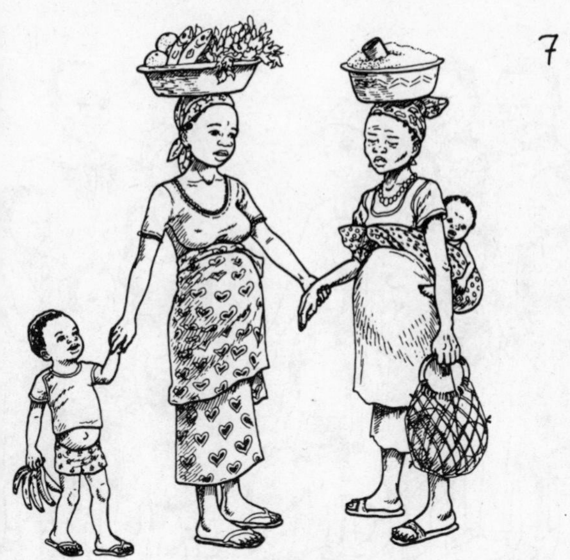

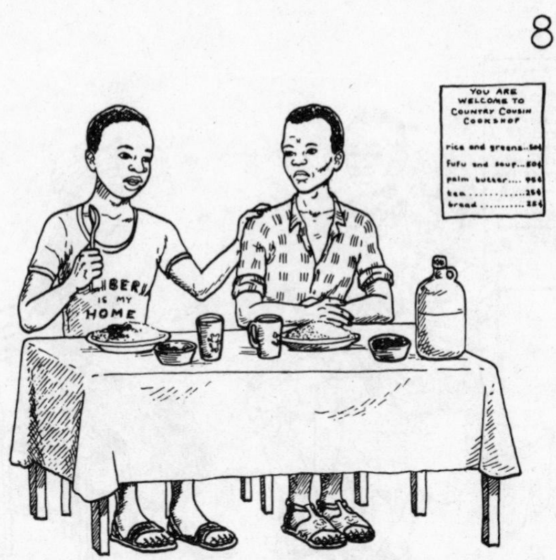

PICTURE 7: One day Musu saw Fatu in the market. Fatu had her fine, fat child on her back. Musu called to her, 'Oh, Fatu, my sister, it's me your old friend Musu!'

Fatu stopped. She said, 'Oh, my sister Musu! I didn't know you. You're looking strange to me. What happened! You haven't been well in body? And, oh, your baby is so small and dry. I'm sorry for you because your first two babies died.'

'Yes, Fatu, it's rough this time. My first baby boy and my second baby, a girl, went back. And now even my third baby is not good. I have belly again, and I am too tired this time. But you, my friend, oh you're looking too fine and your baby is fat and beautiful.'

Fatu said, 'My sister, ever since I bore my boy child, my husband and I have been practising child spacing. Now that my son is almost three years old, and we are both strong in body, I am pregnant again. We thank God for everything this time!'

Musu listened to Fatu explain about the way she and Flomo practised child spacing. Because she was very tired and wanted to rest, Musu was very interested. But she knew that her own stubborn husband would never agree to child spacing and she was discouraged.

PICTURE 8: One day, a few months after the women met in the market, Kerkula and Flomo met inside a cookshop. When Flomo saw his old friend, he said, 'Ah, Kerkula, my man, I haven't seen you for a long time. What news this time?'

'Well, my brother,' Kerkula said, 'I am sorry to say that things are not good with me. The first two babies my wife bore me have already died, and our third child is very weak and dry. My wife, Musu, is not well in body and is looking dry. I am convinced someone is witching me and my family! That is why all my children die and my wife is weak.'

Flomo said, 'What kind of things are you talking, Kerkula? No one is witching you or your family. You are not practising child spacing, so your wife will soon be a tired old woman, if you do not let her rest. I thank God, because my wife and I are well in body, and we have a strong boy child and a fine new baby girl. Ain't I told you before, that we are serious about child spacing medicine? Fatu will not get belly again until the new baby is big. One day, I know our family will be large past your own, because we are taking time to space our children. But you, Kerkula, are suffering! Your children die and your wife is weak because you are a stubborn man! If you would learn about child spacing business, your children would not die. And your wife would have time to get strong again.'

When he heard this, Kerkula was shamed. He decided it was time to learn about child spacing methods, so that he would have a healthy wife and family one day.

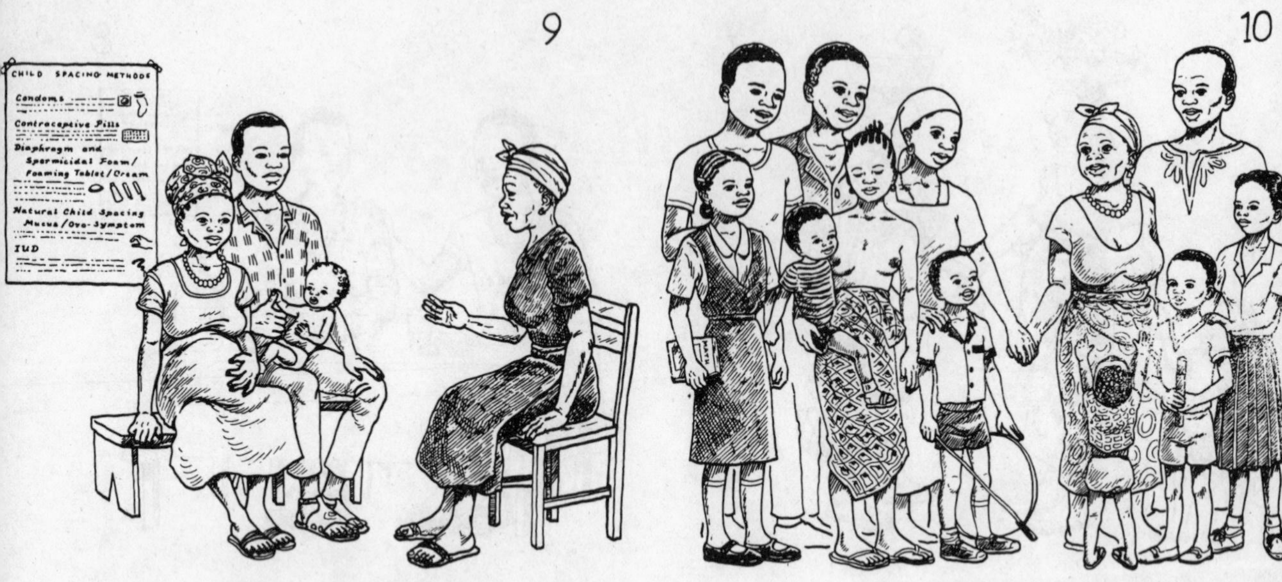

PICTURE 9: So Musu and Kerkula went together to the clinic. The nurse there was kind and patient with the unhappy couple. They listened to the nurse as she told them these important things about child spacing:

'My people, long ago, life was very hard for mothers and children. Few babies lived long enough to become strong healthy boys and girls.

Today, people know that their babies can live and grow up strong and healthy if they practise child spacing and other good health habits.

Too many babies too soon, means that the children will be sick and the mother will be weak. Child spacing means helping mothers and children to be strong and healthy.'

So Musu and Kerkula learned about the different child spacing methods and agreed to use one of the methods together. They also remembered what the nurse told them about caring for their young baby, so it too would not go back.

PICTURE 10: After many years went by, both Kerkula and Flomo were rich men with fine families. Flomo and Fatu had five grown children who all worked hard on the farm and made them proud. They were satisfied because they had taken time to space their children, and all had remained healthy and grew to be adults.

Because Kerkula and Musu were late to practise child spacing, they did not have as many living children as Flomo and Fatu. But after they started to practise child spacing, they found that their babies lived to be healthy, grown children. Kerkula was glad to have a healthy wife again, and his three fine children gave him happiness in his old age.

Unit 3
Planning and Making Your Own Visual Aids

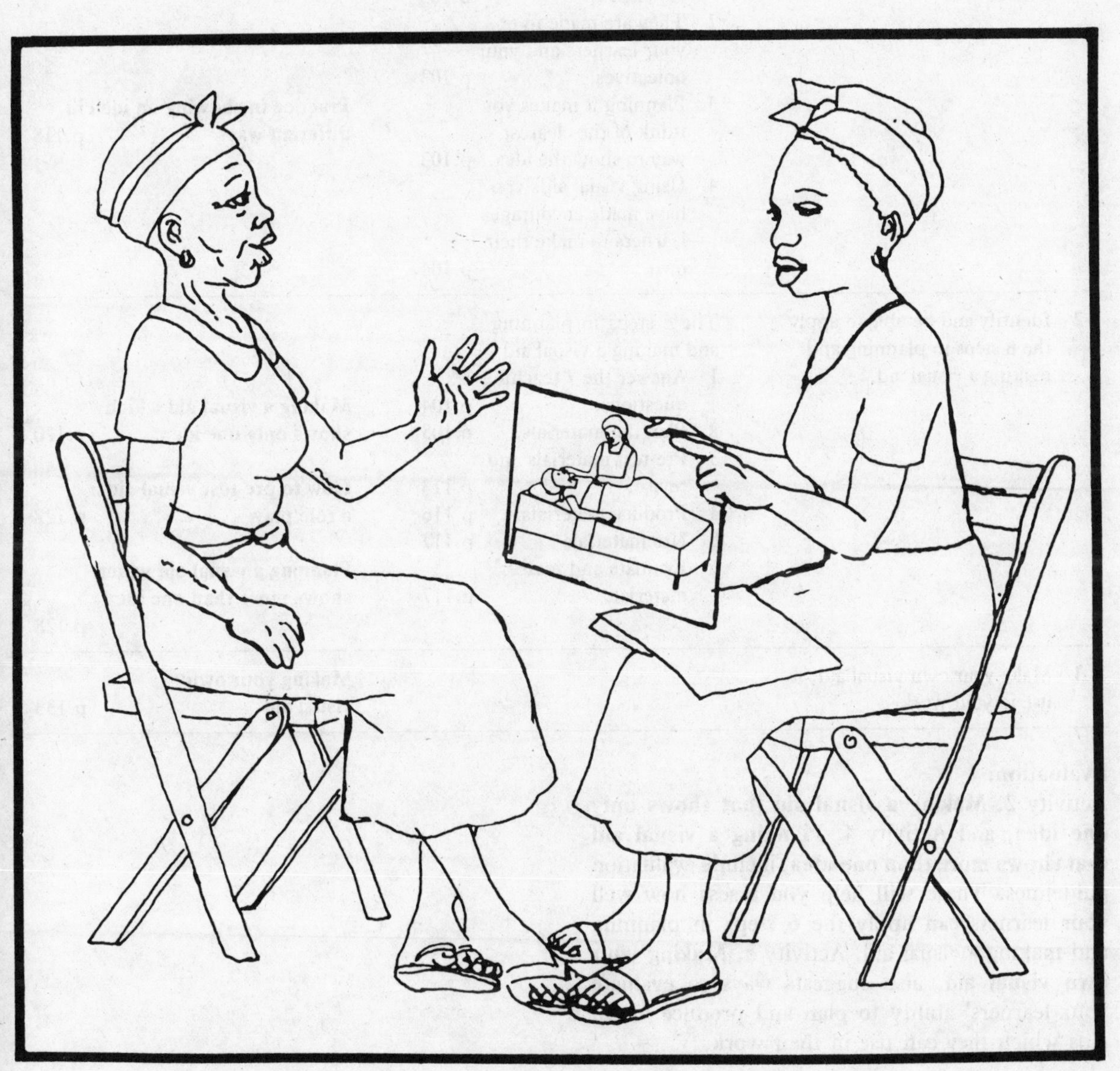

Unit 3 is about planning your own visual aids so they are most effective. You can use the beginning of this unit to discuss with your learners the advantages of making visual aids. Learners apply the guidelines for choosing and designing visual aids that they learned from Unit 2 to planning and making visual aids. They experiment with showing an idea in different ways to see which is best. They also learn how to pre-test a visual aid before using it.

Unit 3: Planning and making your own visual aids

Objective	Information	Activities
1 Describe 3 reasons why making your own visual aid is often better than using a ready-made one.	Visual aids you make yourself are often better than ready-made ones. 1 They are less expensive. p.103 2 They are made to fit your learners and your objectives. p.103 3 Planning it makes you think of the clearest way to show the idea. p.103 4 Using visual aids you have made encourages learners to make their own. p.104	**Practice in showing an idea in different ways** p.118
2 Identify and be able to apply the 6 steps in planning and making a visual aid.	The 6 steps in planning and making a visual aid: 1 Answer the 7 teaching questions. p.104 2 Plan the materials. p.105 3 Pre-test materials and revise. p.113 4 Produce materials. p.116 5 Use materials p.117 6 Evaluate and revise materials. p.117	**Making a visual aid which shows only one idea.** p.120 **How to pre-test visual aids: a role play** p.122 **Planning a visual aid which shows more than one idea** p.128
3 Make your own visual aid, to use in your work.		**Making your own visual aid** p.133

Evaluation:
Activity 2, **Making a visual aid that shows only one idea,** and Activity 4, **Planning a visual aid that shows more than one idea,** include evaluation guidelines. These will help you assess how well your learners can apply the 6 steps in planning and making a visual aid. Activity 5, **Making your own visual aid,** also suggests ways to evaluate your learners' ability to plan and produce visual aids which they can use in their work.

Ask learners to turn to the person on their right. As groups of 2, their task is to think of at least 2 reasons why making their own visual aids can be better than using ready-made ones. Give the groups about 5 minutes.

Have one group at a time suggest the reasons they have thought of. Write these on a chalkboard or large sheet of paper as they are mentioned. Discuss each briefly and be sure that all participants agree before you go on to the next reason.

Your learners may think of other reasons besides the 4 listed here. Discuss all of their suggestions.

If no one mentions these 4 reasons, suggest them for discussion yourself.

Advantages of making your own visual aids

1 Visual aids you make yourself are usually *less expensive*.

If you make visual aids out of locally available materials, you do not have to buy expensive posters made by artists or expensive models which must be imported. Slides and films are expensive. Often they are not very reliable because of equipment problems and the need for electricity.

2 Visual aids you make are *planned to suit your learners and your objectives*.

Making your own visual aids means that you do not have to depend on the Ministry of Health or other such organizations for your visual aids. Sometimes such visual aids are useful, and they are free. But they cannot take the place of a visual aid which you have planned and made especially for *your* learners in a particular situation.

3 *Planning a visual aid makes you think about the information in different ways*. This helps you present the information to your learners more clearly.

Answering the 7 teaching questions and following the 6 steps presented in the next section of this unit requires you to:

(a) know the information very well;

(b) be able to find the clearest way to show it to your learners.

Remind your learners that Unit 1 mentioned that making your own visual aids is a way to learn to discover new information.

4 *Using visual aids you have made yourself encourages your learners to make their own.*

Your learners are also teachers and trainers. Encouraging them to make their own visual aids is useful to both them and their learners. They learn by making the visual aid, and they have something to use in their own teaching or training.

Encourage the people you teach to have *their* learners make visual aids as a way to learn or discover new information.

Do Activity 1, **Practice in showing an idea in different ways.**

Ask your learners to suggest steps they think are necessary in planning and making a visual aid. List them on the chalkboard as they are mentioned.

Add any of the 6 steps that were left out. If there are questions, a brief discussion is all that is necessary at this point. The steps will become clearer as learners do the activities in this unit.

Steps in planning and making a visual aid

The steps listed below are very helpful for planning and making such visual aids as posters, picture series, and flip-books. The basic ideas in the steps are also useful for planning and making flannelboards, models, and displays.

You may want to tell your participants the story of Mrs Luyomba and how she made her visual aid. There are larger versions of the pictures shown here in the Resource Pictures section of this manual.

A Answer the 7 teaching questions.

Always answer the 7 teaching questions before you begin planning or making a visual aid. The 7 questions help you decide what *kind* of visual aid will be best to use in your specific situation and help you to think about how to use it.

Mrs Luyomba gives short in-service training sessions for the nurse aides in her district on the first day of each month when they come to the district office to pick up their pay checks.

The nurse aides requested a training session on the menstrual cycle because they have difficulty explaining to their clients the changes in the ovaries and the lining of the uterus that occur during the menstrual cycle.

When Mrs Luyomba started planning her session she first sat down and thought about the 7 teaching questions. This is what the wrote:

1 **What** is the **problem?**
Nurse aides have difficulty explaining the menstrual cycle to their clients.
2 **Who** are my learners?
15 nurse aides.
3 **What** do I want them to be able to **do**?
Explain the changes in the ovaries and the lining of the uterus that occur during the menstrual cycle.
4 **Where** and for **how long** will the instruction take place?
In a room in the district health centre; 30 minutes.
5 What **teaching method** or methods will I use?
Short lecture/demonstration; group discussion; then have one or two nurse aides explain the menstrual cycle using the visual aids.
6 What **visual aids** will I use?
Large paper or cloth figures with moveable parts, chalk and chalk-board.
7 How will I know how **effective** the instruction was?
Nurse aides will use the visual aids to accurately explain the changes that occur in the ovaries and lining of the uterus during the menstrual cycle.

B Plan the materials

Once you have answered the 7 teaching questions you can begin planning the materials you will develop and use. Mrs Luyomba followed the steps below as she planned her materials.

1 Identify resources such as existing teaching materials, production supplies and/or facilities, people, money. Mrs Luyomba couldn't find any existing visual aids on the menstrual cycle, so she decided to make her own. She had very little money in her budget for visual aids, but she was able to find some supplies in the health centre, such as paper, crayons, cloth, and chalk.
   She knew she could ask the doctor and some of the nurse aides in the district health centre to review and pre-test the draft materials.
2 Prepare a work plan, including budget, schedule, tasks and staff responsibilities. As part of Mrs Luyomba's work plan, she listed the tasks she would have to complete in

order to develop her visual materials. She then made out a schedule for completing the tasks in advance of the session she would give 4 weeks later. She allowed time in her schedule for such things as content review, pre-testing and revision of the materials.

3 Organize the content and list the main ideas or points which the learner needs in order to accomplish teaching question number 3. If you only want to communicate one idea, such as 'Mother's milk is best', then you will only have one idea to list at this step. But if you need to teach nurses how to explain the changes that occur during the menstrual cycle, there are several ideas they must know in order to explain the process correctly. Mrs Luyomba listed the main ideas in her lesson about the changes that occur in the ovaries and the lining of the uterus during the menstrual cycle.

- Menstruation is the shedding of the thick lining of the uterus that takes place each month.
- Every month the lining of the uterus thickens, preparing to receive a fertilized egg that could grow into a baby.
- When an egg matures it leaves the ovary. This is called ovulation. Then the egg moves slowly through the fallopian tube, taking about 6 days to reach the uterus.
- If the egg is not fertilized by a man's sperm while in the fallopian tube, it moves through the uterus and outside the body.
- About 14 days after ovulation the uterus begins to shed the thick lining. This is called menstruation.

4 Make a sketch or 'visual plan' for each main idea. You can use tracing and sketching skills from Unit 4 to make these sketches. Sketches like these can be called a 'visual plan'.

To make the visual plan, you trace or draw the illustrations you want and place them on the paper where you want them. Add any words or numbers you want to show.

Sometimes you may make more than one sketch for one main idea. Then you can pick the one you like best or ask other people which sketch illustrates the idea the best. Making a visual plan like this before you make the final visual aid is very useful. It means that you can ask other people about it and change it, if necessary, before you have spent the time and money to make a final visual aid.

Mrs Luyomba looked at the 5 main ideas and made these sketches to show them.

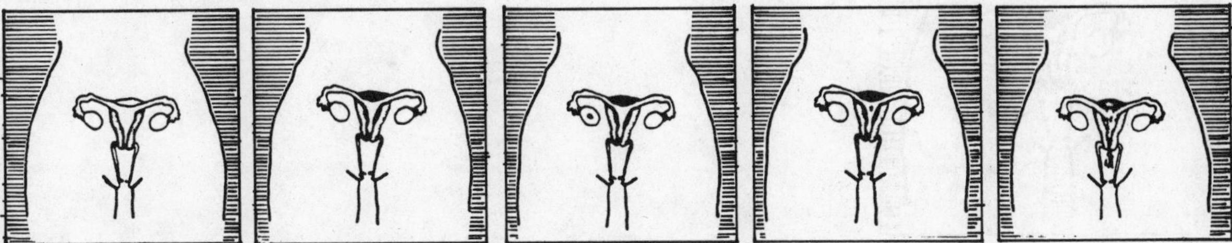

5 Develop the first draft materials. You can continue using tracing, sketching, and enlarging skills from Unit 4 to make your first draft materials. Whereas your sketches can be very rough and small, your first draft materials should be neatly drawn and large enough for other people to clearly see them. Apply the 6 design considerations from Unit 2 as you develop your first draft materials.

Mrs Luyomba looked at her sketches to see if they followed good design guidelines. She found that the background she had put in some of the pictures was distracting. She left out the background lines when she prepared the first draft drawings.

If you make a visual aid that has a story or other explanation with it, it is helpful to write it on the back of the picture. If this is not possible, you can write it on another piece of paper as a note to go along with the visual aid. Mrs Luyomba wrote this explanation on the back of her pictures:

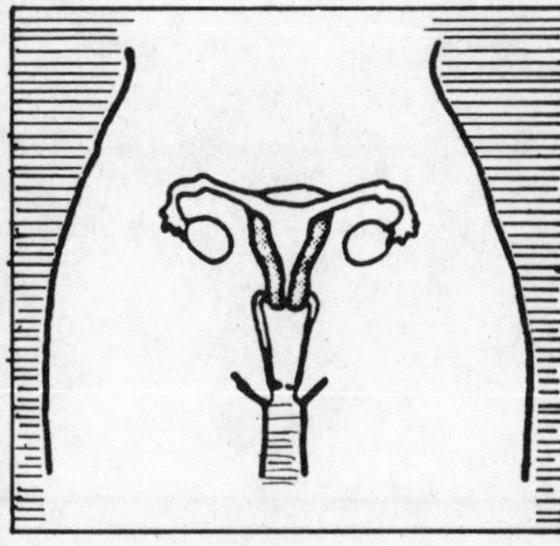

Menstruation is the shedding of the thick lining of the uterus that takes place each month.

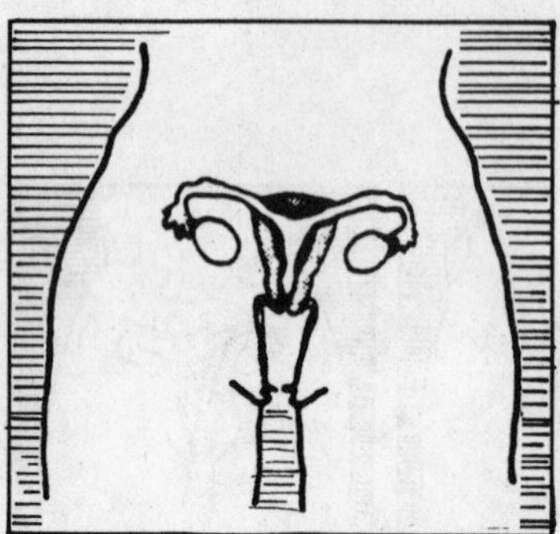

Every month the lining of the uterus thickens, preparing to receive a fertilized egg that could grow into a baby.

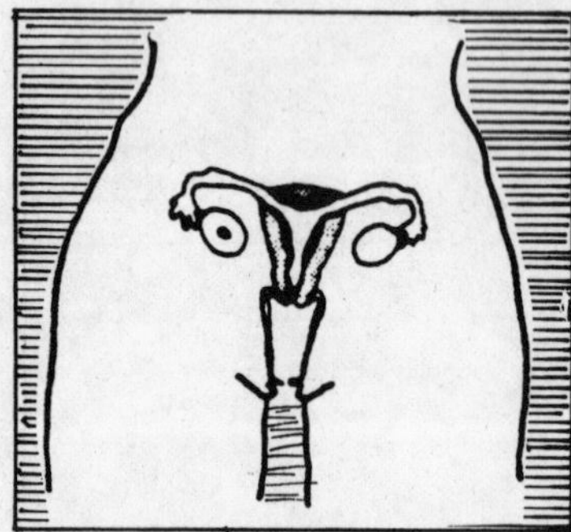

When an egg matures it leaves the ovary. This is called ovulation. Then the egg moves slowly through the fallopian tube, taking about 6 days to reach the uterus.

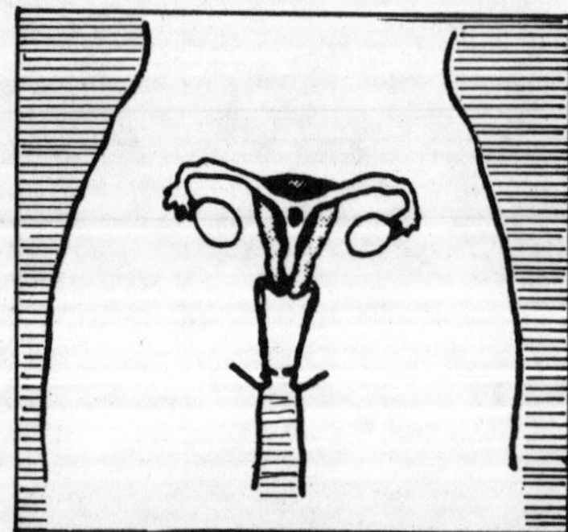

If the egg is not fertilized by a male sperm while in the fallopian tube, it moves through the uterus and outside the body.

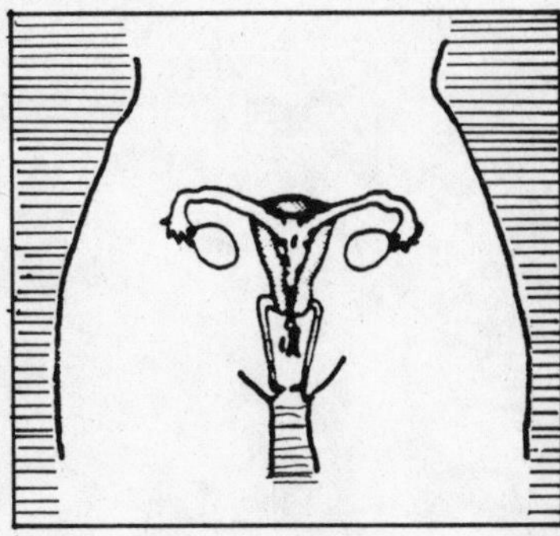

About 14 days after ovulation, the uterus begins to shed the thick lining. This is called menstruation.

6 Have content specialists review the draft materials for accuracy and completeness. These content specialists can be other health workers like yourself. They can suggest changes in the message you are presenting, or in how you are presenting it.

Mrs Luyomba asked the doctor and one of the nurses at the district health centre to look at the pictures and review them for her.

She asked the doctor, 'Do these pictures show the changes that take place in the ovaries and the lining of the uterus during the menstrual cycle?' The doctor looked at the pictures and said 'Yes'.

Use this example to begin a discussion of using open rather than closed questions when you are pre-testing visual aids.

Mrs Luyomba's question told the person who was reviewing her visual aid what he was supposed to see. A question like this is called a 'closed' question because it interprets the pictures for the person who is reviewing the visual aid. After such a question, it was impossible for the doctor to give a completely honest reaction to the pictures.

Ask your learners to think of other closed questions that Mrs Luyomba could have asked. Some other examples are listed here:

- Can you tell that the lining of the uterus has thickened?
- Is it clear that the egg moves from the ovary through the fallopian tube and into the uterus?
- Can you tell that the lining of the uterus is shedding in this picture, causing the monthly bleeding?

Mrs Luyomba then asked the doctor to read what she had written on the backs of the visuals and tell her if the information was accurate and complete. The doctor said the information was accurate, but suggested that a sentence and perhaps a picture be added at the beginning to relate menstruation to a woman of childbearing age.

Then Mrs Luyomba asked a nurse at the clinic to look at the pictures for her. She asked her the same kinds of questions. When she got to the third and fourth pictures, she pointed to them and said, 'Is it clear that ovulation is occurring and that the egg travels from the ovary through the fallopian tube to the uterus?'

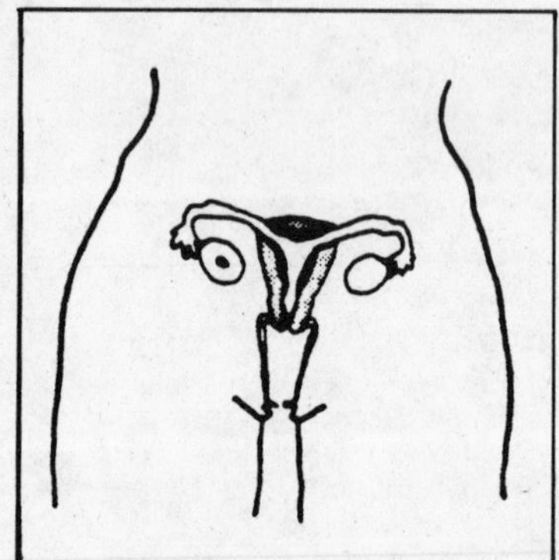

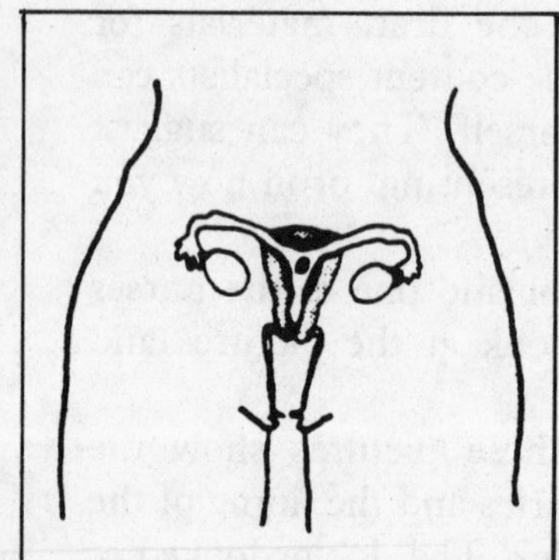

The nurse said, 'If you had not told me this was ovulation, I would not have known. I can barely see the egg in both pictures, and I certainly can't tell from these 2 pictures that the egg moves through the fallopian tube to reach the uterus.' She suggested writing the word 'ovulation' on the board next to the third picture and then using a pointer to trace the movement of the egg from the ovary to the uterus.

She also suggested to Mrs Luyomba that her questions were telling her reviewers things about the pictures.

The nurse said that pre-testing had been very helpful to a friend of hers at a nearby clinic. But her friend had said it was very important to ask the right kind of questions when pre-testing a visual aid, or you will not know if the visual aid really works. She told her what she had heard from her friend.

She said that the closed questions such as she was asking come more easily and naturally to everyone. But they do not permit honest responses. Open questions must be worded more carefully, but they are the only way to be sure that people are telling you what they really see. With closed questions, people may tell you what they think you want to hear.

They talked about some open questions Mrs Luyomba could use when she field-tested the visual aid. Mrs Luyomba went away grumbling, but she decided to try the nurse's suggestions.

Ask learners to suggest some other 'open' questions Mrs Luyomba could ask. These might include:

- 'What is happening in this picture?'
- 'Is there anything in this picture that is confusing to you? What?'
- 'Is there anything in this picture that might confuse or offend you or your friends?'
- 'Can the picture be improved? How?'

Mrs Luyomba then made revisions in her visual aid according to the suggestions the content reviewers made. The next draft of her visual aid looked like this:

Story

Menstruation is the regular bleeding in women during the years when they can bear children.

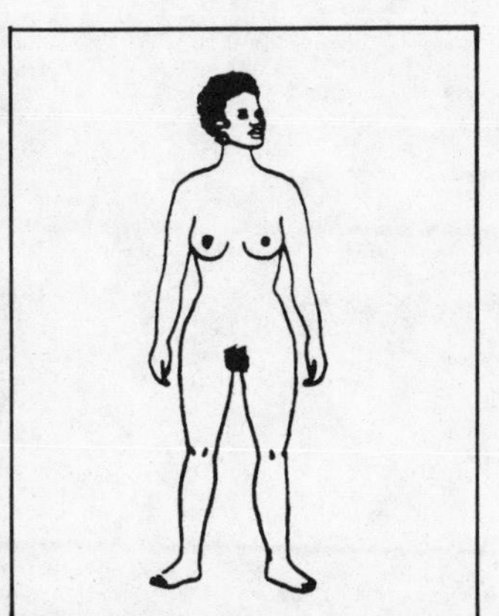

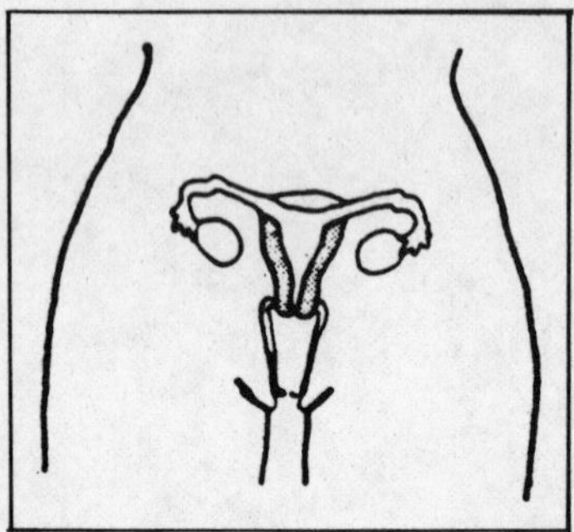

This bleeding is the shedding of the thick lining of the uterus that takes place each month.

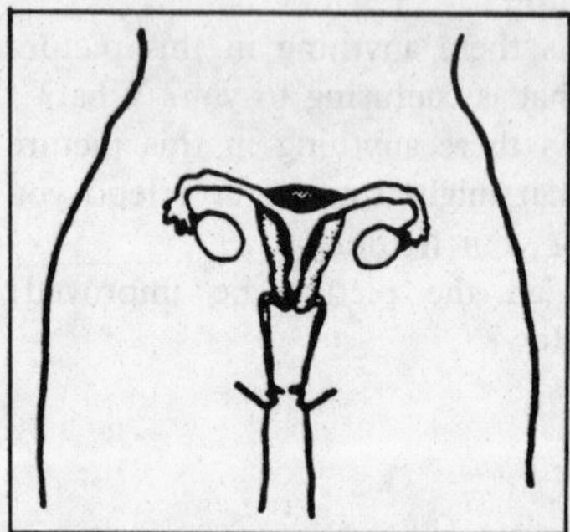

Every month the lining of the uterus thickens, preparing to receive a fertilized egg that could grow into a baby.

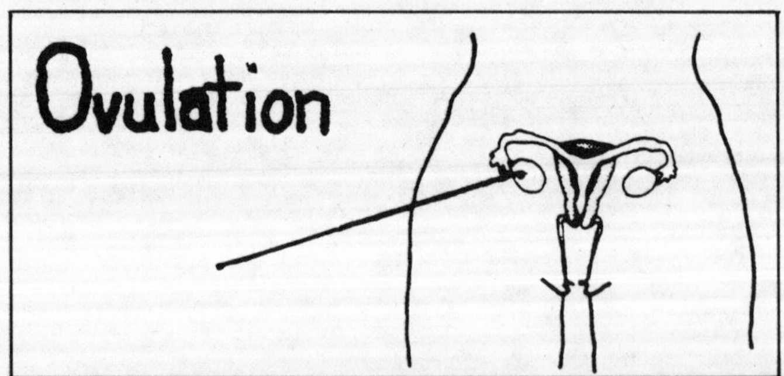

When an egg matures, it leaves the ovary. This is called ovulation. Then the egg moves slowly through the fallopian tube, taking about 6 days to reach the uterus.

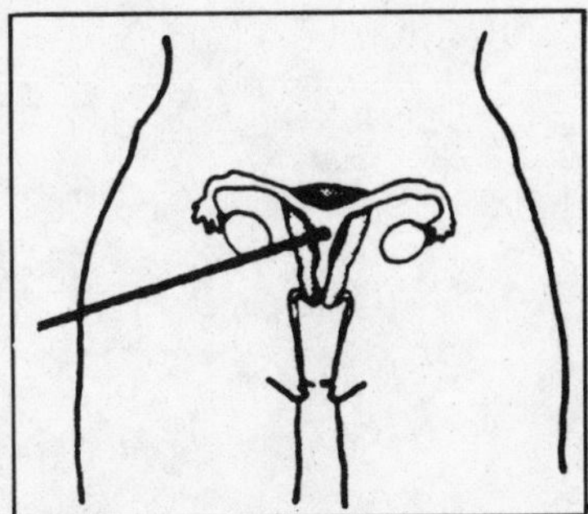

If the egg is not fertilized by a male sperm while in the fallopian tube, it moves through the uterus and outside the body.

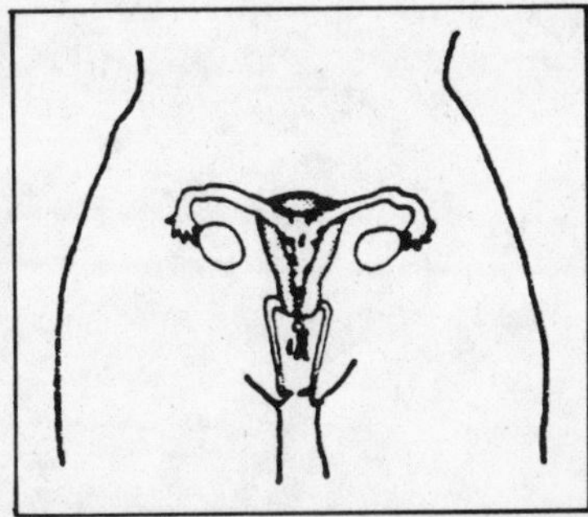

About 14 days after ovulation the uterus begins to shed the thick lining. This is called menstruation.

C Pre-test materials with a sample of intended learners and revise if necessary.

Trying out your materials with several people very much like the people you will be teaching or training is one of the most important steps in the process of developing the materials. Pre-testing can help you discover if the visual aid works the way you want it to; it can help you find out whether your learners can learn and use needed information and skills from the instructional materials.

Mrs Luyomba asked the five nurse aides working at the district health centre individually to look at the next draft. For each nurse aide, Mrs Luyomba showed each visual separately and first found out her understanding of the visual alone, then of the visual with the words that go with it. This time, she asked questions like this:

What do you think this picture is about?

What is the main idea in the picture? Why do you say that?

How can the picture and words be improved?

Mrs Luyomba then showed the entire set of visuals and read the words that go with them. Afterwards, she asked the nurse aide to explain the changes in the ovaries and the lining of the uterus that occur during the menstrual cycle. She also asked them for suggestions on how she could improve the pictures and words in the lesson to better enable them to explain afterwards the changes that occur in the menstrual cycle.

Three nurse aides said that it would be helpful to write the word 'menstruation' beside the last picture which shows the uterus shedding its lining.

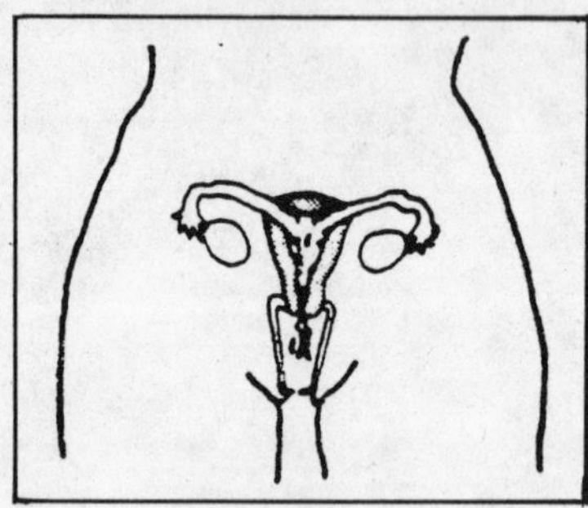

Several of the nurse aides had difficulty relating the second picture to the first in the beginning of the lesson. They suggested that Mrs Luyomba add a picture in between the first two which would show that the second picture was an enlargement of a part of the woman in the first picture.

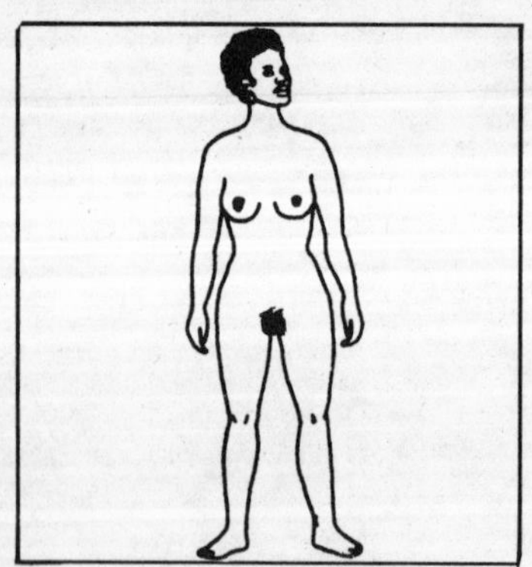

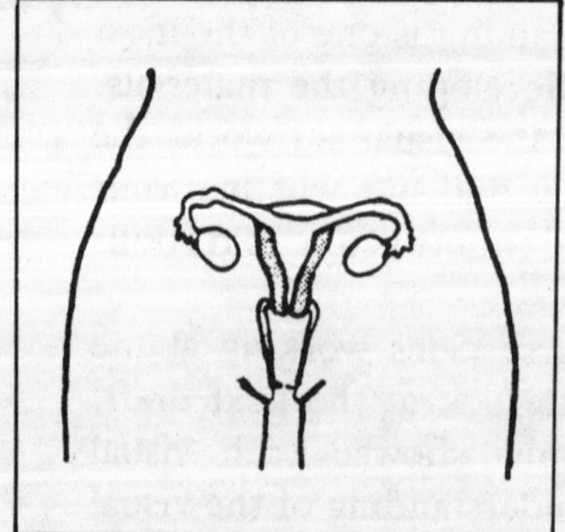

Mrs Luyomba was soon convinced of the value of open questions rather than closed questions because she received a number of helpful suggestions. She was glad she had taken the time to pre-test her visual aid.

According to the information you receive during the pre-testing, decide these things:

- what pictures, words or numbers to keep
- what pictures, words or numbers to omit
- what to add
- what to change

Mrs Luyomba made these changes in her pictures and words as a result of the pre-testing. She added the word 'menstruation' to the last picture.

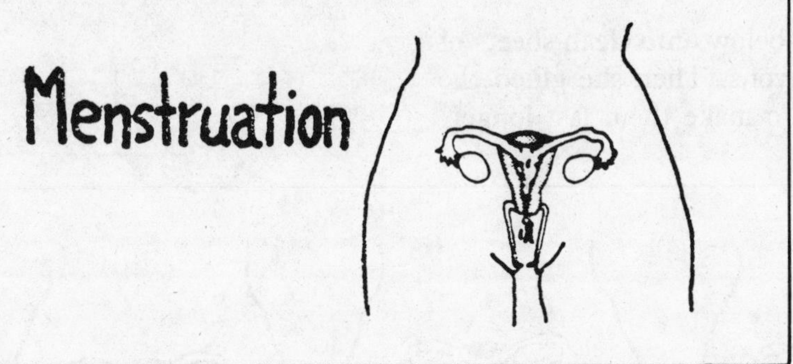

She added a picture and words between the first two pictures.

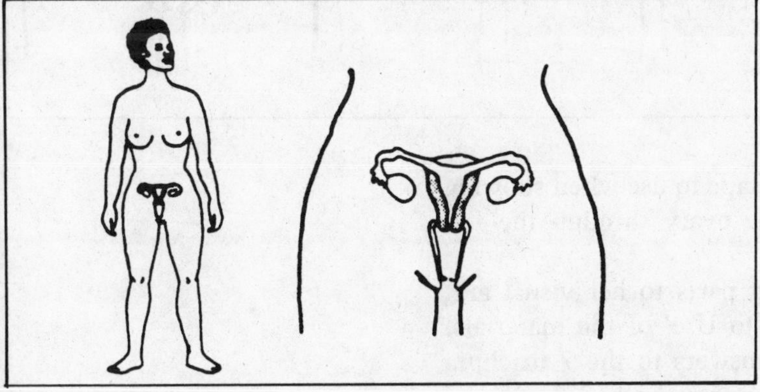

This shows where a woman's reproductive organs, including the uterus and ovaries, are located inside her body. On the right is an enlargement of this area of her body, so you can see the reproductive organs better.

D Produce materials

You may want your finished visual aid to be larger than the visual plan which you pre-tested. Or you may want to make the final visual aid out of a different paper or material.

You will probably have several changes to make as a result of your pre-testing. Do not be discouraged. Many changes mean that you are doing a good job of listening to the responses of other people. These changes also mean that you will have a more effective visual aid.

Unit 4 is a collection of production skills which you and your learners can use in making your visual aids. Refer to the Trainer's Guide at the beginning of the manual for ways to combine the information in these two units.

Mrs Luyomba traced the drawings below onto clean sheets of paper and coloured them with crayons. Then she glued the pictures onto pieces of cardboard to make them last longer.

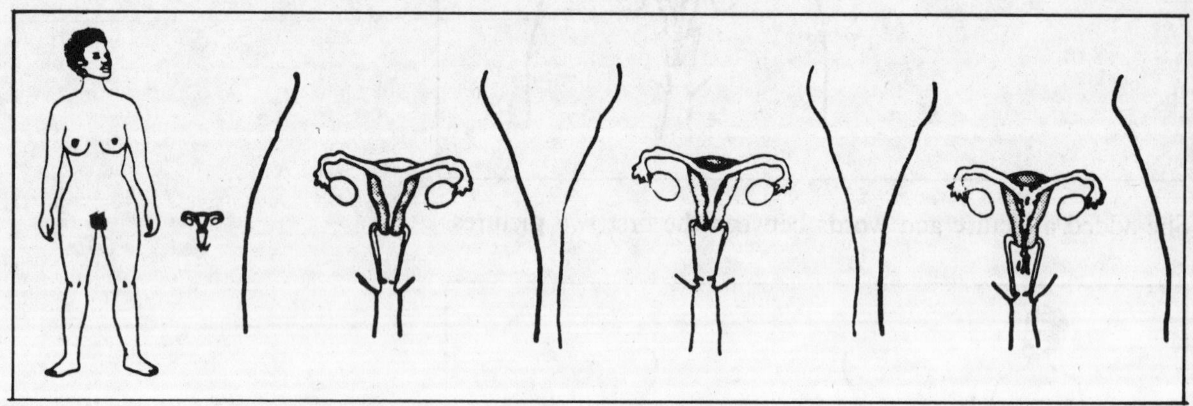

She made a pointer out of wire and tape to use when showing the movement of the egg from the ovary through the fallopian tube to the uterus.

Because there are several moving parts to her visual aid, Mrs Luyomba developed a 'Guide to Use' of the materials. The 'Guide to Use' included her answers to the 7 teaching questions, small drawings of the pictures she had developed along with the words to go with each picture, and instructions on how to use the moveable parts during the lesson.

See Mrs Luyomba's 'Guide to Use' along with the larger versions of the pictures in the Resource Pictures section.

Information	Training ideas and your notes

E Use materials

When you have finished your visual aid, use it in a training or educational session. Unit 5 may help you plan how you will use your visual aid in a session. During the session, be sure to note how well your learners are accomplishing your answers to teaching question number 7.

When Mrs Luyomba used her visual aid in her next in-service training session, she noticed that the nurse aides looked carefully at the visual aids as she used them. Also, the learners she asked to come forward at the end of the session were able to use her visual aid to clearly and accurately explain the changes that occur during menstruation.

F Evaluate and revise materials

Based on your use of the materials with an actual group of learners, you may again want to update or revise them and the way you use them.

Mrs Luyomba's nurse aides thought her visual aid was so useful that they asked if they could have copies to use when explaining menstruation to their clients. So, Mrs Luyomba decided to copy the drawings and have the nurse aides colour them, paste them on cardboard and make the pointer sticks when they came for their next in-service training session.

When learners have a basic understanding of these 6 steps, let them do Activity 2, **Making a visual aid which shows one idea.** This activity asks them to apply these steps to planning and making a poster.

After they complete Activity 1, do Activity 3, **How to pre-test visual aids: a role play.** Then they can practise what they have just learned when they pre-test their group projects.

Ask your learners to do Activity 4, **Planning a visual aid which shows more than one idea,** next. This activity asks them to work in small groups to plan and pre-test a visual aid which shows more than one idea.

After the group project is completed, have learners do Activity 5, **Making your own visual aid.** This activity will help you assess what they have learned from Units 1, 2, 3, and 4.

Activity 1

Practice in showing an idea in different ways

Time

45 minutes

Objective

Learners will sketch 4 pictures, showing how one of the ideas listed can be shown in 4 different ways.

Materials

Drawing paper, pencils, and erasers.
Thin paper for tracing.
A collection of resource pictures that learners can use to trace.

Instructions

1 Be sure your learners have done the tracing and sketching in Unit 4 before doing this activity. They need to be comfortable with tracing and sketching.

2 Introduce this activity by presenting the example. You may need to enlarge these pictures so that everyone can see. Use another example if you prefer, but it is important that you *show* participants what they are expected to do.

3 Explain that this exercise is to give learners practice in thinking of different ways to show information in pictures. Emphasize that sketching skills are not as important as the things they can think of to draw in this activity.

4 Write the list of possible topics on the chalkboard.

5 Have each person choose one of the items on the list. Ask everyone to make 4 different sketches of ways that they could show the idea in a visual aid.

6 Let learners work on their sketches individually. Let them talk with each other, but they should not do each other's work.

7 Meet as a large group again. Have everyone show their sketches of the idea they chose. Ask which sketch they would choose to make a final visual aid. Ask why that one is better than the others. Ask if the group agrees, or if they think another is better.

8 Ask your learners if this activity was easy or hard for them. Point out that thinking of the best way to show an idea in pictures means that you must know the information very well, and you must think of the best way to show it. This is sometimes difficult, but it is very useful, as mentioned at the beginning of this unit.

Possible adaptations

1 If time is limited, have everyone work on the same idea. Ask each person to do only 3 sketches. Then when you have the group discussion, your learners can see how many different

ways others have thought of to show the same thing.

2 You can also use this activity as part of the activity on making a poster. Ask each person to sketch 4 different ways to show their topic in a poster. Then have them choose the one they think is best to pre-test and make.

3 If the ideas on the list are not appropriate for your learners, make up your own list. The ideas need to be things your learners work with often.

Possible topics for visual aids which show only one main idea

1 Breast-feeding is healthier for baby than bottle-feeding.
2 Child spacing leads to healthier mothers and healthier babies.
3 A pregnant woman needs to eat healthful foods.
4 Visit the clinic before your baby is born (pre-natal check-ups).
5 Feed children high-protein foods to prevent kwashiorkor.

Example of four different ways to show one idea

Main idea: Take your pill everyday.
Learners: Women coming to a family planning clinic who have decided to take oral contraceptives for the first time. Some of the women cannot read.
Possible ways to show the idea:

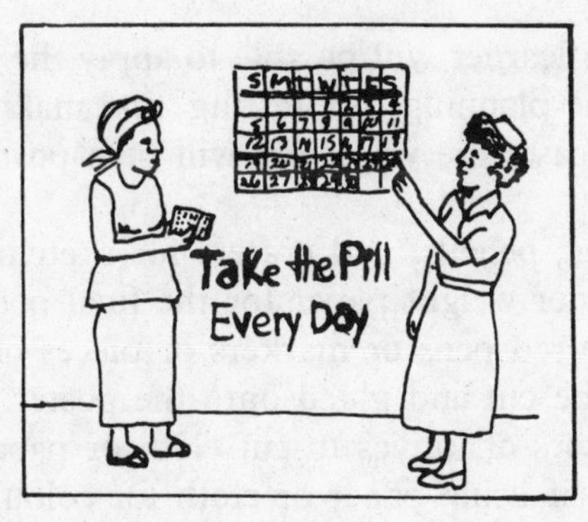

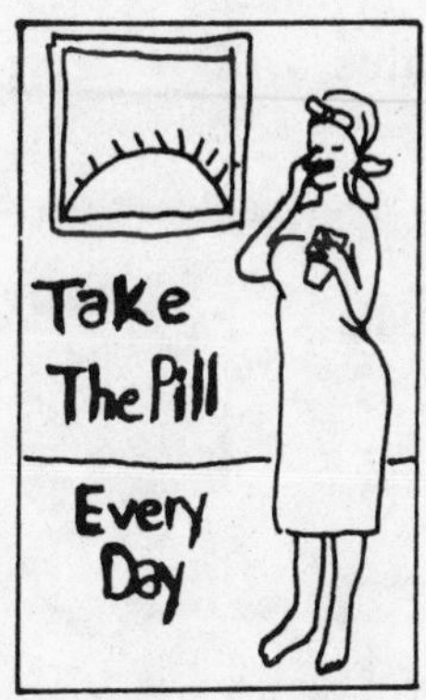

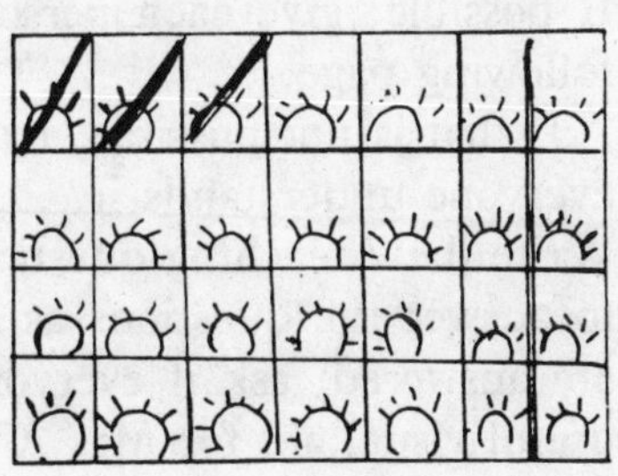

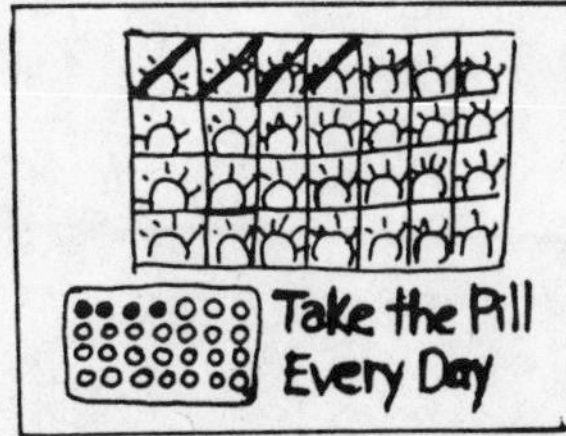

Choosing the best sketch to use:

The picture with the sun calendar, the pill pack and words is best. It requires learners to do something with it (cross off each day when they take their pill). The pill pack picture reminds them why they are crossing off the days. The words also remind those who can read to 'take the pill everyday'.

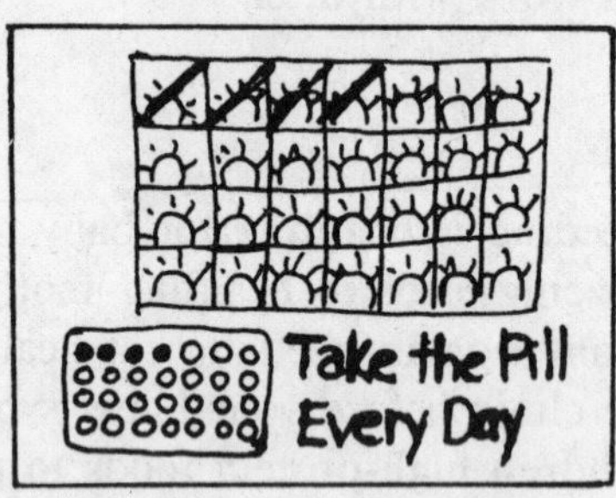

Activity 2

Making a visual aid which shows only one idea

Time

3 hours

Objective

Each learner will be able to apply the 6 steps in making a visual aid to the planning, pre-testing, and making of a one-idea visual aid. In this case, the visual aid will be a poster.

Materials

Paper, pencils, and erasers for sketching.
Heavier weight paper for the final posters.
Coloured pens or markers or pieces of coloured cloth or paper that can be cut and glued onto the poster.
Scissors or knives to cut cloth or paper.
Glue if using paper or cloth for colours.

Instructions

1 If possible, give each person a copy of the case study on the following page.
If that is not possible, read the case study out loud. Be sure everyone understands it.

2 Write the 7 teaching questions on the chalkboard. Ask learners to answer the questions as a large group. When the questions are answered, ask if everyone agrees that a poster would be a useful visual aid for Mrs Abubaber.

3 Be sure everyone has a copy of the 6 steps in making a visual aid. The steps should either be written on the chalkboard or posted on a wall throughout the activity. If this is not possible, be sure learners have the steps copied into their notes.

4 Tell learners that in this activity, each person will be making a poster as a solution to this case study. They can refer to the 6 steps for guidance on how to make the poster. Tell them you will also be going from person to person to answer questions and check their progress.

Give participants paper and pencils for sketching. Let them ask you for other materials when they need them.

5 Help each person work with the topic and the 6 steps. This part of the activity is like a workshop. Learners work individually, except when they need help. Allow people to help each other, but not to do each other's work.

6 When a person is ready to pre-test the visual plan, have him ask 3 other participants to look at it for him. Suggest to participants that they will gain much from this activity by helping and co-operating with each other in this way.

7 If you do not have coloured pens or markers, participants can draw figures on the poster paper and then cut pieces of coloured cloth or paper to fit.

8 When the posters are finished, have participants take turns presenting them to the large group. Then display the posters on the wall.

At the end of each person's presentation ask the group to respond to the questions in the guidelines included with this activity. After the first few presentations these questions can be answered very quickly and briefly.

Possible adaptations

1 You can make up your own case study if you like. If you do this, be sure that you have a list of answers to the teaching questions for your own reference. Also be sure that a poster or other one-idea visual aid is the best solution for that case study problem.

2 You can have participants pre-test their posters with each other as an overnight homework assignment.

Case study

Mrs Abubaber works in a regional clinic which serves the surrounding rural area. Most of the women who come to the clinic are not literate. Many of the children she sees have diarrhoea and vomiting, worms, or bilharzia. She talks to the mothers of these children about good sanitation practices. She also wants to make a visual aid to put in the waiting room of the clinic. She wants to use the visual aid to help the women remember to wash their hands thoroughly with soap and water before they prepare food for the family.

Guidelines for evaluating visual aids that show only one idea

1 Have the 7 teaching questions been answered well?
(1) **What** is the **problem**?
(2) **Who** are my learners?
(3) **What** do I want them to be able to **do**?
(4) **Where** and for **how long** will the instruction take place?
(5) What **teaching method** or methods will I use? (There may be none, as when a poster or display is used by itself.)
(6) What **visual aids** will I use?
(7) How will I know **how effective** the instruction was?

2 Is the main idea pictured clearly?

3 Does the picture follow the guidelines for good design as presented in Unit 2? Can this picture be used with illiterate learners?
(1) The words and pictures should be **easy to see.**
(2) The words and pictures should be **easy to understand.**
(3) The information should be presented **clearly and simply.**
(4) The visual should be **well organized.**
(5) The viewer's **attention** should be **directed to the important information.**
(6) The visual should be **interesting** to the people for whom it is intended.

4 Was it clear that the person knew exactly what he or she wanted to say when presenting the visual aid to the group (if there was any story or background information to give)?

5 If pre-testing showed that changes should be made, were these changes made?

Activity 3

How to pre-test visual aids: a role play

Time

1 hour

Objective

Learners will pre-test visual aids without influencing the reactions of the people who are looking at the visual aid.

Materials

Roles for the health worker and for the people looking at the visual aid.

Sample visual aid plan to be pre-tested (a sample is provided).
Large sheet of paper and marker or chalk and chalkboard.

Instructions

1 Choose 2 people to play the roles of the health worker and the person looking at the visual aid. You may want to play the role of the health worker yourself.

2 Explain the roles to the people who will be involved in the role play. You can use the role descriptions included in this activity or make up your own. If you make up your own role descriptions, see item 2 under 'Possible adaptations' for guidelines.

3 Allow the people who will take part in the role play to think about their roles. You may want to give them their role descriptions the day before, if you want them to think about their characters. But if you want them to react more spontaneously, only give them a few minutes. They can read their role descriptions while you are explaining the situation to the others. Remind the role players that pre-testing is one of the most important parts of planning and making visual aids. They should not discuss their roles together before the role play.

4 Tell the group that in this activity, 2 people will do a role play on how to pre-test visual aid plans. Tell them they are to watch and listen for answers to these questions:
(a) What steps does the health worker go through to pre-test the visual aid?
(b) What does the health worker do to obtain honest reactions from the person who is looking at the visual aid?
(c) What does the health worker do that prevents the person from reacting honestly?

5 Set up the scene for the role play. If available, use simple objects that make the situation more realistic, such as chairs and small pieces of health equipment for a clinic setting.

6 Begin the role play. During the role play, you may need to give suggestions to the learners who are in the role play to help them to follow their roles.

7 Stop the role play when the health worker has completed the pre-test of the visual aid plan.

8 Lead a discussion about the role play. Ask the learners who were involved in the role play to describe their *feelings* about playing their roles. Were they comfortable or uncomfortable? What was easy and what was hard about playing the roles of the health worker and the person? How did they *feel* as the people they were representing in the role play?
Ask the other learners for their answers to the questions you asked them before the role play:

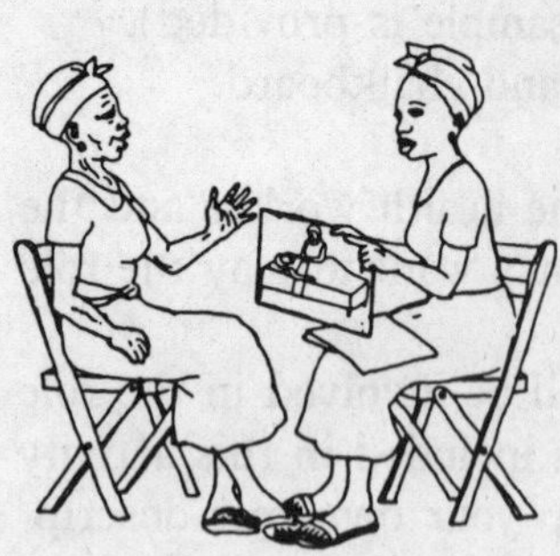

(a) What steps did the health worker go through to pre-test the visual aid?
Answer:
(1) Put the other person at ease.
(2) Asked open questions about the pictures, one at a time.
(3) Showed pictures again in the correct order and said the words that go with the pictures.
(4) Asked open questions about the person's understanding of the pictures and words.
(5) Thanked the person for his help.

(b) What did the health worker do to encourage honest reactions from the other person?
(Some possibilities are: asked open instead of closed questions; encouraged the other person to talk; was friendly.)

(c) What did the health worker do that prevented the person from reacting honestly?
(Some possibilities are: used closed questions; was defensive; looked angry or upset.)

9 Ask the learners why it is important to get honest reactions to a visual aid they have planned.
(Some reasons are: honest reactions tell the health worker what needs to be changed in the plan for the visual aid to make it more understandable; honest reactions to a visual plan allow the health worker to make changes before he or she spends more time and money making a final visual aid.)

10 Explain that in the next activity participants will plan and pre-test their own visual aids. It will be important to remember the steps for pre-testing and the ways that a health worker can encourage honest reactions.

Possible adaptations

1 You can also add the role of recorder to the activity if you think this will be useful for your learners. The role is described after the other roles.

2 If you make up your own role descriptions, be sure that you answer the following questions in the descriptions of the person looking at the visual aid:
(a) Who is the person? (village mother? community leader? nursing student?)
(b) Can this person read?
(c) Where is this person from? (the city? a remote village?)
(d) What situation has made it possible for the health worker to interview this person? (a mother has brought her child to the clinic? a visit by the health worker to the community?)

3 You can use a visual aid plan that you have developed instead of the sample plan provided in this activity.

4 If time allows, give everyone some time to practise pre-testing plans for visual aids with other learners.

5 If time allows, after your learners have practised pre-testing with each other, have them pre-test plans for visual aids with people like their intended learners.

Role descriptions

Health worker

You are a nurse-midwife who works in a health centre in a remote area of the country. You are responsible for supervising a nurse, a nurse's aide, and 2 traditional birth attendants. The traditional birth attendants deliver many of the babies born in your area. You have been teaching them the correct methods for delivery, pre-natal care of the mothers, and post-natal care of the mothers and newborns.

You want the traditional birth attendants to know what to do before the actual delivery of a baby. You have planned a series of visual aids to help the traditional birth attendants learn and remember what to do before time for the delivery. You want to pre-test your plan with one of the traditional birth attendants.

Use the following steps to pre-test the visual aid:

(1) Introduce yourself and try to put the other person at ease. Explain that you want her to help you by looking at some pictures and telling you what she sees.

(2) Show each picture, one at a time. Ask *open* questions about the picture, like 'What is happening in this picture?', 'Is there anything in this picture that might embarrass you or your friends?', 'Is there anything confusing in this picture?', 'If yes, what is it?', 'Who would be most interested in this picture?' Be sure you do not influence the person's answers by your words or gestures.

(3) Show the pictures again, this time saying the words that go with each one. Go through the whole series of pictures with the person before you ask any questions.

(4) Ask open questions about the person's understanding of the pictures and words, such as 'Please explain to me in your own words what happens in this series of pictures' or 'What are some important ideas you remember from this series of pictures?' Pay attention to any misunderstandings the person might have about the ideas in the picture series.

(5) Thank the person for helping you to make a better visual aid.

Person looking at the visual aid

You are a traditional birth attendant who lives and works in a remote rural area of the country. The nurse-midwife at the health centre has been teaching you about correct methods for delivery, pre-natal care of mothers, and post-natal care of mothers and newborns. You have never been to school and cannot read or write.

The nurse-midwife has asked you to look at some pictures she has drawn. You do not mind looking at the pictures, but you hope you are not going to be tested as if you were a child. You do not have too much time to spend looking at the pictures because you have to see Mrs Lankaounde. She is almost ready to have her baby.

Some of the pictures that the nurse-midwife shows you are confusing to you. You also do not understand some of the words she uses when she shows the pictures.

Recorder

You are a nurse's aide. You have helped the nurse-midwife teach traditional birth attendants correct methods of delivery, pre-natal and post-natal care. You have helped the nurse-midwife plan a series of visual aids to help traditional birth attendants learn and remember what to do before time for the delivery. You are assisting the nurse-midwife in pre-testing the plans with one of the traditional birth attendants. You will carefully record the answers given by the traditional birth attendant. Do not ask questions. Do not draw the attention of the traditional birth attendant to your writing. Avoid making her nervous. If she appears to be upset by your note taking, remember her comments and write them after she leaves.

Sample visual aid plan: preparing for delivery

Note to the trainer

We know that there are some things about these pictures and the words that go with them which need to be improved. That is why the picture series is useful for this activity. The person playing the traditional birth attendant in the role play may say some of the following things:

(1) What do you mean by the bag of waters or the vagina?
(2) You cannot hear the baby's heartbeat through a folded blanket.
(3) The TBA in the last picture does not look very reassuring. She is sitting where the mother cannot see her.

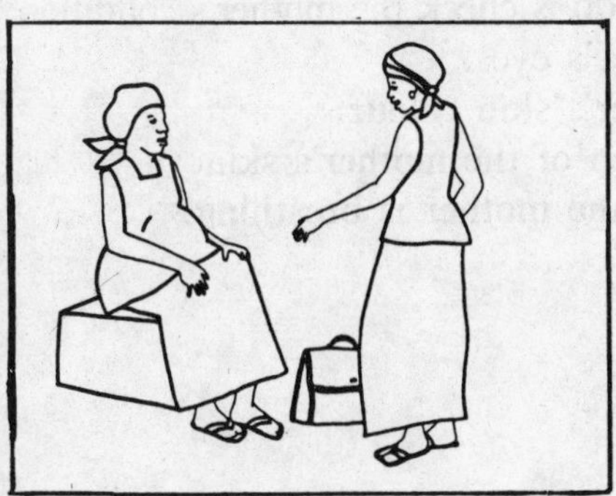

When you are called to the home of a woman in labour, greet her in a friendly way.

There are 5 things to do before the baby is born. We will talk about the 5 things to do.

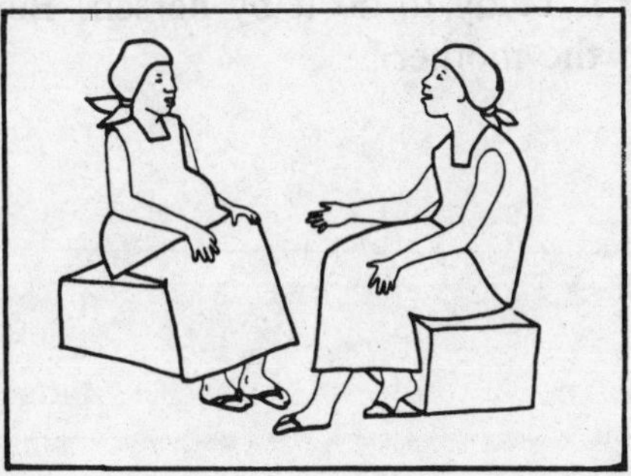

The first thing you do is talk to the mother. Ask her the following questions:

- How many babies have you had?
- Have you had any problems having your other babies?
- When did labour start?
- Has the bag of waters broken? (Have you seen any fluid coming from your vagina?)

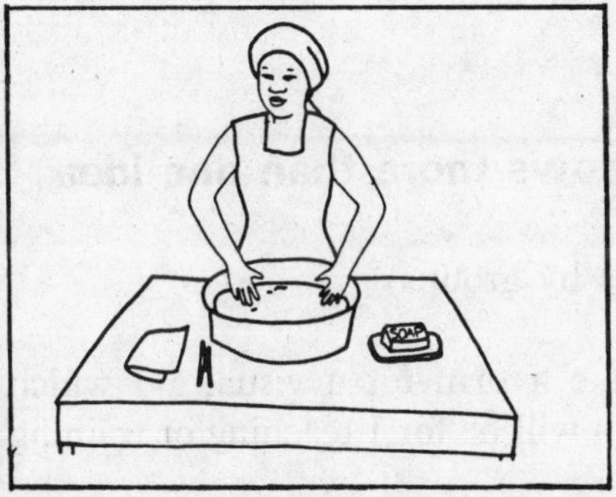

The second thing to do is wash your hands in clean water. Use soap. Clean your fingernails with a stick. Also wash the mother's belly and between her legs.

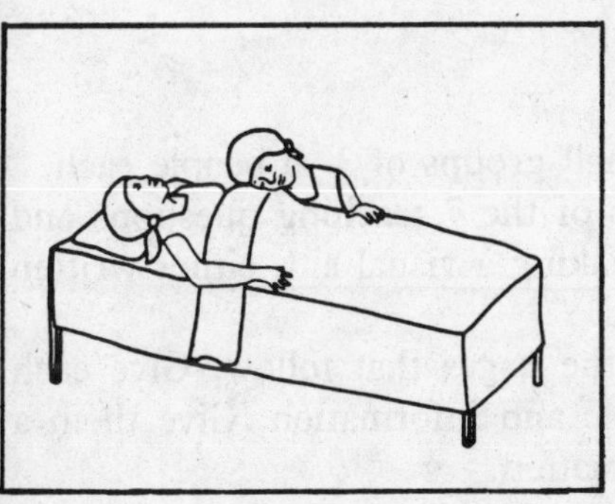

The third thing you do is to listen to the baby's heart beat. Do this to find out the baby's position in the mother's belly.

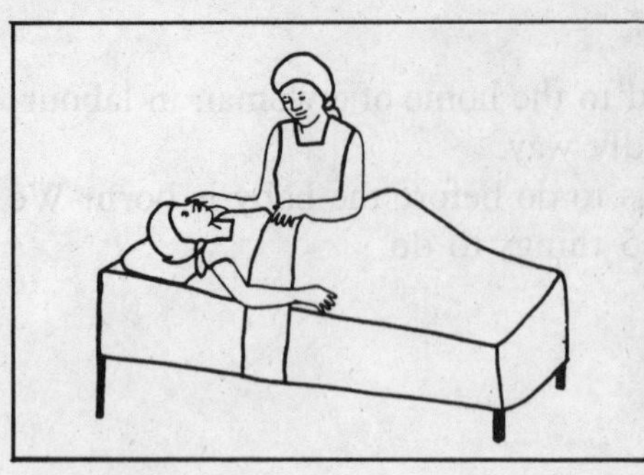

The fourth thing you do is check the mother's condition:
- Look at the mother's eyes.
- Look at the mother's skin colour.
- Check the condition of the mother's skin.
- Observe how fast the mother is breathing.

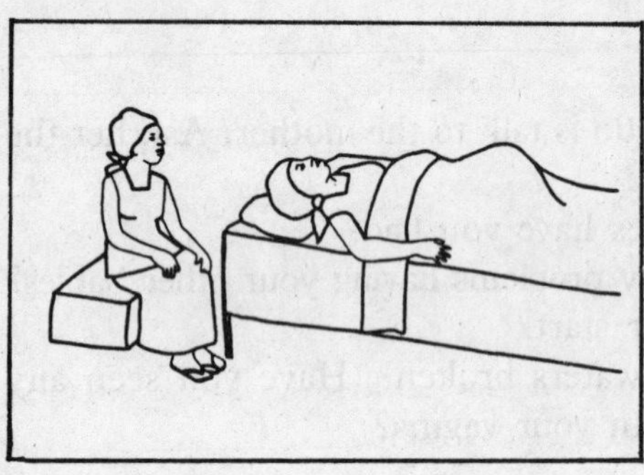

The fifth thing to do is be patient. Do not make the mother push until she is ready to do it by herself. Be calm and reassuring to the mother.

Activity 4 **Planning a visual aid that shows more than one idea**

Time 7–8 hours (including presentations by groups)

Objective In small groups, learners will make a plan for a visual aid which shows more than one idea. The plan will be for 1 teaching or training session.

Materials Paper and pencils for sketching.
Coloured pens or markers.

Instructions

1. Tell learners to divide into small groups of 3–6 people each.
2. Make sure groups have copies of the 7 teaching questions and the 6 steps in planning and making a visual aid, either written on paper or on the chalkboard.
3. Choose one of the topics on the pages that follow. Give each group a copy of the same topic and information. Give them a few minutes to read the information.

4 Explain that the assignment is for each group to plan a visual aid for one teaching or training session on the topic given to the group. (You may want to specify a time limit, such as 15 minutes, for the session.) The groups will follow only the first 3 steps in planning and making a visual aid. They will not actually produce, use or evaluate the visual aid (steps 4–6).

5 Point out that the information does not actually answer the 6 teaching questions. Each group will have to decide how they want to answer the teaching questions based on the information, and limit the information about the topic according to the time limit for the session they are planning.

6 The groups will work separately on planning their sessions and visual aids and can decide how they want to work as a group. For example, a group may work together to answer the teaching questions and define the main ideas, and then assign each individual to make sketches of one or more main ideas.

7 Explain that for step 3 (try out, or pre-test, your visual plan) each group will present their visual plan to the large group for review and suggestions for revision.

8 Tell participants that they will have about 6 hours to prepare their visual plans before presenting them to the large groups. Ask if participants have any questions about the assignment or the topic.

9 Go from group to group. Help each group work with the information and the 6 steps in making a visual aid. Usually, the most difficult steps are listing the main ideas and making a sketch for each main idea. These are part of step 2: plan the materials.

10 When the groups have finished their visual plans, have learners arrange their chairs so that everyone can see. Ask one person from each group to pre-test their visual plan with the large group. The person conducting the session with the visual plan must tell the others *who* the intended learners are and *what* the learners will be able to do after the teaching session. Then the large group will pretend to be these learners. The presenter can use the guidelines suggested in Activity 3, **How to pre-test visual aids: a role play.**

11 At the end of each session, ask the large group to respond to the first 6 questions on the guidelines included with this activity. (15–20 minutes for each session and discussion by the large group.)

12 When the sessions have been conducted, ask the small groups to revise their visual plans based on the suggestions made by the

large group. (This is step 3 of the 6 steps in planning and making a visual aid). (30 minutes)

13 Go from group to group to help them make the necessary changes.

Possible adaptations

1 You can write up your own topic and content, if you like. If you do this, try to pick a topic that would benefit from a visual aid and that includes 3–6 ideas.

2 You can assign different topics to each group. If you do this, the groups may not feel so competitive, but they will not realize that there often can be different ways to communicate an idea using a visual.

Guidelines for evaluating visual aids that show more than one idea

1 Were the 7 teaching questions answered well?
(1) **What** is the **problem?**
(2) **Who** are my learners?
(3) **What** do I want them to be able to **do**?
(4) **Where** and for **how long** will the instruction take place?
(5) What **teaching method** or methods will I use?
(6) What **visual aids** will I use?
(7) How will I know **how effective** the instruction was?

2 Does the work plan include a schedule for all the tasks that must be completed to develop the materials?

3 Does every main idea in this lesson have a picture? Did the group leave out any main ideas?

4 Is the picture for each idea clear?

5 Do the pictures follow the guidelines for good design as presented in Unit 2? Can they be used with illiterate learners?
(1) The words and pictures should be **easy to see.**
(2) The words and pictures should be **easy to understand.**
(3) The information should be presented **clearly and simply.**
(4) The visual should be **well organized.**
(5) The viewer's **attention** should be **directed to the important information.**
(6) The visual should be **interesting** to the people for whom it is intended.

6 Was it clear that the group knew exactly what it wanted to say when presenting the visual aid (if there was any story or narration to go with the pictures)?

7 If pre-testing showed that changes should be made, were these changes made?

Topics for small group visual aid planning

1 Wean your baby slowly and with the right foods. (A 15–minute session for mothers in a clinic waiting room)

Breast milk is the best food for a baby. After the baby is 6 months old, breast milk by itself is not enough for proper growth. The baby needs extra protein and nutrients from other foods, as well as breast milk. Weaning is the process of gradually introducing new foods, while continuing to breast-feed as long as possible. It is important to introduce new foods to the baby's diet one at a time and gradually, to allow the baby's system to adjust.

The food given to the baby should be available locally and should not interfere with the family's customs and beliefs. Usually, babies are first given locally available mashed carbohydrates such as banana or porridge made from maize, millet, cassava or another grain. After several weeks, other foods are added one at a time. These foods should include protein foods, vegetables, and fruits. The amount of food can be gradually increased as the baby gets older. It is very important that the baby gets enough protein. The best sign that the baby is getting enough of the right kinds of food during weaning is a monthly increase in weight.

2 What is natural family planning? (A 20-minute session for nursing students)

Natural family planning is the term used to describe methods of contraception in which a woman observes the natural changes taking place in her body during the menstrual cycle. These changes indicate when she is likely to be ovulating. As conception can only take place during ovulation, a woman can reduce the chance of pregnancy by avoiding sex at that time.

There are four methods that a woman can use to determine when she is ovulating:

(1) Because there is a rise in body temperature at the beginning of ovulation, a woman can take her temperature each morning to see when it begins to rise. This is called the basal body temperature method (BBT).

(2) Because ovulation generally takes place about 14 days before the start of the next menstruation, a woman can record her days of menstruation on a calendar over a period of 6–12 months to know when ovulation is likely to occur. This is called the calendar method.

(3) Because there are certain changes in the consistency of the cervical mucus during the menstrual cycle, a woman can observe her mucus daily to detect when it is clear, wet, slippery, and stretchy. This indicates the actual time of ovulation. This is called the mucus method.

(4) A woman can combine taking her temperature with the observation of her cervical mucus. This is called the symptothermal method, (S–TM).

3 The importance of child spacing for the health of the family. (A 30-minute session for parents in a rural village meeting place)

Infants and young children are less likely to die from malnutrition and gastro-enteritis caused by abrupt weaning if babies are not born too close together. Mothers will have time to devote to preventive health measures such as:

- regular visits to MCH/FH centres for well-baby care and immunizations
- cleanliness of the home
- preparation of nutritious meals
- supervision of infants and young children and prevention of home accidents

4 How breast-feeding can reduce the chances of pregnancy. (A 20-minute session for nursing students)

After a baby is born, breast-feeding can delay the onset of ovulation and menstruation. When the baby sucks on the mother's nipple, impulses are sent from the areola (surrounding the nipple), along a nerve pathway to the anterior pituitary in the brain. The anterior pituitary secretes the hormone *prolactin* into the bloodstream. This stimulates the glands in the breast to produce milk. It also decreases the level of the luteinizing hormone (LH) which is necessary for ovulation and menstruation to occur. The increased intensity, frequency and duration of breast-feeding, accomplished by feeding on demand, are necessary to delay ovulation in this way.

5 How to tie, cut, and wrap the baby's cord after a home delivery. (A 30-minute session for traditional birth attendants in a home)

Wash your hands very well.

Wait until the cord is not beating any more. The colour will change from blue to white, which means that the blood has stopped flowing. Tie the cord in two places (about 3 cm and 7 cm from the baby) with very clean, dry strips of cloth, string, or ribbon. Use a new or sterilized razor blade or sterilized knife or scissors to cut the cord between the ties. Cover the navel with sterile gauze or freshly washed and ironed cloth. You can wrap and pin a piece of thin, light cloth around the baby's belly to hold the gauze in place. Make sure the bandage is loose enough to let air in under it, to keep the navel dry.

Activity 5 Making your own visual aid

Time

Learners will vary in time taken. Plan for at least 6–8 hours of individual working time.

Objective

Learners will make their own visual aids, which they can use in their work.

Materials

Thin paper for tracing.
Paper, pencils, and erasers for sketching.
Poster paper or cardboard.
Coloured pens, markers, coloured cloth, paint or dyes.
Scissors or knives.
Glue, rubber cement, or paste.
Rope, twine, yarn.
Real objects related to family planning and family health.
Any other available supplies you feel are appropriate (see 'Possible adaptations').

Instructions

1 Let your learners choose a topic from their own work situation.

2 Allow learners to work on choosing a topic and answering the 7 teaching questions. Give them a few guidelines to work with such as:
 – choose a topic which has only 3–5 main ideas; or
 – this visual aid will be for use in a 10-minute session.
 Go from person to person, helping them to choose topics they can do in the time allowed without too much frustration. Also help them answer the 7 teaching questions, if they need help.

3 Tell learners they can make any kind of visual aid they want as long as it fits with their answers to the teaching questions. What they make also depends on what supplies you have available. They may choose to make a picture series, model, display, flannelboard, or whatever they want that you have supplies for.
 Ask people not to make visual aids which have been used as examples in the manual. It will be more useful for them to have to work with one of their own teaching problems, and decide for themselves what the most important information is.

4 Give your learners time to make a visual plan for their visual aid. Tell them to follow the 6 steps in planning and making a visual aid. If they are making a model or display, they will have to make one to pre-test it.

5 Require that learners do both content, review and pre-testing, if this is at all possible.

Ask learners to review each other's plans individually. Everyone should ask at least 3 other people to review their visual aid before taking it out to pre-test.

Help all learners arrange to pre-test their visual aids with at least a small group of learners like the ones they will be teaching.

6 Schedule individual conferences to assess each person's final work on this project. Use the visual introduction the person did for Unit 1 to help you assess how much progress the person has made since then. Learners also may be pleased to see how much they have learned since doing their visual introduction.

7 If time permits, have a large group discussion on problems which arose during this activity and how people solved them. Ask learners to share their pre-testing experiences with the group.

This is often one of the most valuable parts of the activity. It gives people a chance to share their experiences and learn from each other.

Possible adaptations

Remember that when you are gathering the materials for this activity you are determining what visual aids learners can make. Think about what your learners do at their jobs and what supplies are normally available to them. Try to use supplies that they can also find later. Help them discover that they can make useful visual aids with very common supplies.

Unit 4
Production Skills

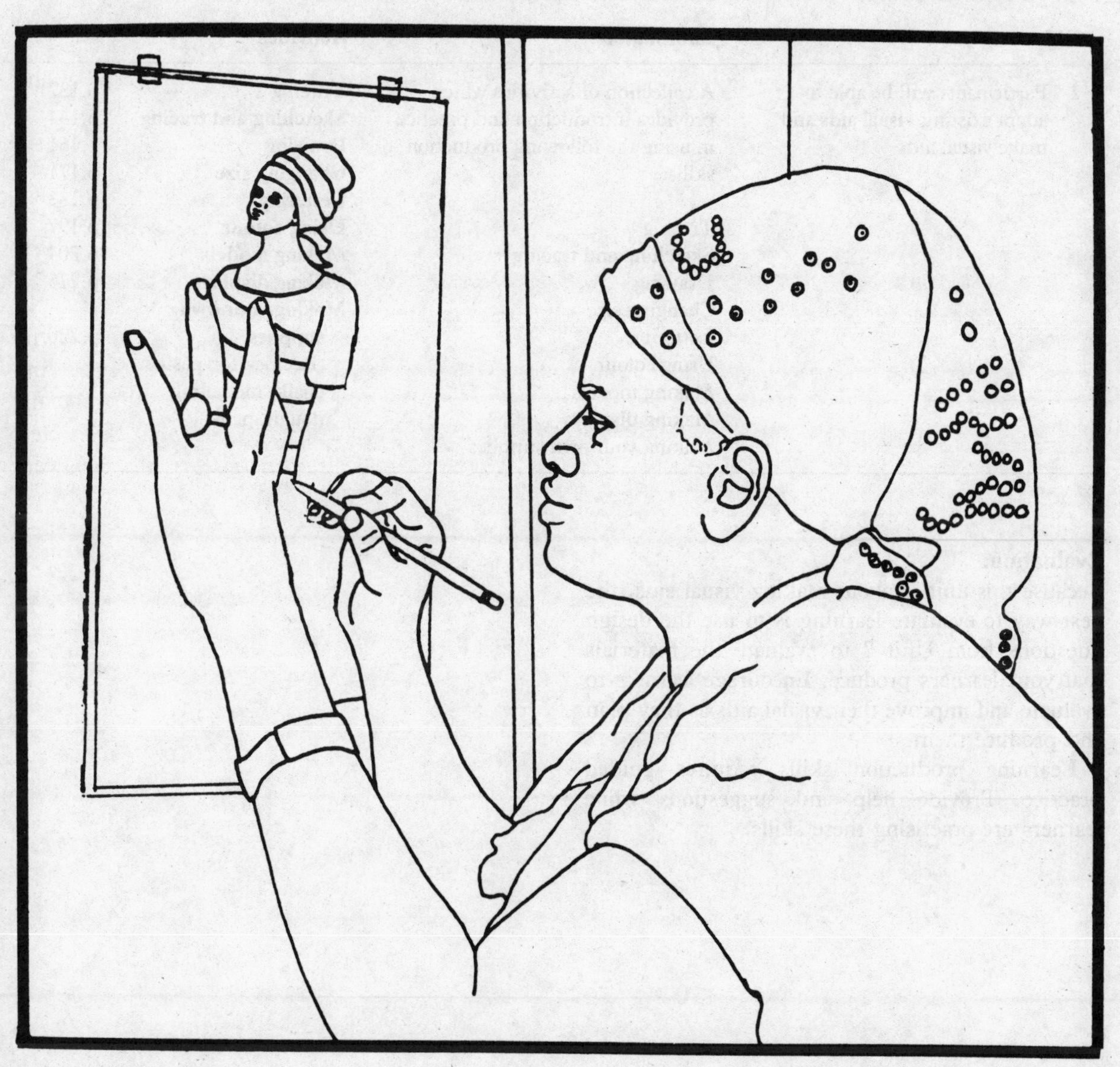

Unit 4 is a reference unit. It is a collection of instructions for developing skills needed for making simple low cost visual aids, such as tracing, sketching, changing the size of pictures, lettering, and using colour. It also includes instructions for making simple models and displays as well as recipes for making supplies such as paste, chalk, modelling dough, and paint. Trainers and teachers often combine these production skills with lessons from the first three units. See examples of this in the sample curricula included in the Trainer's Guide at the beginning of the manual. You may want to duplicate this unit for your learners to use as a reference book. It is very important to practise the skills presented in these activities before you demonstrate them to your learners.

Unit 4: Production skills

Objective	Information	Activities	
1 Participants will be able to adapt existing visual aids and make visual aids.	A collection of activities which provides introduction and practice in using the following production skills: Tracing Sketching and tracing Drawing Changing size Lettering Using colour Making models Making displays Making your own supplies	**Tracing**	p.137
		Sketching and tracing	p.144
		Drawing	p.161
		Changing size	p.171
		Lettering	p.183
		Using colour	p.197
		Making models	p.204
		Making displays	p.215
		Making your own supplies (Recipes for paste, chalk, modelling dough, paint)	p.220

Evaluation:
Because this unit is about making visual aids, the best way to evaluate learning is to use the design questions from Unit 2 to evaluate the materials that your learners produce. Encourage learners to evaluate and improve their visual aids as they plan and produce them.

Learning production skills requires guided practice. Provide help and suggestions while learners are practising these skills.

Tracing skills for making visual aids

Objective

These activities should enable learners to prepare shapes, simple line drawings, and detailed line drawings using two tracing techniques.

Information and notes to the trainer

Many health care trainers know that visual aids can make new information easier to understand. Unfortunately, visual aids which fit the needs of your learners are not always available.

You can use tracing techniques to make visual aids which do not require many materials or any special skills in drawing. Magazines, books, posters, and many other materials contain photographs and drawings which can be used to make visual aids for health training and public health education.

For example, a health worker in a rural clinic may need a poster on child spacing that shows a family with two or three children who are obviously happy and healthy. The only available and suitable pictures show only larger groups of people. By using tracing techniques, the health worker can make the needed poster by combining tracings of individuals from different pictures to create a family group, as shown below.

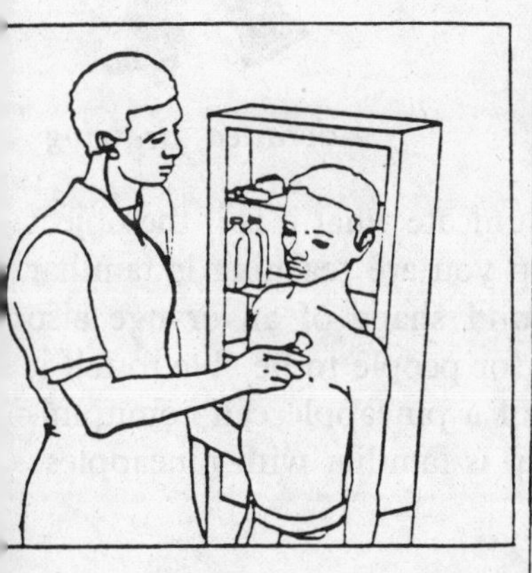

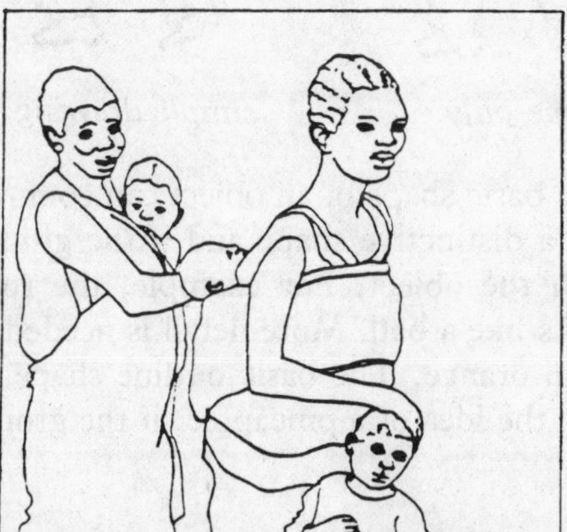

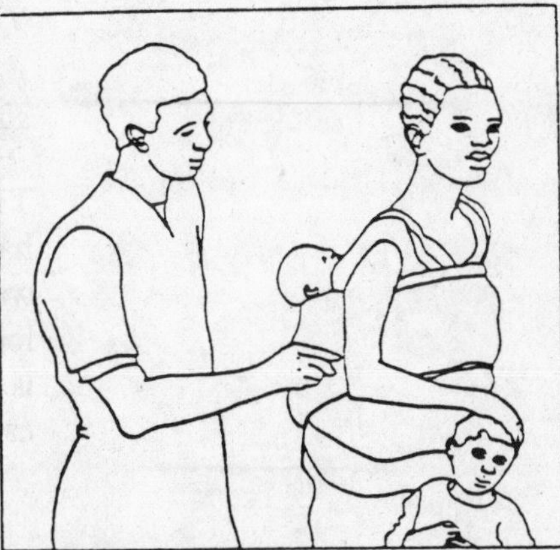

There are two activities on tracing: one to practise simple tracing and one to practise transferring a picture using carbon. The skills taught in these two activities will be necessary to do other activities in this unit, so we recommend that you do both of them.

You may want to demonstrate all of the skills before beginning the activities. The skills which need to be demonstrated are:

(1) Simple tracing

(2) Tracing using a light source
(3) Making your own carbon paper
(4) Transferring a picture to another piece of paper using the carbon transfer technique
(5) Outlining the figures in black and colouring them in, using available colouring materials.

See Unit 5, Demonstrations, for tips on giving a good demonstration.

Share the following information with your participants before beginning the activities.

Before using one of the tracing or transfer techniques that you will learn, decide which pictures to trace and how much detail to copy from those pictures to communicate your message. The amount of detail can range from only an outline of the shape of the picture to a very detailed drawing.

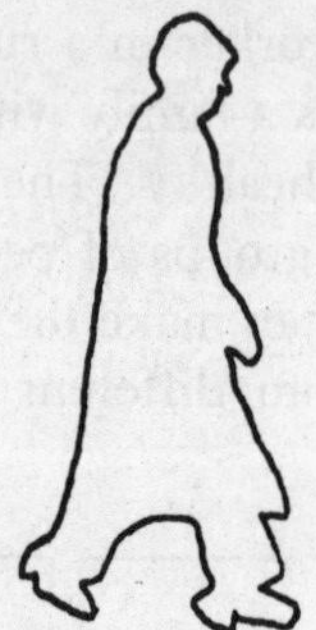
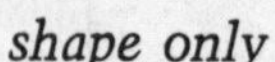
shape only

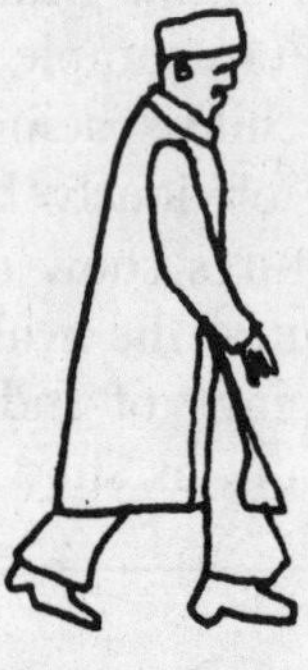
simple drawing

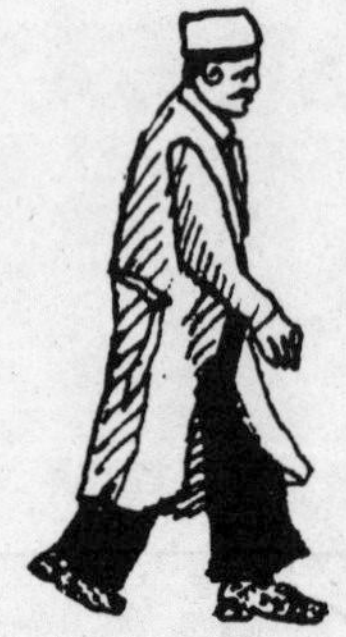
detailed drawing

The basic shape of an object can communicate what it is if the object has a distinctive shape and if the group you are teaching is familiar with the object. For example, the round shape of an orange also looks like a ball. More detail is needed for people to be able to tell it is an orange. The basic outline shape of a pineapple can communicate the idea of a pineapple, if the group is familiar with pineapples.

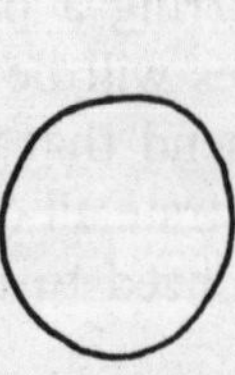

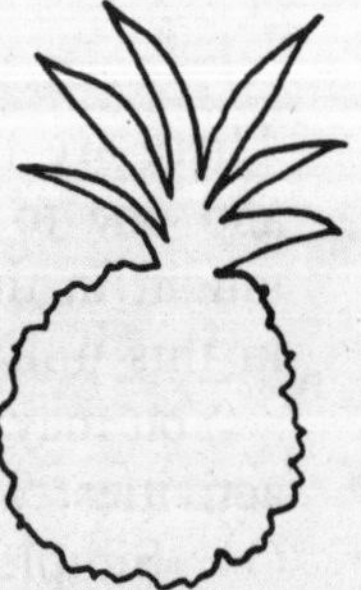

More detail provides more information about the real object or person the tracing represents. Too much detail can be distracting. The person looking at the picture may pay more attention to the background or details of costumes than to the central subject.

It is important to try out your drawings with the people for whom they are intended. You should choose shapes, simple drawings, or detailed drawings carefully based on the idea you want to show and the group of people you want to teach.

Evaluation

After each activity, ask your learners to:

1 Compare their traced drawing with the original picture. Did they trace enough of the person or object to communicate what it is? Did they copy too many details so that the drawing is cluttered and confusing or possibly distracting?

2 Show the drawing to a few people from the group with which they plan to use it or to people with similar background and interests. Ask them what they see. If these people are confused in any way by the picture, ask them why. Make changes in the picture until it does communicate your message.

Activity 1

Simple tracing technique

Time

20 minutes

Objective

Learners will use simple tracing to trace one figure from a picture showing several people.

Materials

Soft lead pencil.
Eraser.
Materials for colouring, such as crayons, paints or inks.
Paper clips.
Thin white paper.
Pictures for tracing. (You can use the example following or find your own.)

Instructions

1 Choose a picture from a magazine, poster, or some other source, or use the enlarged drawing of the picture on the next page (included at the end of this activity).

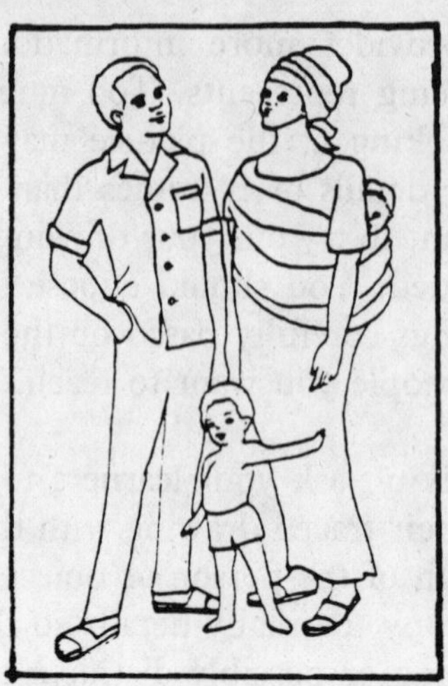

2 Place a piece of thin paper (paper you can see through) over the picture. Use paper clips or pins to hold the two pieces together. Do not use tape because it may damage the original picture.

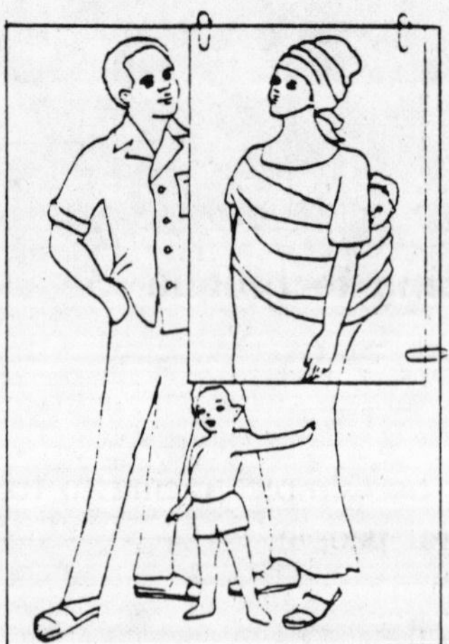

3 If you cannot see the picture through the paper, hold both pieces against a light source such as a window or on an overhead projector.

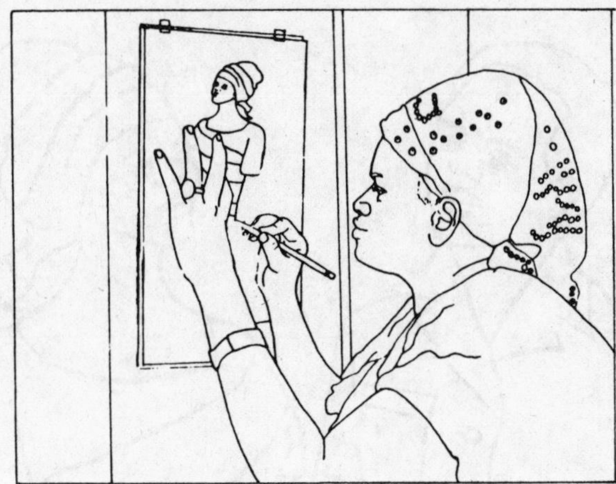

4 Using a pencil, carefully trace the parts of the picture you wish to use. Use only as much detail as you think is needed. In the example, you may wish to copy only the part of the picture that shows the woman and baby.

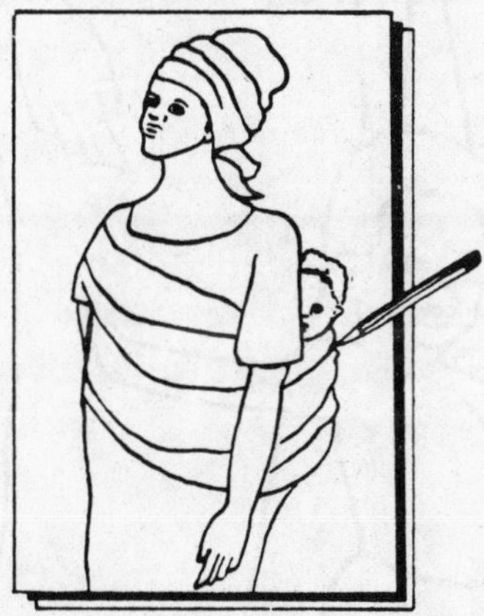

5 You can finish the drawing on the thin paper by covering your pencil lines with ink, paint, crayon, or coloured marking pens. Erase any pencil marks not covered by colour or ink. The figures will show up better if you outline them with black and then colour inside the black lines. (See **Using colour** in this unit.)

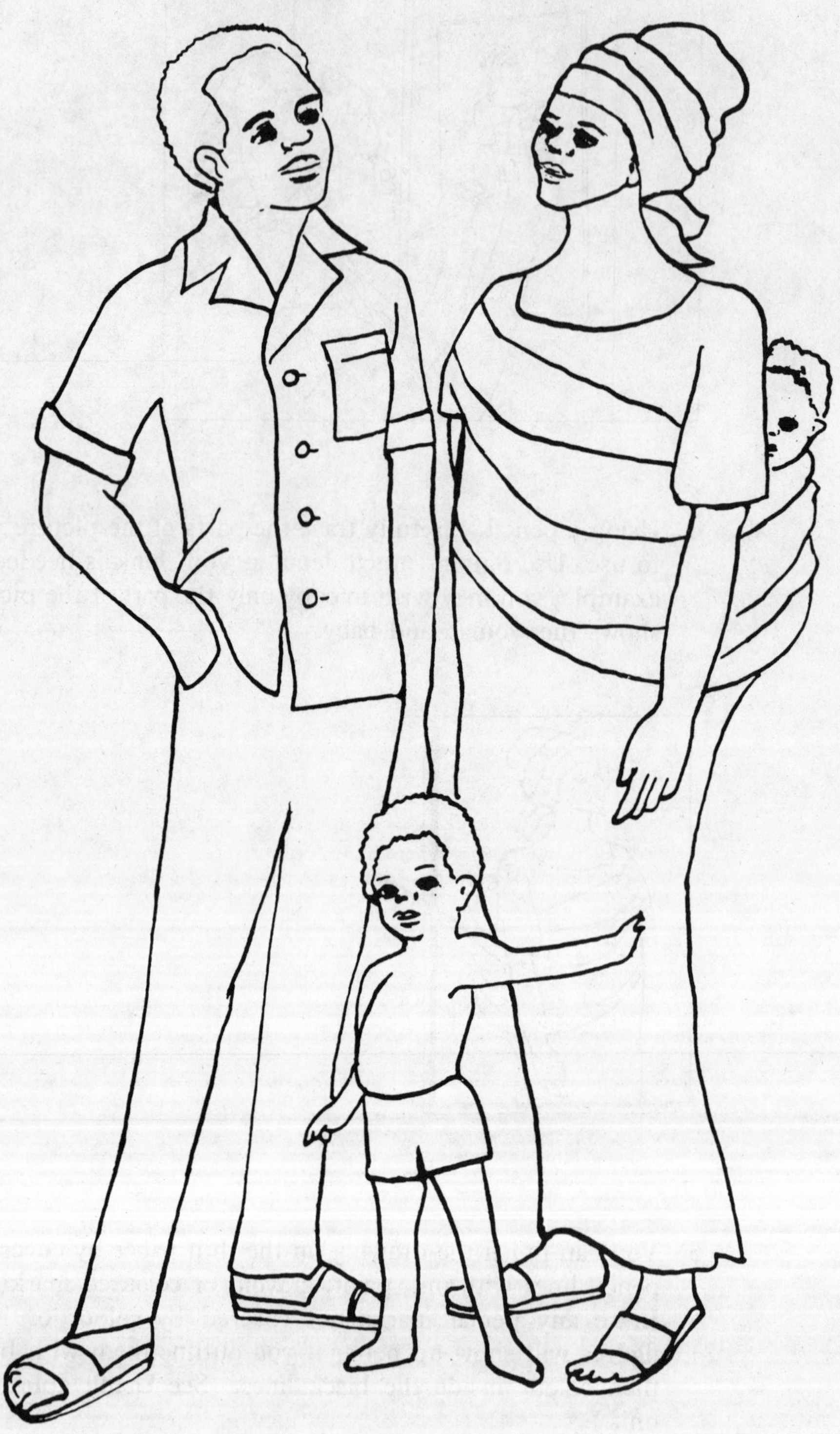

Activity 2

Carbon transfer technique

Time

30 minutes

Objective

Learners will transfer a tracing to a sheet of drawing paper by using the carbon transfer technique.

Materials

Soft-lead pencils and erasers.
Crayons, paint, ink or other colouring materials.
Thin white paper and paper clips.
Pictures for tracing. (You can use the example in Activity 1.)
Carbon paper (or make your own with the instructions below).

Instructions

To use the tracing technique explained in Activity 1, you need to use thin white paper so that the picture will show through the paper. The thin paper will not last a very long time, so you may want to transfer your tracing to a thicker piece of paper, such as drawing paper. This activity explains how to transfer your tracing from one piece of paper to another.

1 Trace any picture on thin, white paper. You can use the tracing you made for Activity 1.

2 Use a piece of carbon paper or make your own, like this: Cover the back of your tracing with pencil lead by using the side of a soft-lead pencil. You can use a piece of charcoal from your kitchen fire, if pencils are scarce. You could also rub the pencil lead into a separate piece of paper and use it like you would use carbon paper.

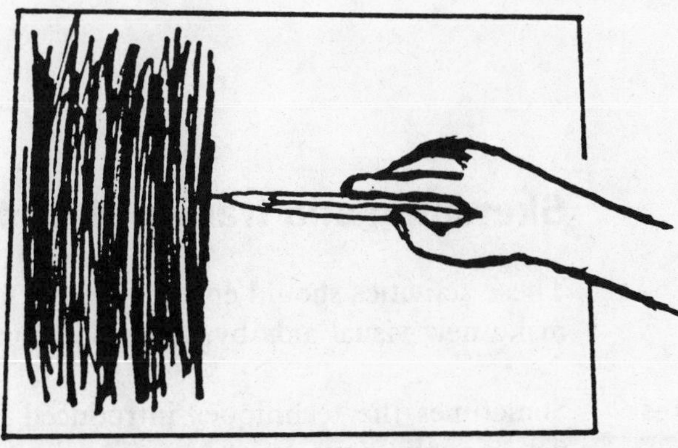

3 Place the paper with carbon (bought or made) on top of a sheet of drawing paper. The carbon side should be touching the drawing paper.

4 If you are using a separate piece of carbon paper, place your tracing on top of the carbon paper.
5 Fasten the 2 or 3 pieces of paper together with paper clips or pins.
6 Trace over the lines of the drawing using a soft-lead pencil with a fairly sharp point. As you trace the lines, the pressure of the pencil will transfer the picture onto the drawing paper (see illustration below left).

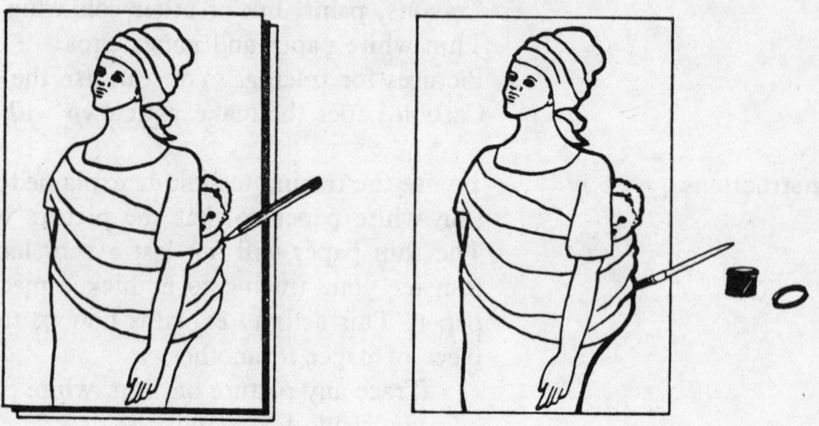

7 You can complete your drawing by using pen and ink, crayons, paint, or coloured markers to colour the visual aid. Remember to outline the lines in black and then to colour inside the lines (see illustration above right).
8 Erase any carbon or pencil line that is not covered.

Sketching and tracing skills for adapting pictures

Objective

These activities should enable learners to adapt existing visual aids to make new visual aids by using sketching and tracing techniques.

Information and notes to the trainer

Sometimes the techniques introduced in the **Tracing** activities are not enough. Your learners may have found the pictures they need but they need to put them together in a new way. They may need to change or adapt figures. For example, they may have found a good photograph of a woman, but she is dressed in city clothing and they need a picture of a woman dressed in rural clothing. They may have found a drawing of a happy, smiling child, but they need a picture of a crying child.

These **Sketching and tracing** activities show your learners how to make simple changes in pictures so that they can adapt them to their needs. Learners will practise combining tracing skills with some new sketching skills. They will be able to make greater use of the pictures they find if they can adapt them to fit the specific needs.

Four activities are included here. Activities 1, 2, and 3 each focus on one type of adaptation. Activity 4 combines the skills learned in the first 3 activities with those from the **Tracing** activities. In Activity 4, learners must create a complete drawing. If time permits, do all 4 activities in the order they appear here. If time is limited, you may want to leave out Activities 1 and 2 and do only Activities 3 and 4.

The following example provides an introduction to the activities.

We have already seen how pictures can be taken from different sources and combined to create a new visual aid by using tracing techniques. Look at the example (Drawing 1). What changes were made in the first two pictures to make the 'Space Your Family' poster?

The man:

stethoscope left out
legs added
left arm left out

The woman and children:

woman's dress lengthened
child's lower body and legs added
baby's hair added

In this example, the tracing techniques have been used to draw the basic shapes and lines of the people. Small changes have been made to adapt the pictures for use as a poster. These changes were made by *sketching*. A *sketch* is a rough drawing that represents the main features of an object, a person, or a scene. By completing these activities, you will be able to combine your skill in tracing with a new skill in sketching to adapt pictures for visual aids.

Drawing 1

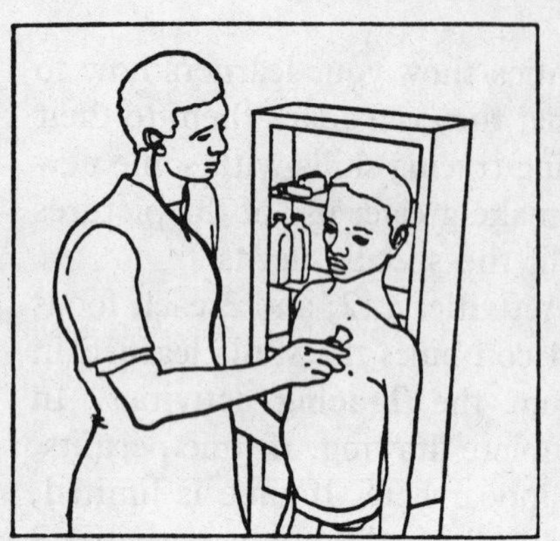

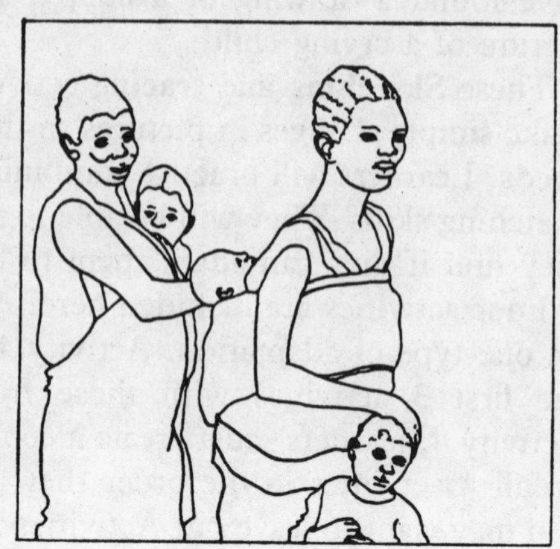

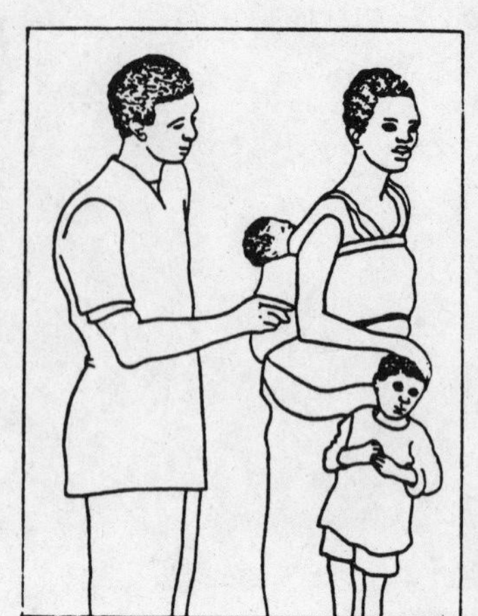

Materials needed for all activities

Thin, white paper.
Pencil.
Eraser.
Ruler or straight edge.
Tape.
Pictures that trainer and learners need are listed for each activity.

Evaluation

You can use Activity 4 to assess the skills in (1) combining pictures from different sources, (2) using tracing and transfer techniques, and (3) sketching.

Activity 1

Adapting clothing

Time

30 minutes

Objective

Learners will adapt clothing using sketching techniques.

Materials

Large drawing of the 'Space Your Family' poster (Drawing 1).

Instructions

1 Use the 'Space Your Family' poster (Enlarged part of drawing 1).
2 Trace the poster on thin, white paper, using one of the tracing techniques. (Do not forget to trace the lines that mark the edge or 'space' for the poster. A ruler or a straight edge will be helpful.)

3 Make the changes listed below by *sketching*. To sketch, lightly draw in new lines for the needed changes and erase lines you no longer need. You will probably not make a perfect drawing the first time you try. Just keep sketching and erasing until the changes are made. Remember, as with most skills, practice makes perfect.

Changes to make in the woman:

(a) Add a scarf to the woman's head. Think about how a scarf looks. Lightly sketch the lines of the scarf on the woman's head. Erase and draw again until it looks like a scarf. Erase the woman's hair that cannot be seen under the scarf.

(b) Change the woman's dress so that it covers her shoulders. Again, lightly sketch the new lines to your tracing to extend the woman's dress over her shoulders.

4 Show your drawing to a friend and ask for suggestions for improving it. Try to make the changes by your friend's suggestions.

There is no one right drawing. You may have added short sleeves or long sleeves. The neckline of the dress may be a round opening or it may have a collar. The scarf may be tied at the neck or on top of the head. It may cover all of the woman's hair or it may leave some hair showing. Here are some examples of how your drawing may look.

Drawing 2

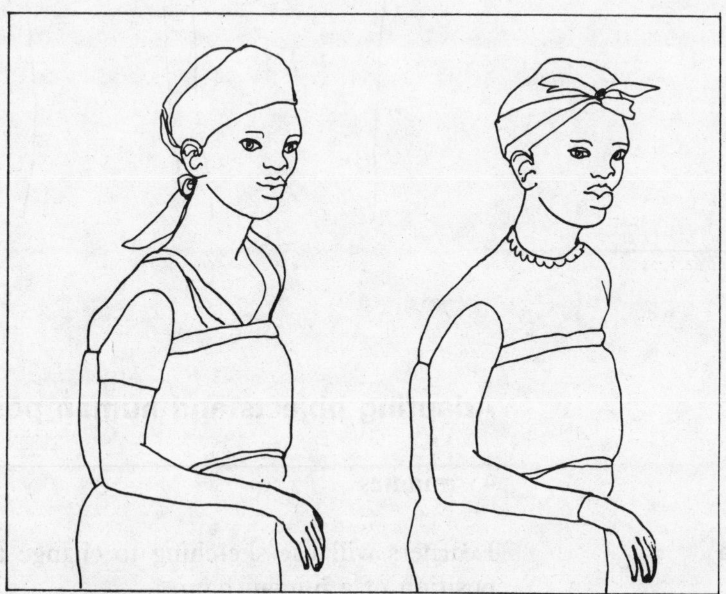

Enlarged part of drawing 1

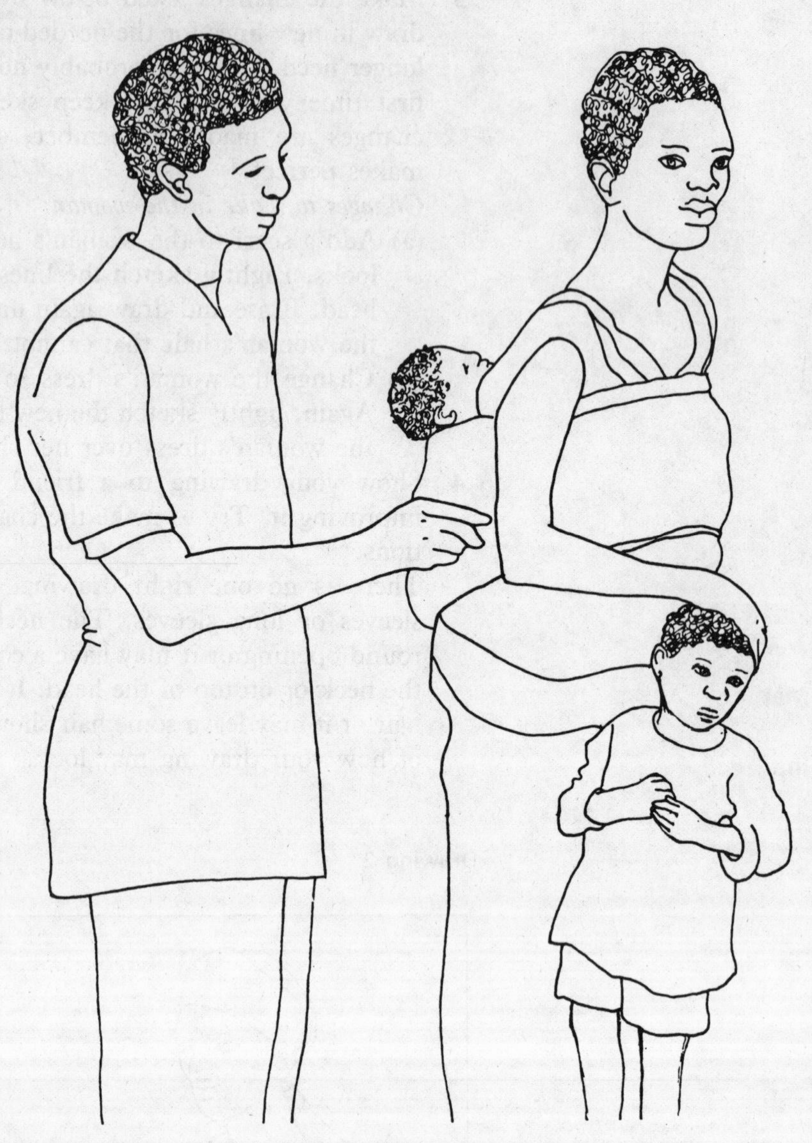

Activity 2 **Adapting objects and human positions**

Time 45 minutes

Objective Learners will use sketching to change an object and to change the position of a human figure.

Drawing 3

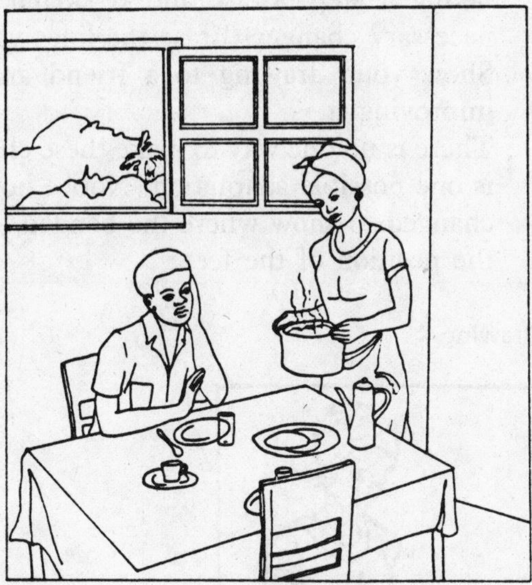

Materials

Large drawing of the family scene in Drawing 3.

Instructions

1 Use the picture of the family at mealtime. (Enlarged version of drawing 3).
2 Trace as much of the woman as is possible.
3 Change the pot or dish she is holding to a woven basket. The basket can be of any size or shape you want to make it as long as it still fits into the woman's hands. You can use the lines of the pot or dish to begin the shape of the basket. Add lines to make the basket look like it is made of woven grass.
4 Continue the lines of the woman's dress so that it reaches to her feet.
5 Now the woman is standing and holding a basket.
6 Change the drawing so that the woman is taking a step forward.
7 Ask someone to take a step forward and to hold the position. Look for the answers to these questions:
(a) How will her dress look if she is taking a step forward instead of standing still? If she is stepping forward, the leg in front will have a bended knee.
(b) How much of the woman's feet will show below the dress?
(c) What position will her feet be in if she is taking a step forward? The foot that is stepping forward will be flat on the ground. The heel of the other foot will be slightly off the ground.

8 Lightly sketch new lines onto your tracing to show the woman taking a step. Erase and re-sketch until you have made the necessary changes. Erase the lines you no longer need.

9 Show your drawing to a friend and ask for suggestions for improving it.

There is no one way to make these changes in the drawing. Here is one possible adaptation. Notice how the shape of the dress is changed to show where the bended knee would be. Notice also the position of the feet.

Drawing 4

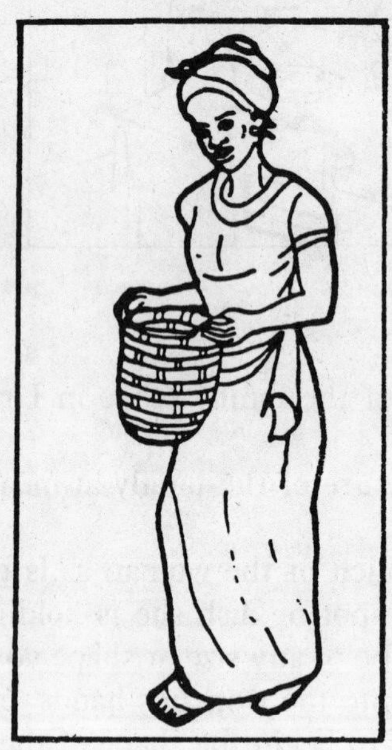

Englarged version of drawing 3

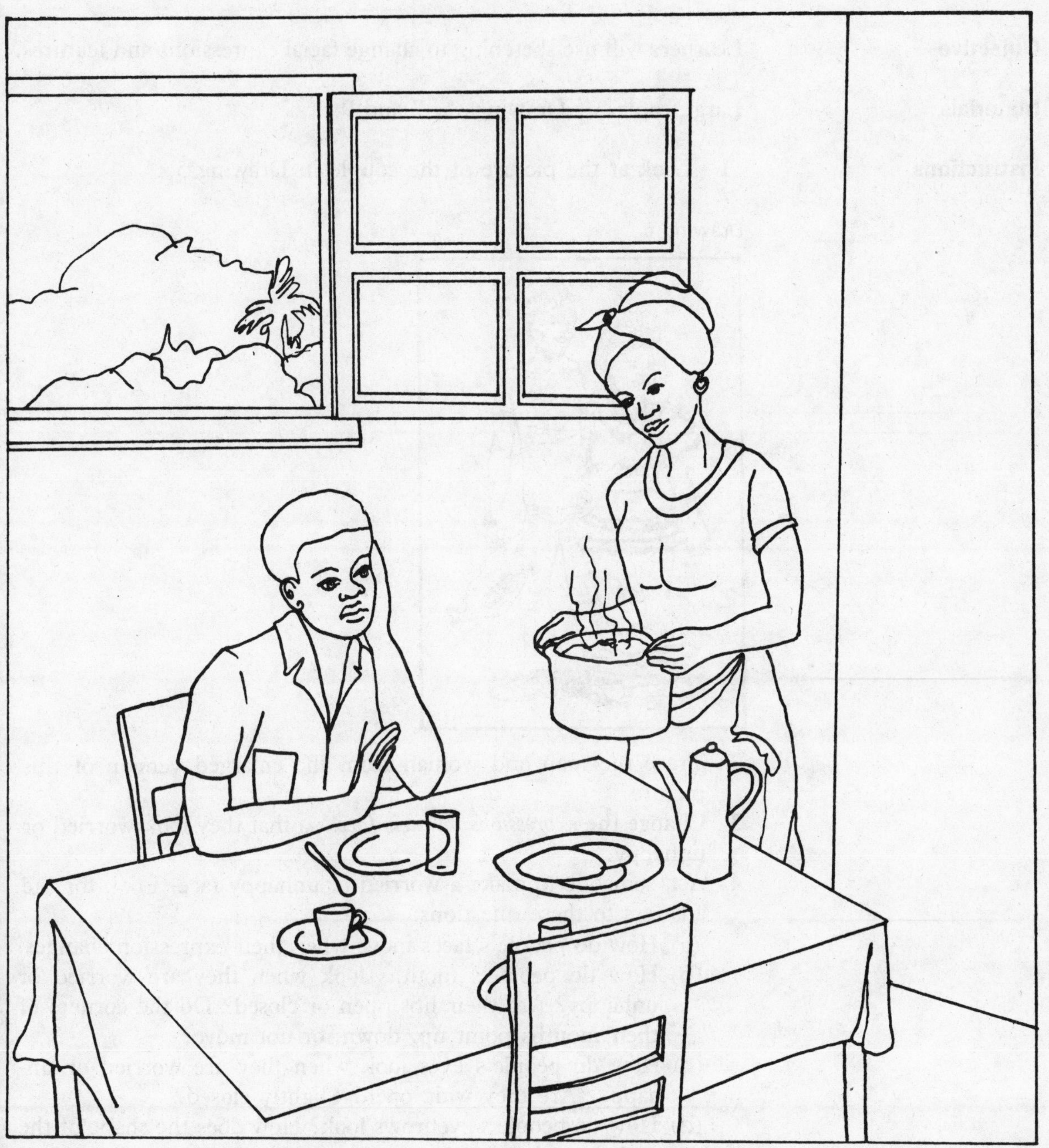

Activity 3

Adapting facial expressions and features

Time

45 minutes

Objective

Learners will use sketching to change facial expressions and features.

Materials

Large copies of Drawings 5, 7 and 9.

Instructions

1 Look at the picture of the couple in Drawing 5.

Drawing 5

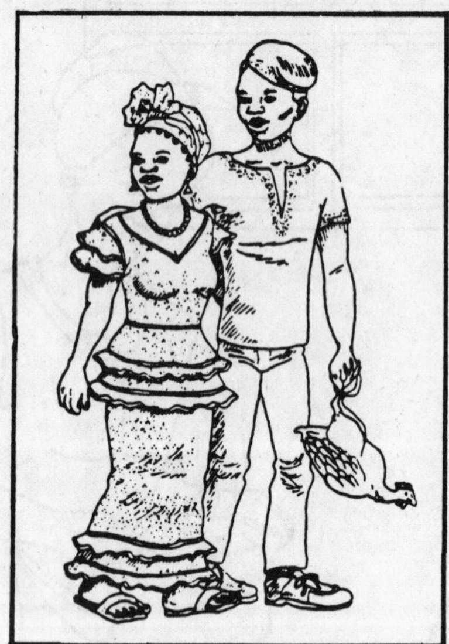

2 Trace the man and woman from the enlarged version of this picture.
3 Change the *expressions on their faces* so that they look worried or unhappy.
4 Ask someone to make a worried or unhappy face. Look for the answers to these questions:
   (a) How do people's faces move when their expression changes?
   (b) How do people's mouths look when they are worried or unhappy? Are their lips open or closed? Do the corners of their mouths point up, down, or not move?
   (c) How do people's eyes look when they are worried or unhappy? Are they wide open? Slightly closed?
   (d) How do people's eyebrows look? How does the shape of the eyebrows change when someone is worried or unhappy?
   (e) How do people's foreheads change when they are worried or unhappy?

5 Begin making changes on the pictures. Start with one part of the face. Use the lines which are already in your tracing. For example, start with the eyebrows. Lightly sketch new lines for the eyebrows to show worry or unhappiness. Erase unnecessary lines. Go on to another part of the face and continue the changes.

Your new expressions will look something like this:

Drawing 6

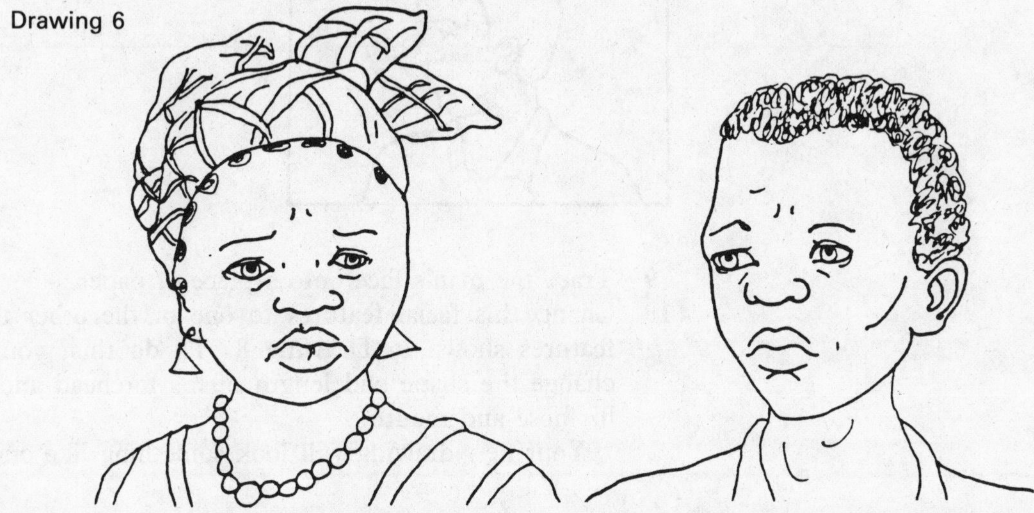

6 Can you identify the three facial expressions in Drawing 7? Notice the differences in the eyebrows, eyes, and mouths.

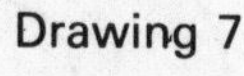

Drawing 7

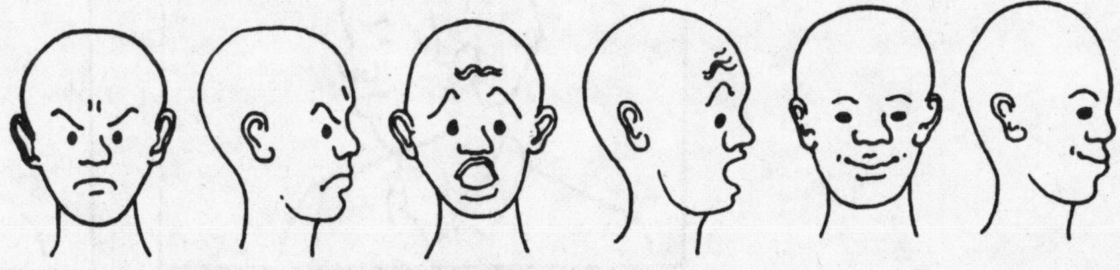

7 *Facial features* can also be adapted so that the people look more like the ones in your area. You will need to pay special attention to the shapes of the forehead, nose, and lips. Look at the examples in Drawing 8. Which facial features look most like the people in your area?

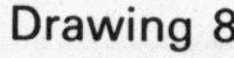

Drawing 8

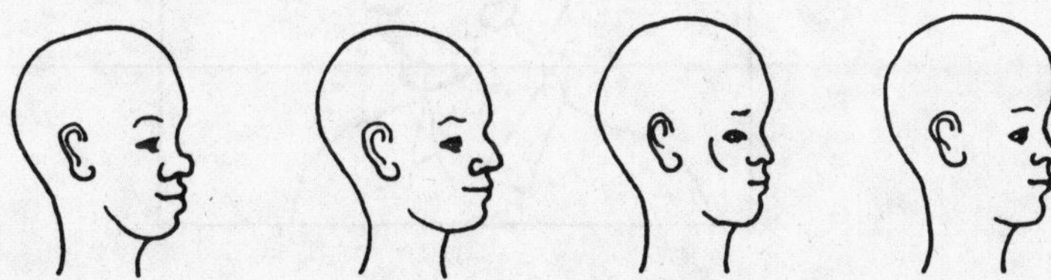

8 Change the facial features of the man in Drawing 9 to another type.

Drawing 9

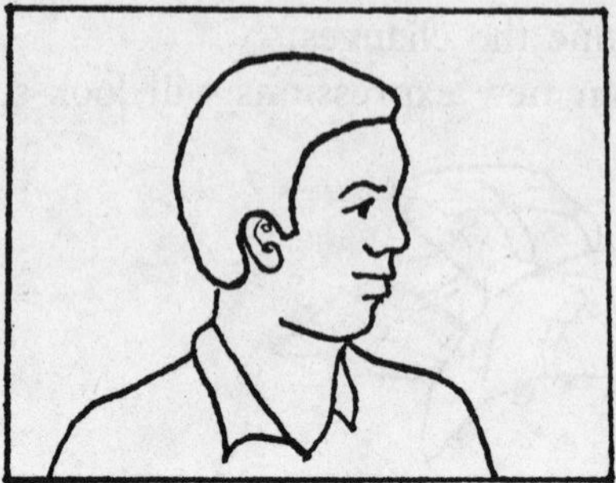

9 Trace the man's face onto a piece of paper.

10 Change his facial features to one of the other types of facial features shown in Drawing 8. To do this, you will need to change the shape and length of his forehead and the shape of his nose and mouth.

Your new drawing will look something like one of these:

Drawing 10

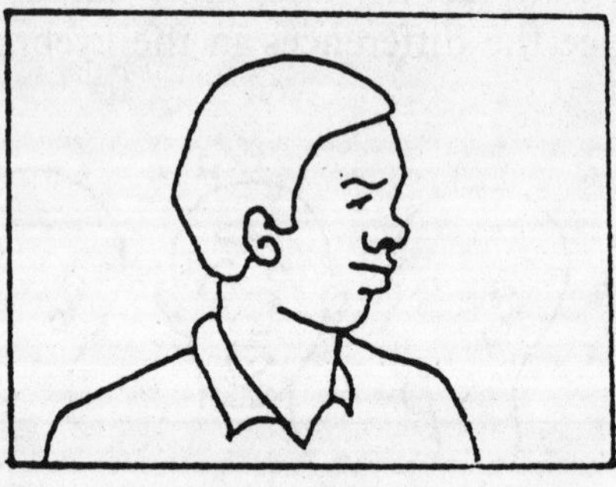

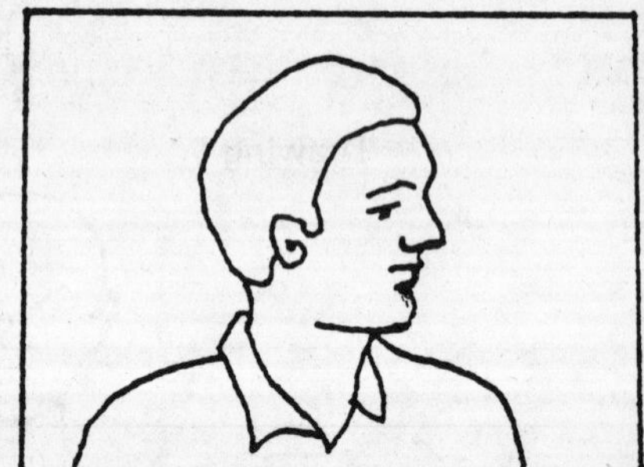

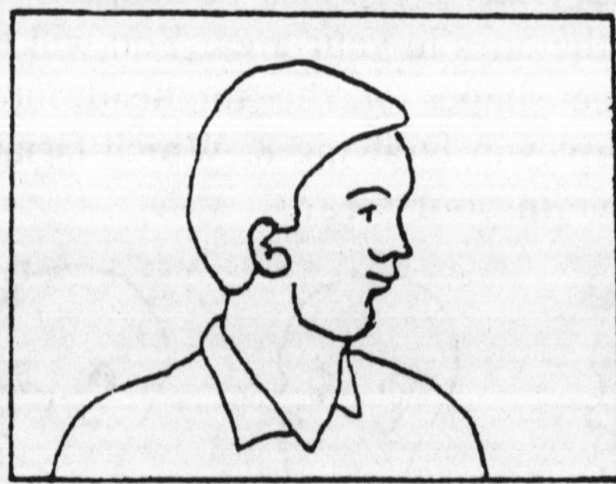

Enlarged version of drawing 5

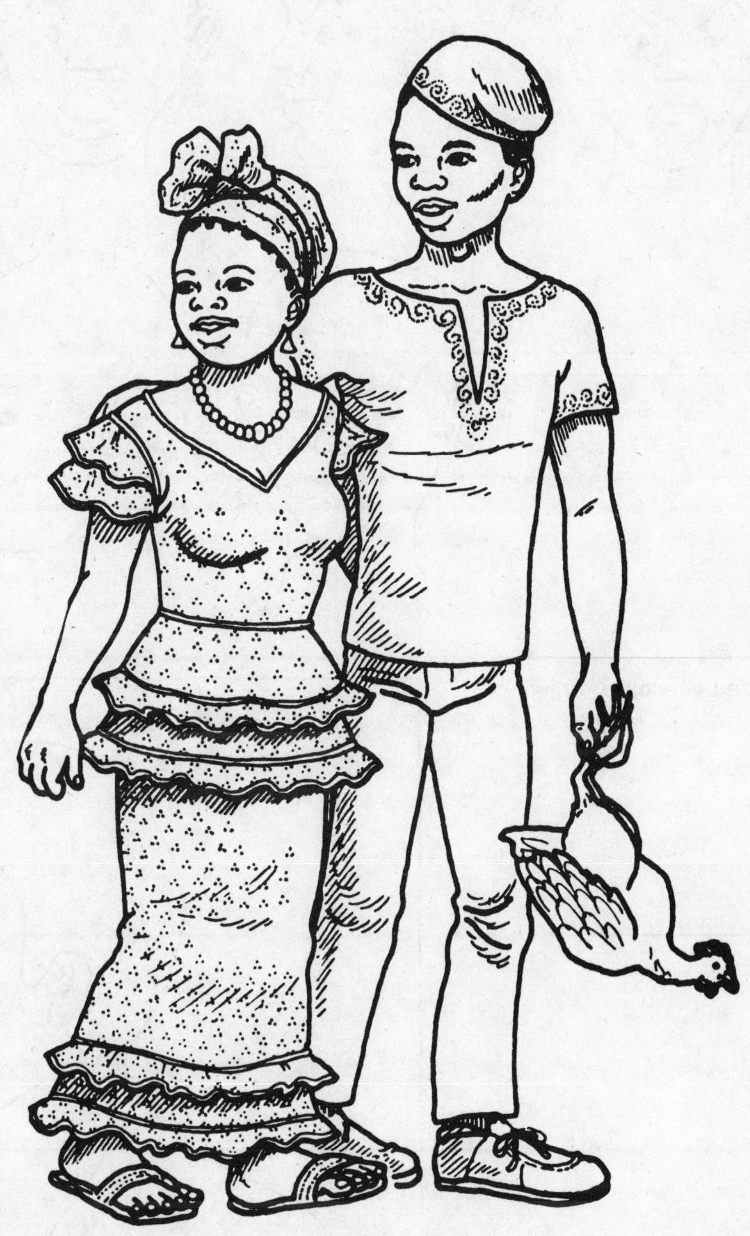

Enlarged version of drawing 7

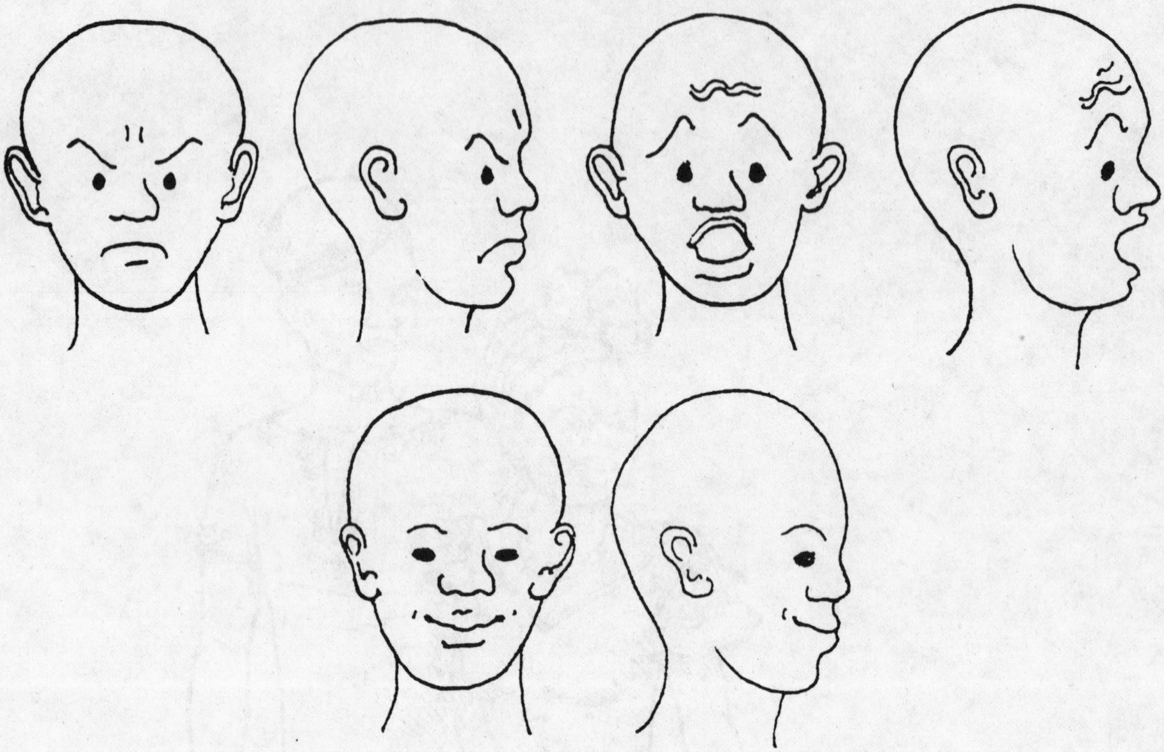

Enlarged version of drawing 9

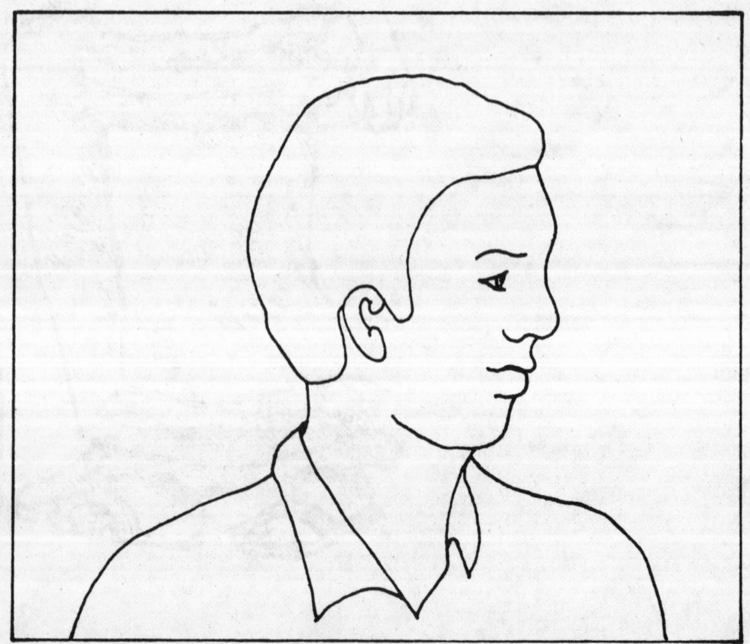

Activity 4 **Making a complete visual aid through adaptations**

Time If Activity 3 has been completed – 45 minutes
If Activity 3 has not been completed – 1 hour

Objective Learners will make a picture of a family by (1) combining pictures from different sources, (2) using tracing and transfer techniques, and (3) using sketching.

Materials Large versions of Drawings 5 and 11.

Instructions

1 Use the full body tracings you have already made of Drawing 5 (the man and woman).

2 Add the little boy in Drawing 11 (use the enlarged version) to the tracing of Drawing 5 so that the child is holding his father's hand.

Drawing 11

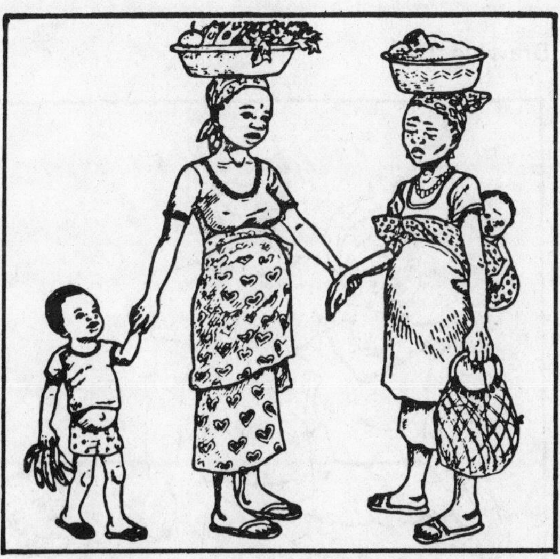

To do this, you must change the direction in which the little boy is facing and change the position of his arm so that his hand will reach his father's. (You could change the father's arm instead of the boy's but that would be more difficult.)

3 *Step one:* Change the little boy so that he is facing his father.
 (a) Trace the drawing of the little boy onto a separate sheet of thin white paper.

(b) Turn the tracing over so that the clean side of the paper is facing you.

(c) Use either the carbon transfer technique or a window as a light source to make another tracing of the little boy onto another sheet of paper. (See **Tracing** for how to do the carbon transfer technique and how to use a window as a light source for tracing.)

You should now have a tracing of the little boy facing in the direction of his father.

4 *Step two:* Add the little boy to the drawing of the mother and father.

(a) Put the paper on which you have traced the little boy *under* the paper which has the tracing of the mother and the father.

(b) Move the tracing of the little boy around until he is in the correct position to hold his father's hand. Be sure that he is not stepping on his father's foot! The little boy's feet should be at the same level as his father's.

(c) Tape the corners of the two pieces of paper to either a table top, a window, or another hard surface. The tape will prevent the tracings from moving out of place.

Drawing 12

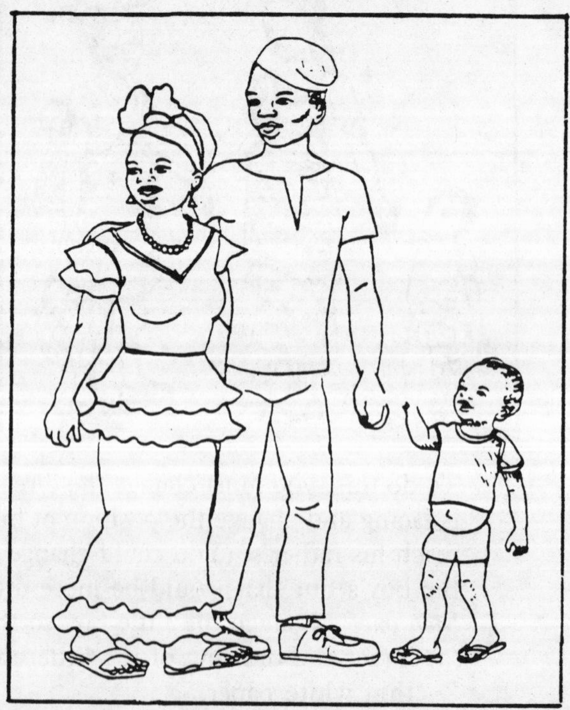

(d) You will see that the little boy's arm is raised too high to meet his father's hand. (See Drawing 12.) You will need to change either the position of the little boy's arm or the position of his father's arm. The little boy's arm will be easier to change because you will have to move it less than the father's arm.

(e) Lightly sketch the new position for the child's arm so that his hand is inside his father's hand. Sketch and erase until you have the child's arm in the correct position.

5 *Step three:* Sketch the fingers to the father's hand so that it looks like he is holding the child's hand.

You should now have a new picture of a man, woman, and child! It will probably look something like this:

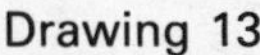

Drawing 13

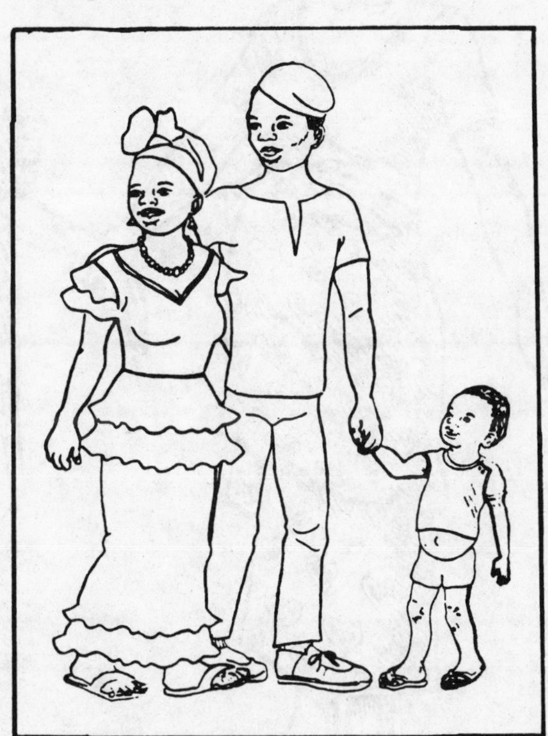

Enlarged version of drawing 11

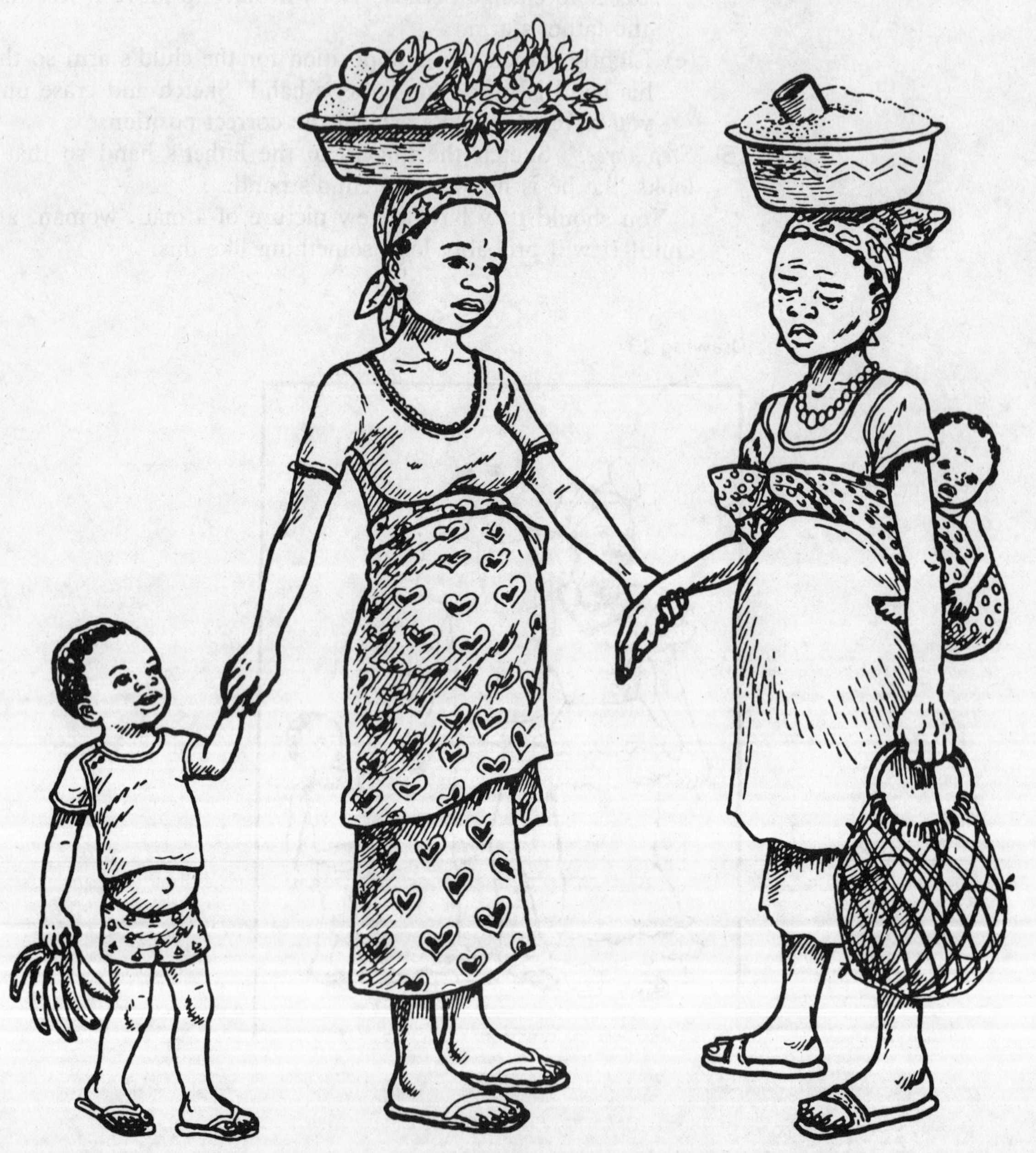

Drawing

Objective

Learners will be able to draw human faces and bodies both while they are at rest and in motion.

Information and notes to the trainer

Almost everyone can learn to draw people. All it requires is looking carefully at people, practising drawing people, and learning the sizes and positions of the different body parts as compared to each other. The three activities that follow give guidelines for drawing facial features and body parts in the right positions. Activity 1, **Drawing faces,** Activity 2, **Drawing pictures of people** and Activity 3, **Drawing pictures of people as they move**, enable the learner to develop skills for drawing good pictures of people. Emphasize to your learners the only way to learn to draw people well is to practise drawing.

Evaluation

You can evaluate learners' sketches by comparing the proportions with those on the sketches included in Activity 2 of this group.

It is important to give suggestions while individuals are sketching to help them improve their work.

Encourage learners to evaluate their own work by looking at facial features and the position of body parts compared to each other.

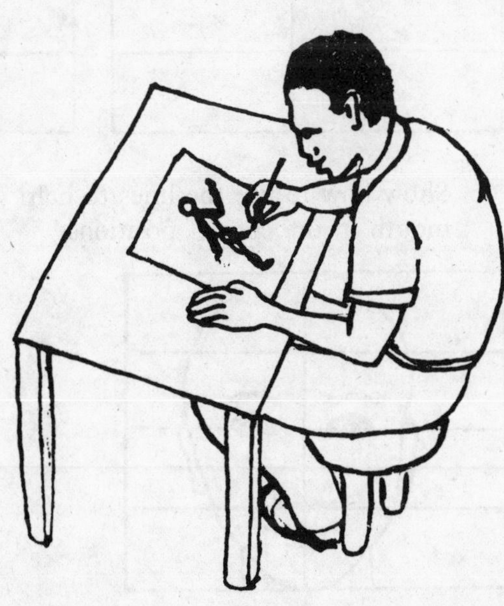

Activity 1 **Drawing faces**

Time 45 minutes

Objective Learners will be able to draw the head of an adult in the correct proportions.

Materials Paper and pencil for each participant.
Chalk and chalkboard.
Drawing of a person's face, large enough for the group to see.
Good large photographs of faces, or an adult from the group who will model for drawing activity. If your learners need to know how to draw children, you will also need a good photograph or a child as a model.

Instructions

1 Demonstrate how to draw a face by drawing a line down the middle of a piece of paper or on a chalkboard. Show how to locate the middle by folding the paper in half. Then divide the line into four equal parts and draw an oval as shown below.

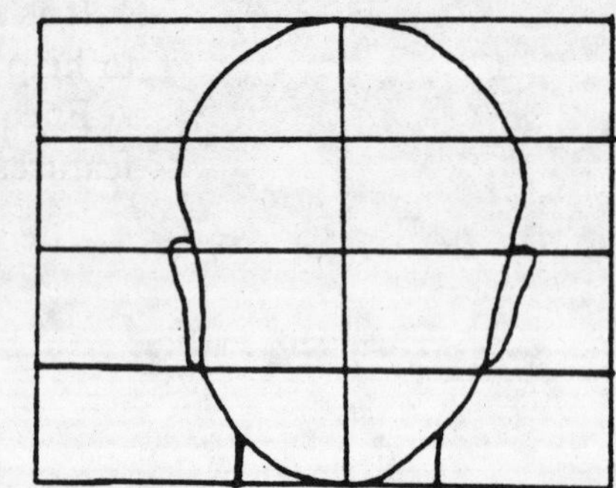

2 Show how to use the lines to help you draw the eyes, nose and mouth in the correct positions.

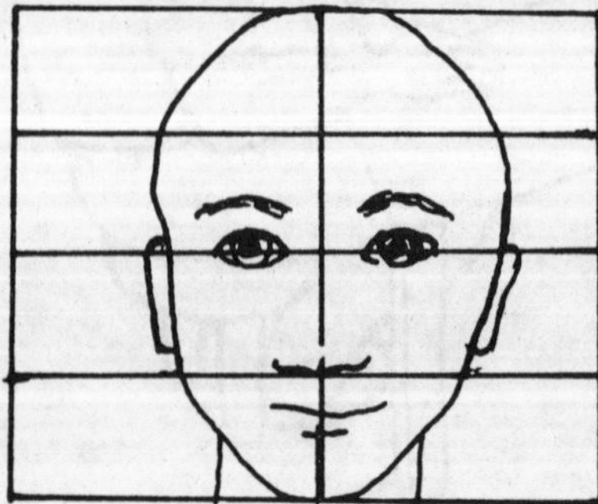

3 Hold up a large picture of a person's face, with the lines drawn on it, next to a real person's face.

4 Notice that a person's eyes are at the middle of his head. The ears are even with the eyes. The distance between the eyes and the bottom of the nose is about the same as the distance between the bottom of the nose and the chin. The width of the mouth is the distance between the centres of the eyes. The nose is about as wide as the space between the eyes.

5 Hand out pencils and paper. Tell learners to split into pairs and ask them to sketch each other's faces. Have them draw a line down the middle of the paper and divide it into four equal parts with lines as shown in the drawing that follows instruction 1. Encourage them to look at each other closely to sketch the size and positions of the facial features accurately. Watch each person sketching and assist anyone having difficulty.

Possible adaptations

1 If some people want to learn more about drawing, you can also include drawings of children.

2 Have a child stand beside a seated adult and ask learners to compare the 2 faces. They should notice that the child's face is smaller compared to the whole head than the adult's face. The child's eyes and ears are lower on his head. Point out that a child's eyes come well below the halfway line.

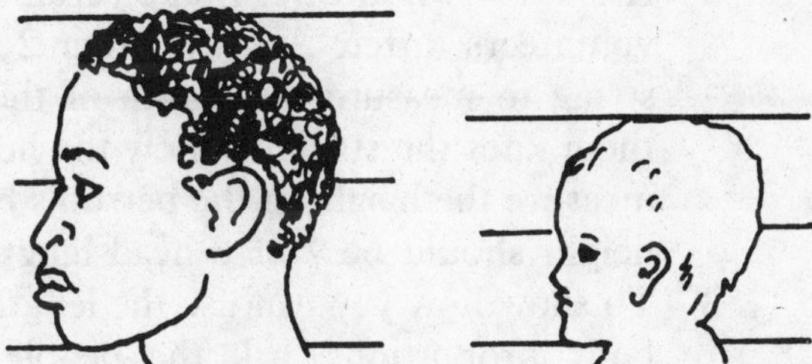

3 Ask them to draw the child's head using guidelines. Help them, if needed.

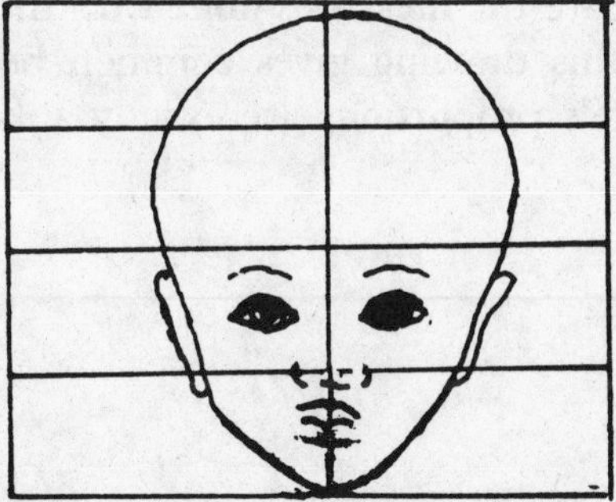

Activity 2 Drawing pictures of people

Time

1 hour

Objective

Learners will be able to draw a picture of a person showing correct relative sizes of head, arms, legs and body.

Materials

Paper and pencil for everyone.
Chalk and chalkboard.
Drawings prepared by the trainer showing the body proportions of an adult.
4 pieces of string at least 12 inches (30.5 cm) long.

Instructions

To draw the parts of human bodies the correct size, there are three things to remember:

(a) Using the head to measure other parts of the body;
(b) The correct size of the head compared to the body's height;
(c) The correct length of arms and legs compared to the body's height.

1 Explain to the learners that accurate drawing is based on *looking* very carefully to see the relative sizes and positions of different parts of the body.

2 Ask for 4 volunteers. Make certain that the heights of 2 of the volunteers differ. Ask the other 2 volunteers to use a piece of string to measure the length of the head of a volunteer. Have them knot the string to show the head length. Then ask them to measure the height of the person's body using this measure. The height should be 7 or 8 head lengths.

3 To show how you can use the length of the head as a measure of body proportions, ask the people measuring to measure the length of the arms and legs, using the same knotted string.

4 Show a larger version of the drawing at the top left of the opposite page, showing the body measured in head lengths. Compare the measures done with the knotted string. Emphasize that this drawing gives common body proportions but not all people's proportions are exactly alike.

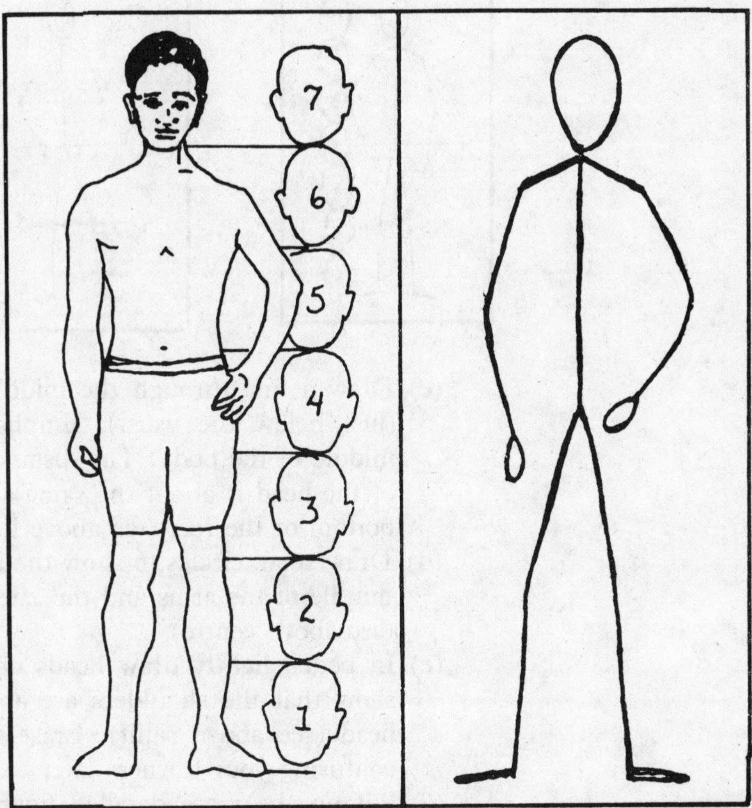

5 Draw a simple stick figure the same size as the drawing and place it beside the drawing of the person as shown above.

(a) Explain that the stick figure makes it easier to think about the sizes and positions of body parts because it leaves out confusing details.

(b) Take down the other drawing. Leave only the stick figure. Draw 7 ovals beside the stick figure to show the height measured in heads.

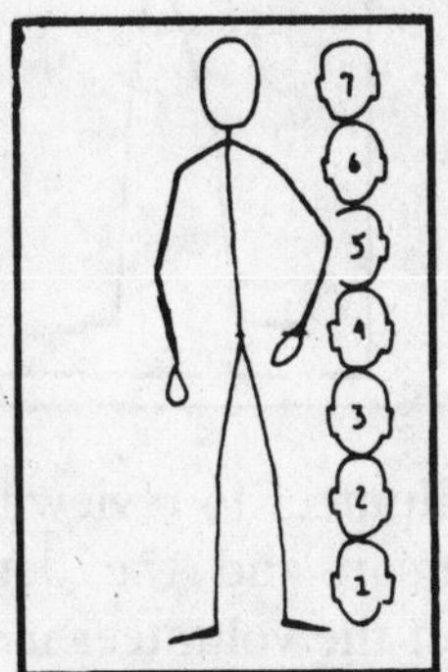

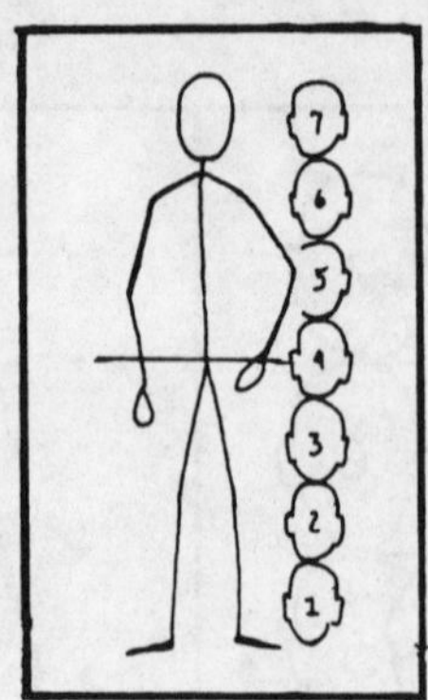
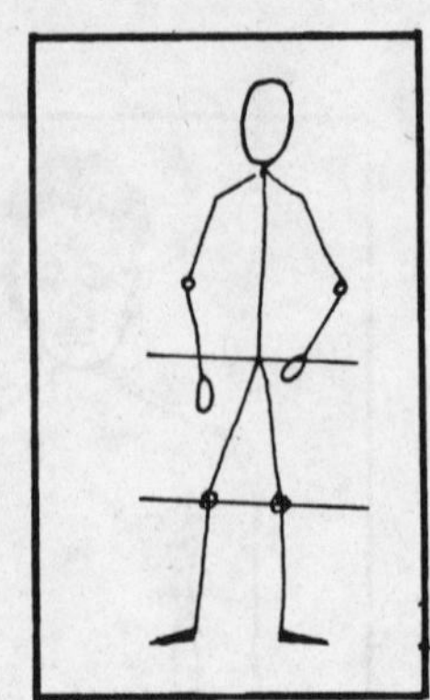
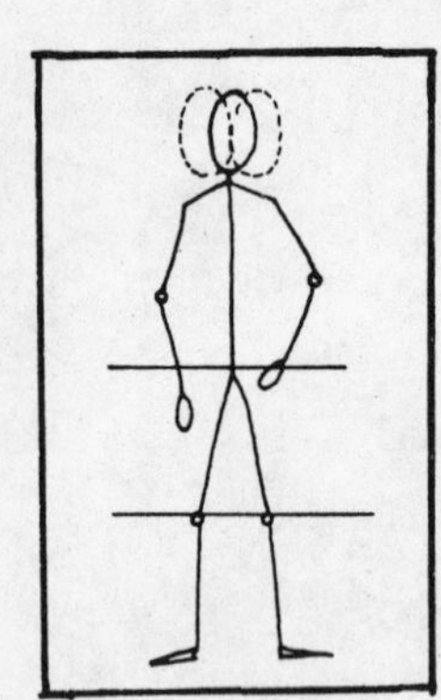

(c) Draw a line through the middle of the body at the navel (just below the waist). Emphasize that the navel is the middle of the body. The distance from the navel to the top of the head is about the same as that from the navel to the bottom of the feet (see above left).

(d) Draw small circles to show the location of the elbows in the middle of the arms and the knees in the middle of the legs (see above centre).

(e) In pencil lightly draw heads on both sides of the head to show that the shoulders are about twice the width of the head (see above right). Erase the 2 extra heads to avoid confusing your learners later.

(f) Put up the more detailed figure drawing beside the stick figure and ask a volunteer to stand beside the drawing.

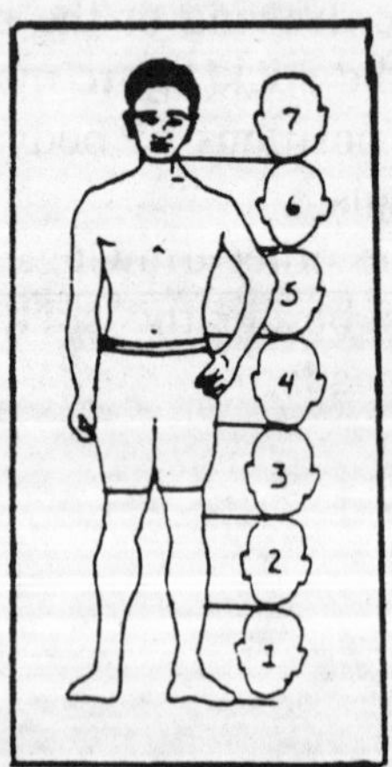
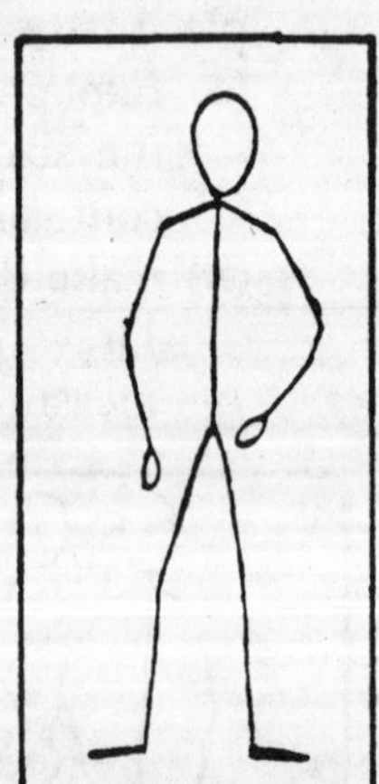

(g) Ask another volunteer to review the body proportions pointing to the person and the detailed drawing. Encourage others to correct the volunteer if she or he makes a mistake.

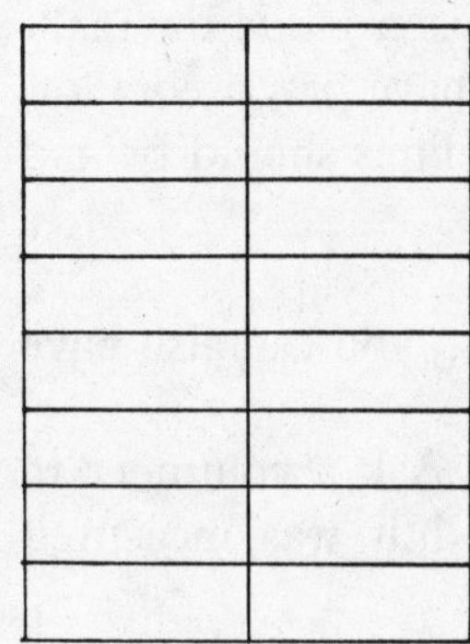

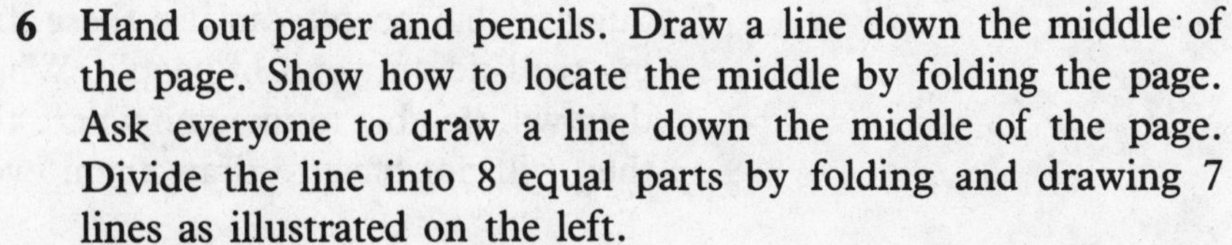

6 Hand out paper and pencils. Draw a line down the middle of the page. Show how to locate the middle by folding the page. Ask everyone to draw a line down the middle of the page. Divide the line into 8 equal parts by folding and drawing 7 lines as illustrated on the left.

7 Ask people to draw a stick figure. Help anyone who has difficulty.

8 Draw another stick figure on a sheet of paper. Show how you can fill in the body parts to make a drawing of a body from a stick figure as shown in the six diagrams below:

(a) Draw a large oval between the waist and the shoulders to show the chest.

(b) Draw a circle to show the hips.

(c) Draw long thin ovals to fill in the arms. Make sure the upper arms are wider than the lower arms. Remind learners that upper and lower arms are about the same length.

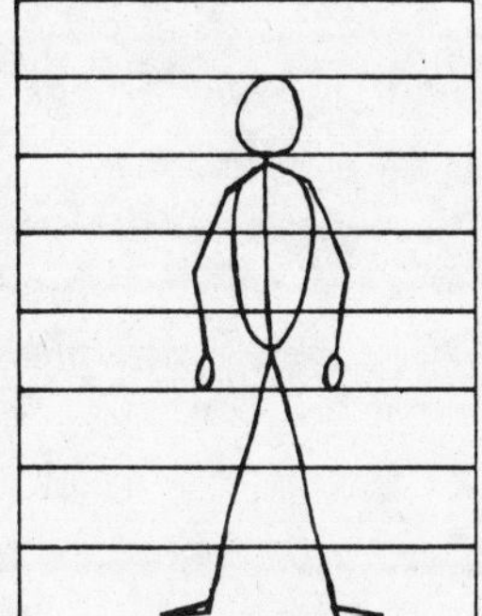

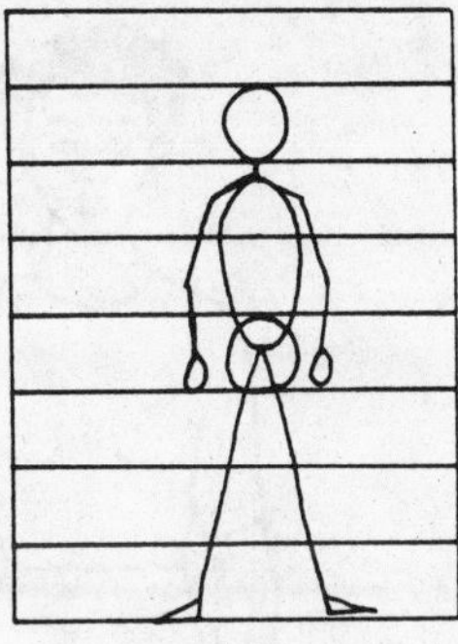

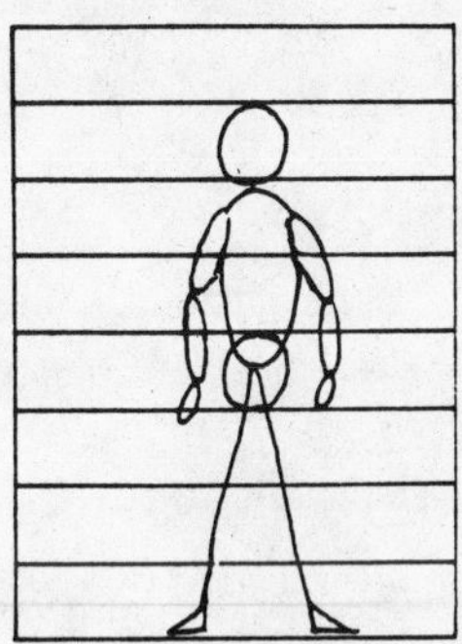

(d) Do the same for the legs and feet. Make sure the upper leg is wider than the lower leg.

(e) Add facial features following the instructions given in Activity 1.

(f) Add clothing.

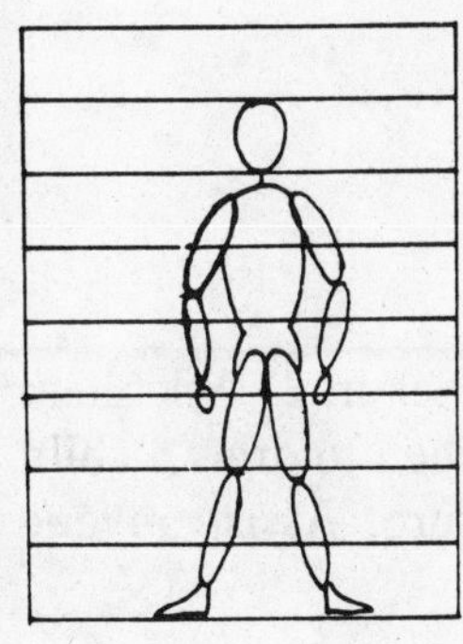

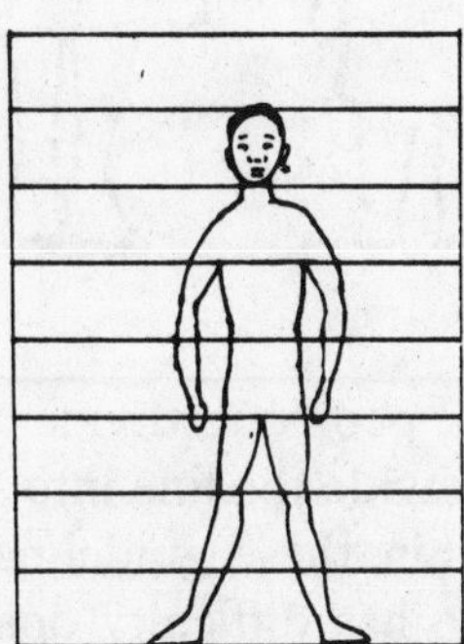

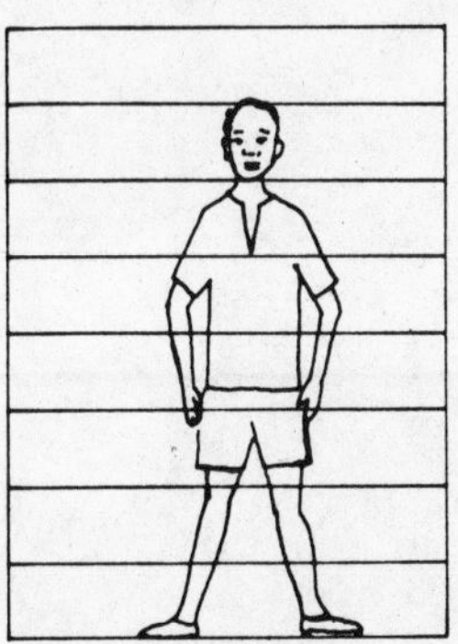

9 Suggest that people can use these drawings as a guide for making realistic drawings of people. When they have practised a lot, they will be able to imagine where the guidelines should be and they will not have to draw them every time.

Possible adaptations

1 If learners want to learn more about drawing, you can also have them practise drawing children.

(a) Bring a child to the front of the group. Ask a volunteer to measure the child the same way the adult was measured (instructions 3 and 4).

(b) Ask learners to discuss the differences between the bodies of children and adults. They should notice that the child's head is larger compared to body length than an adult's head. The child's legs are shorter compared to body length than an adult's legs. Use the drawing of a child's body proportions to summarize this discussion.

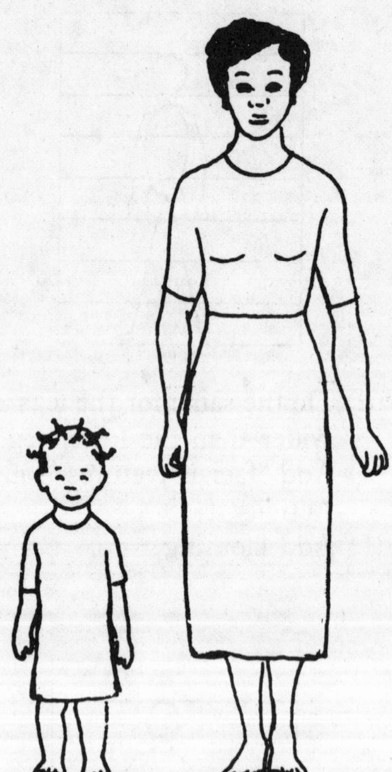

(c) Ask people to divide another sheet of paper in 2. Ask them to divide the line into 4 equal parts, and then to draw a child within these guidelines, using your picture. Assist anyone who has difficulty doing this.

Activity 3

Drawing pictures of people as they move

Time

20–45 minutes. The amount of time will depend on the number of different motions that you ask learners to draw.

Objective

Learners will be able to use a stick figure to make a drawing of a person in motion.

Materials

Enlarged drawings of the pictures below, prepared by the trainer.
Pencil and paper for each learner.
Chalk and chalkboard.

Instructions

1 People are usually moving. To show motion correctly it is important to look carefully at where and how arms and legs bend, how the head bends, and the angle of the body. You can use stick figures to emphasize these lines of body motion with a group that is familiar with stick figures.

2 You may want to review briefly the instructions for drawing stick figures in Activity 2, particularly the body proportions. Examples:

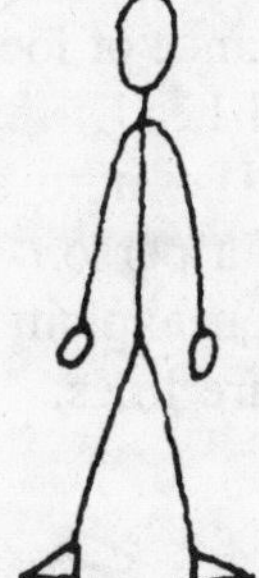

The standing figure is not bending head, arms, legs, or body.

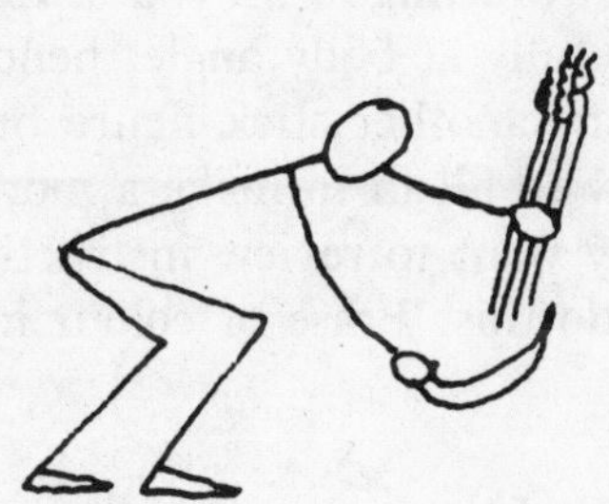

The figure cutting grain is bent at the knees, arms and back bent, head down.

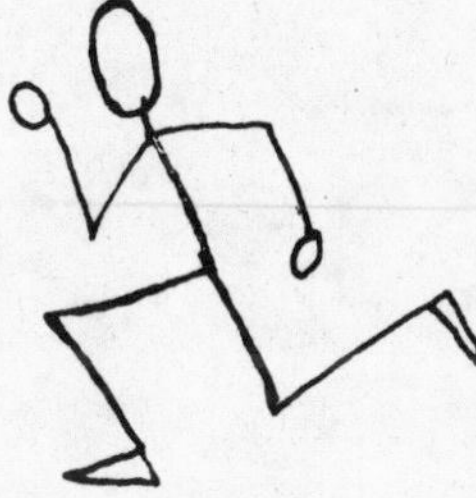

The running figure's body is bent forward, arms and legs back.

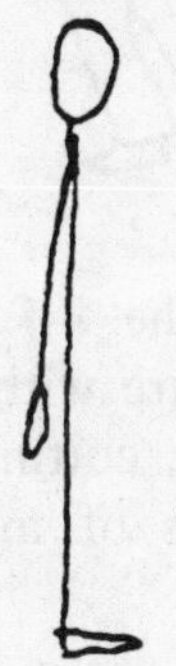

(a) Ask a volunteer to stand in front of the group with his side to the group. Draw a stick figure to show the lines of the figure standing still. Point out the lines on the person. You can draw an imaginary line with your finger. Or you can pin a narrow piece of white cloth on the side of the person. When the person bends the cloth will show the lines of motion.

(b) Ask him or her to bend forward to pick up something. Draw a stick figure showing the motion. Place it beside the stick figure showing the person standing. Point out the lines.

(c) Ask the person to lean back as far as possible without falling. Again make a stick figure to show the motion.

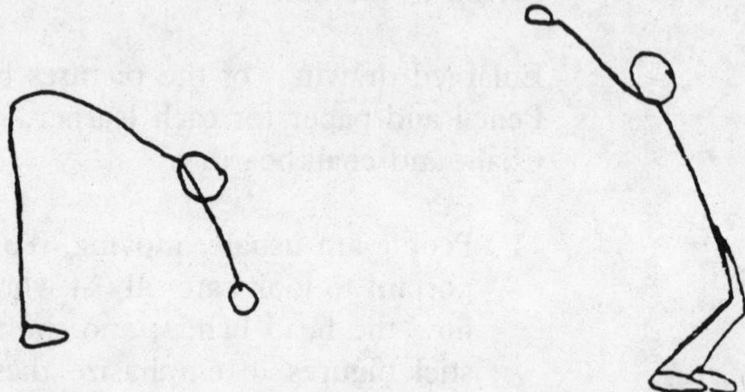

3 Ask the volunteer to reach up to a tree or a shelf. Ask the participants to draw a stick figure showing the lines of motion.

4 Draw the figure yourself so that everyone can see and compare their drawings with yours. Emphasize the importance of looking carefully at body angle, bending arms, legs, and head.

5 Draw another stick figure beside the first one. Use it to show how to fill in to make a more realistic sketch of a person. You may want to review instructions in Activity 2 that explain how to do this. Erase or colour in over the stick figure lines.

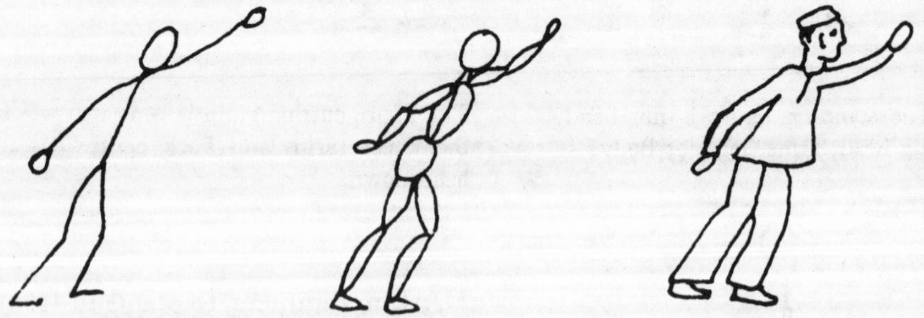

6 Ask everyone to fill in their stick figures. Give help if needed.

7 If time allows, have people repeat this procedure with figures running, sweeping, carrying a child on the hip, cutting grain. Encourage them to continue looking for lines of motion in people working around them.

Changing the size of pictures

Objective

These activities should enable learners to change the size of pictures using 3 different methods.

Information and notes to the trainer

Sometimes your learners find pictures they need for their teaching, but the pictures are the wrong size. Often the pictures will be too small for their learners to see necessary details. Other times they will need to trace figures from a number of pictures that are different sizes so they need to know how to make pictures larger or smaller so all their final figures are the same size.

These activities will show your learners 3 different ways to enlarge pictures. Two of the methods can also be used to make pictures smaller. The first activity shows how to use a projector to enlarge pictures. The other two activities do not require any equipment. Decide how much time, equipment, and other supplies are available. Then demonstrate one or more of the 3 methods for your learners to practise. For these activities, it is very important for the trainer to practise the techniques and carefully prepare the demonstration before the session.

Evaluation

Check to see if the enlarged drawing looks like the original picture.

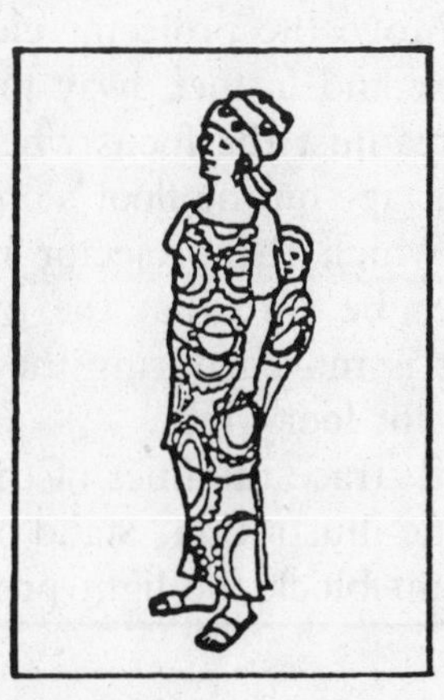

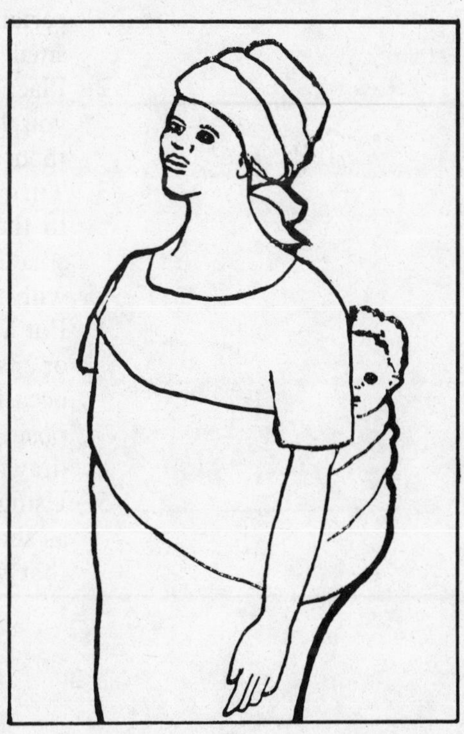

Activity 1 — Using a projector to enlarge a picture

Time 20 minutes

Objective Learners will use a projector to enlarge a picture.

Materials
Slide, overhead, filmstrip, or opaque projector.
Picture(s) to be enlarged.
Large sheets of blank paper and tape.
Pencils.
Ink, paint, crayons, or other colouring materials.

Instructions

Most projectors–slide, overhead, filmstrip, and opaque types–can be used to make a picture larger. Slide, overhead, and filmstrip projectors require that pictures be on film, in the form of slides, overhead transparencies, and filmstrips. The opaque projector uses flat pictures or objects and is often the easiest to use to enlarge a picture.

1 Tape a sheet of paper (the size you need for your visual aid) on the wall. You may need to make the figure a specific size to match other parts of a drawing. If so, draw the other figures on the paper before you do this enlarging. That way you can make certain that the enlarged figure does not look too large or too small compared with the rest of the picture.
2 Place your picture on the platform of the opaque projector. If you have slides, filmstrips, or overhead transparencies, place them in the appropriate type of projector.
3 Turn on the projector and focus the picture on the paper taped to the wall. Move the projector closer to the paper to make a smaller picture and farther away to make a larger picture. You will have to readjust the focus when you move the projector.
4 Put a piece of tape on the floor along the front edge of the table or stand on which the projector is placed. Look at the tape occasionally to be sure that the projector is still in the right position. If it is moved during the time you are copying, your drawing will not look right.
5 Using a pencil, trace the lines of the picture you want to copy, as shown in the illustration. Stand off to the side of the paper so that you do not block the light projecting the picture.

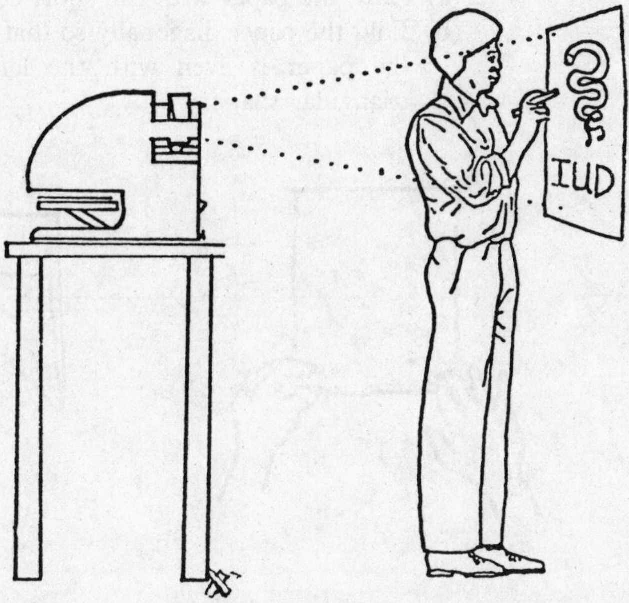

6 Turn off the projector and remove the picture you have just copied.
7 Go over the completed drawing in ink, paint, crayon, or coloured marker. Erase unwanted pencil lines.

Activity 2

Using squares to make a picture larger or smaller

Time

45 minutes

Objective

Learners will make a square grid and use it to enlarge a picture.

Materials

Picture(s) to be enlarged.
Tracing paper or thin paper.
Scissors.
Large sheets of blank paper.
Pencils and erasers.
Ink, paint, crayons, or other colouring materials.

Instructions

1 Use a *square* piece of thin paper that can be used for tracing. The square of paper should be roughly the same size as the figure or picture that you want to trace and enlarge. If the paper is not square, make it into a square as follows:

(a) Place the paper with the short edge at the bottom.
(b) Fold the paper diagonally so that the bottom (short) edge of the paper is even with the left (long) edge, forming a triangular shape.

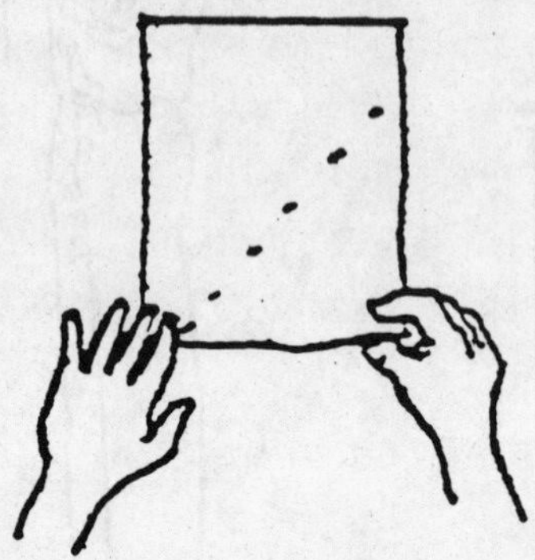

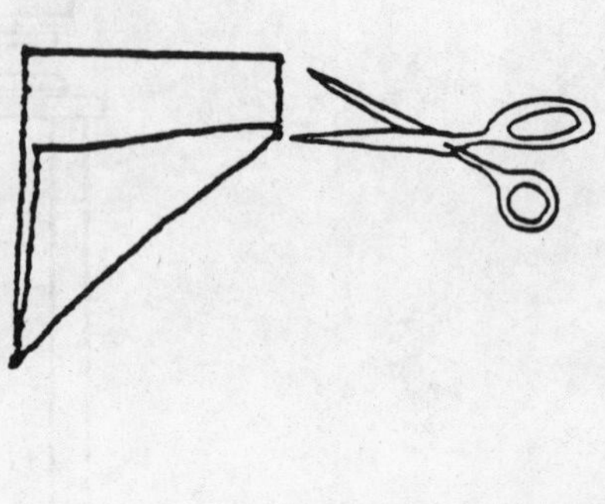

(c) Cut off the paper that is not part of the folded triangles.
(d) Unfold the triangles. Now you have a square.

2 Place the bottom edge of the paper on the top edge and fold it to form a rectangle.

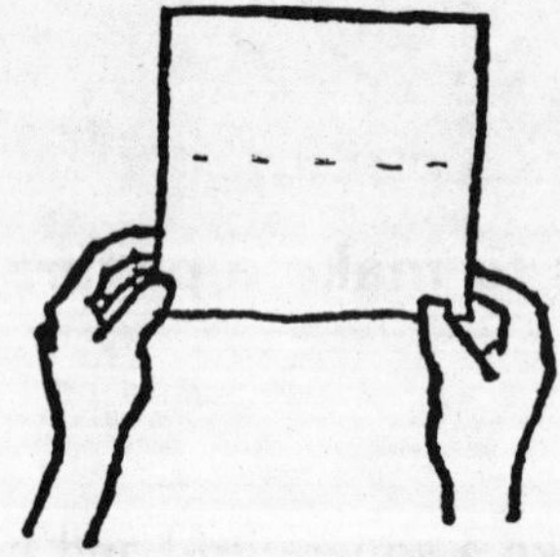

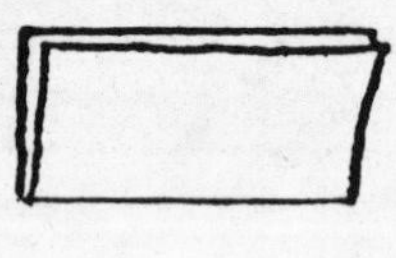

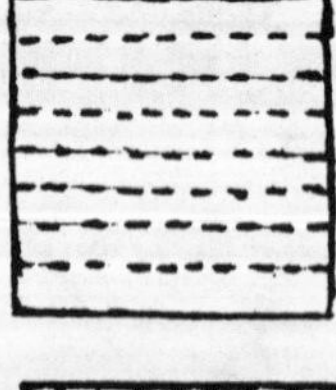

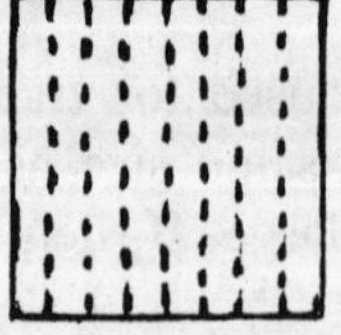

3 Crease the folded edge with your thumbnail to make a sharp fold.
4 Place the bottom (folded) edge on the top edge of the paper, fold it to form a narrower rectangle, and crease the edge with your thumbnail.
5 Fold and crease the paper in the same way 1 or 2 more times to form a narrow strip of folded paper. The more times you fold the paper, the smaller the squares you will eventually make.
6 Unfold the square (see above left).
7 Turn the paper so that the creases run up and down (see below left).

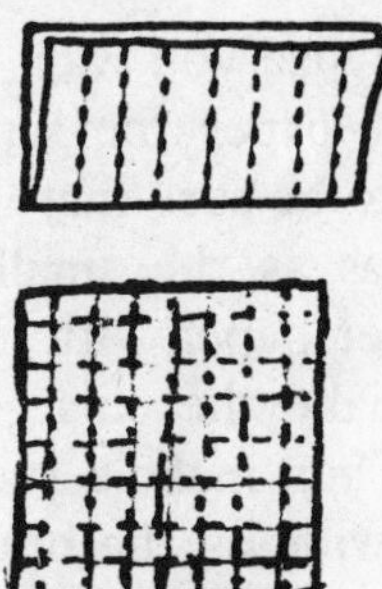

8 Place the bottom edge of the paper on the top edge and fold it to form a rectangle (see above left).
9 Continue folding and creasing the paper the same number of times that you folded it from the other side.
10 Unfold the square (see below left).
11 Look at the picture carefully and decide which lines you need to trace to make a large version of the picture. The example shows the decision to leave out the pattern on the dress.

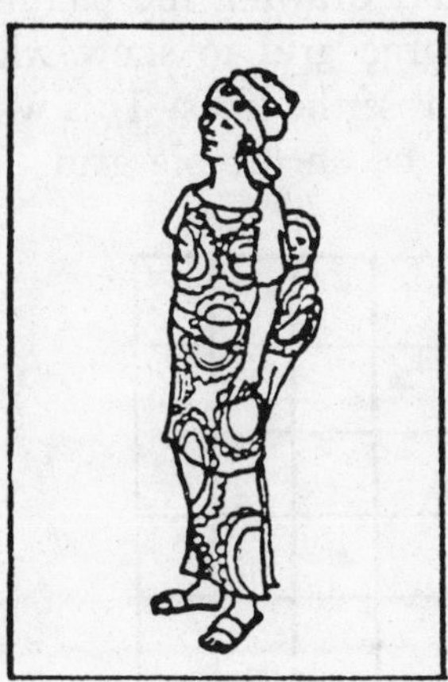

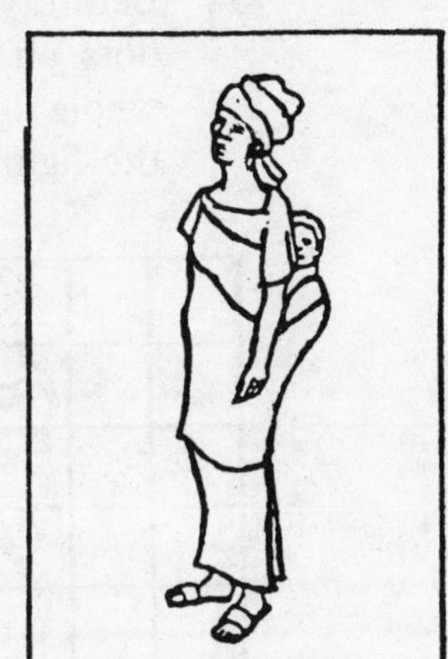

12 Place the sheet with squares over the picture and trace the important lines as shown in the example below.

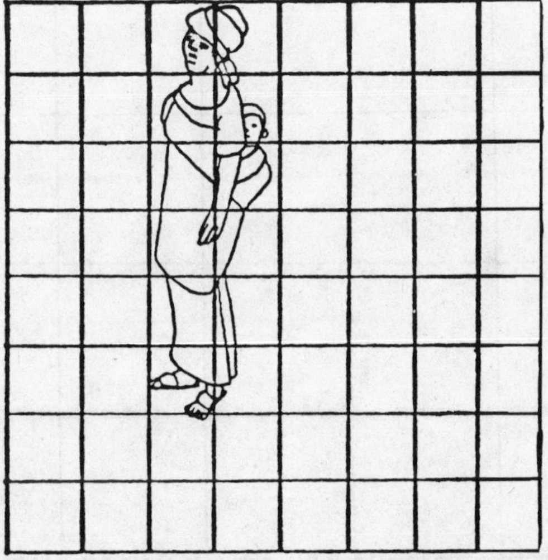

13 Make another larger sheet with squares – the size you want to enlarge the picture. Fold the larger sheet of paper the same number of times you folded the smaller sheet to be sure that the larger sheet has the same number of squares as the smaller sheet. Place the larger paper beside the smaller paper with the tracing of your picture. You may need to make the enlarged picture a specific size to match other figures. Then make certain that the large sheet of paper is as high and wide as the other figure that is the correct size.

14 Before you start drawing the picture, use your pencil to make dots on the large grid to show where important parts of the whole figure cross the lines. This will give you an idea of where the figure will be on the big grid.

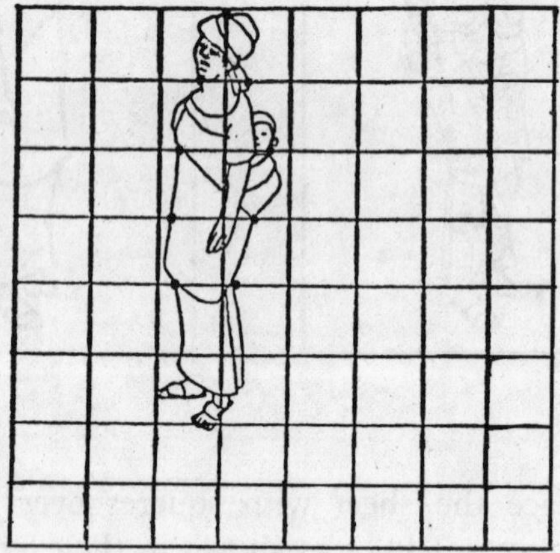

15 Start drawing one part of the picture, such as the woman's face in the example below. On the tracing on the smaller sheet of paper, count the number of squares from the top of the paper and the number from the side of the paper to the point on the picture where you will begin drawing. In the example below, the left side of the woman's face is one square down and 3 squares across from the top left corner of the paper.

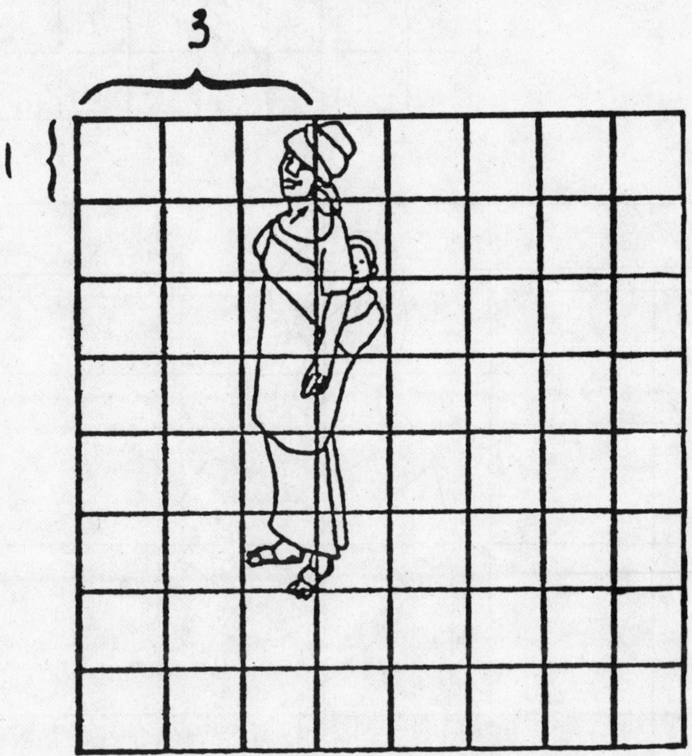

16 Starting at that point, look carefully at the way the line crosses each square on the paper on the smaller picture that you wish to enlarge.

- Does it cross the middle?
- Does it go along the edge?
- Does it cut across the corner of the square?
- Is the line straight?
- Does the line curve? In which direction does it curve?

17 To enlarge the small picture, look at the way the lines cross each square on the small grid and copy them the same way on the larger grid. This is shown in the drawings below.

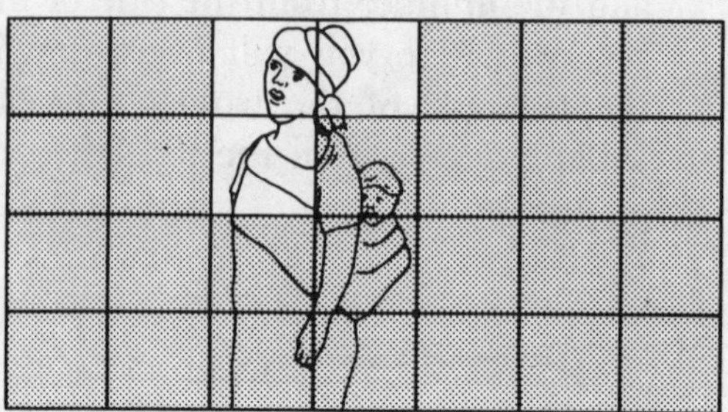

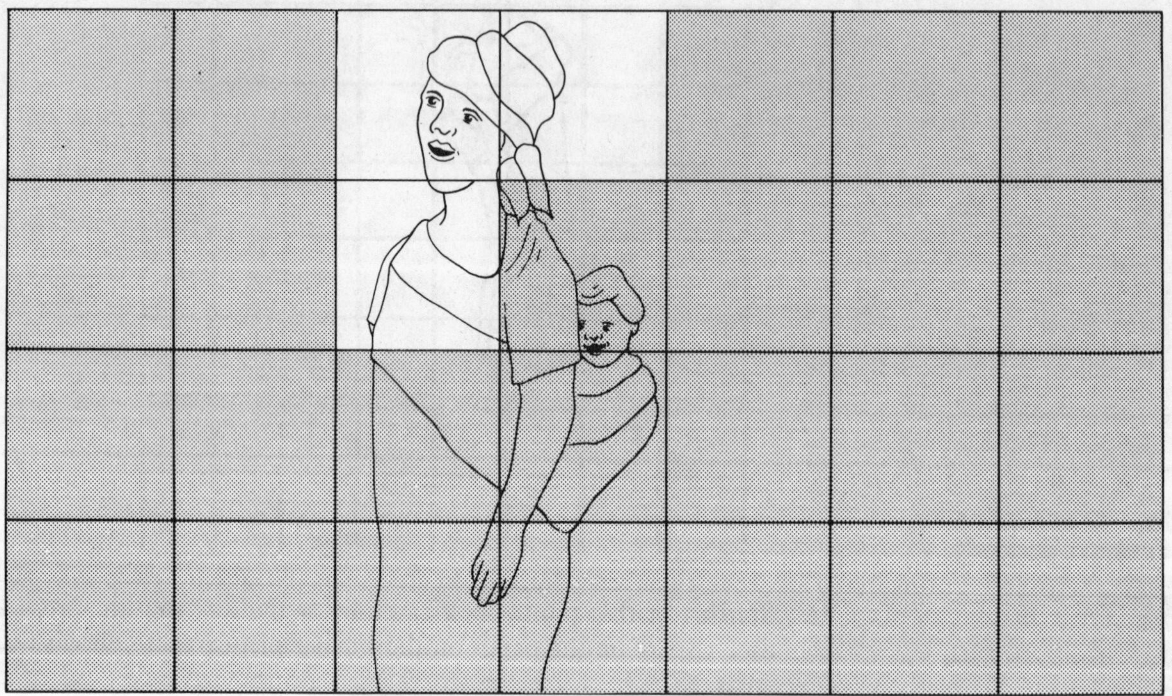

18 Continue in the same way to copy the rest of the drawings on the large grid one square at a time until the drawing is complete.

19 Erase the grid on the enlarged picture or transfer the large picture to another sheet of paper using the transfer technique described in the **Tracing** activities.

20 Use ink, paint, crayon, or other colouring materials to cover the pencil lines. Erase any pencil lines that are not covered.

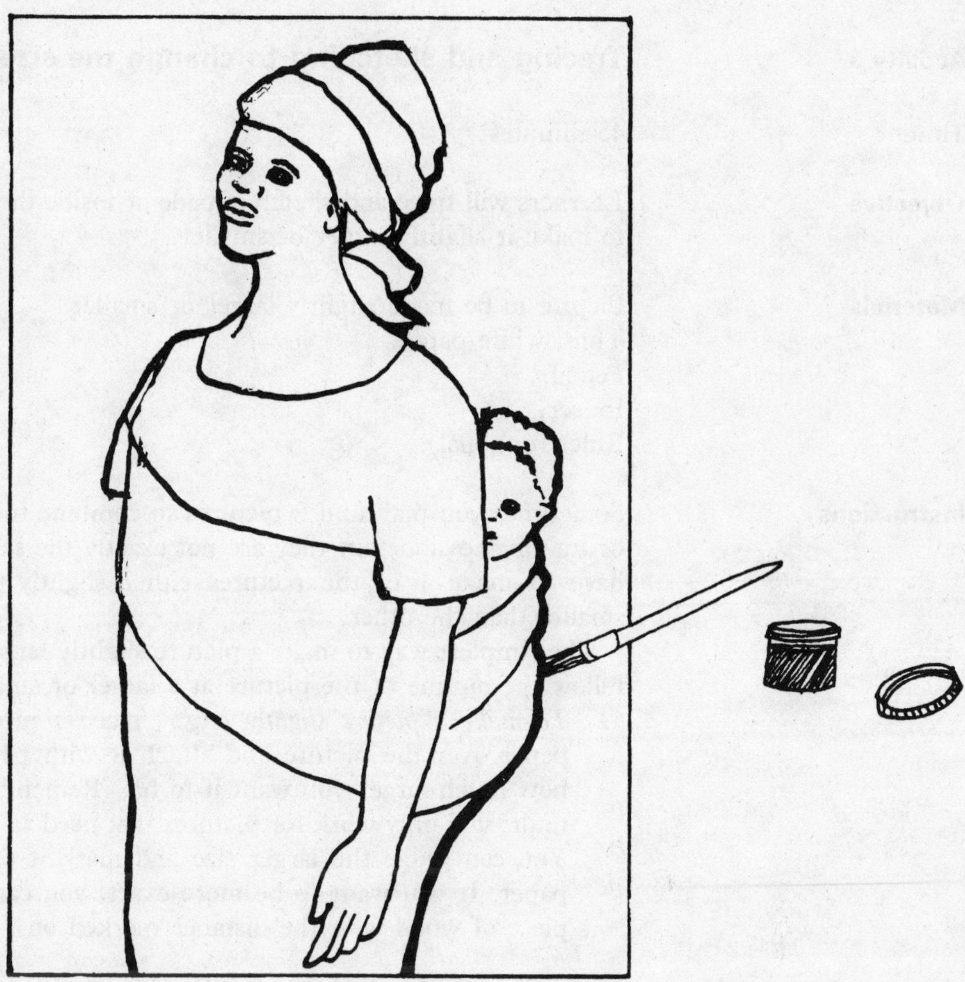

Possible adaptation

You can also use squares to make large pictures smaller. In step 12 you will trace from a large picture instead of a small one. In step 13 you will make a smaller sheet with squares instead of a larger one.

Activity 3

Tracing and sketching to change the size of a picture

Time

45 minutes

Objective

Learners will trace and sketch outside or inside the lines of a picture to make it slightly larger or smaller.

Materials

Picture to be made slightly larger or smaller.
Thin, white paper.
Pencil.
Eraser.
Ruler (optional).

Instructions

Sometimes you may find 2 pictures to combine to use in a teaching or training session, but they are not exactly the same size. You will have to make 1 of the pictures either slightly larger or slightly smaller than the other.

The simplest way to make a picture slightly larger or smaller is to follow the outline of the picture at a larger or smaller size.

1 *To make a picture slightly larger*, place a piece of thin, white paper over the picture and attach it with paper clips. Decide how much larger you want it to be. (Remember that this technique will only work for pictures that need to be *slightly* larger.) You can judge the larger size and mark it on the thin, white paper. If you want to be more exact, you can use a ruler or a piece of wood with the distance marked on it.

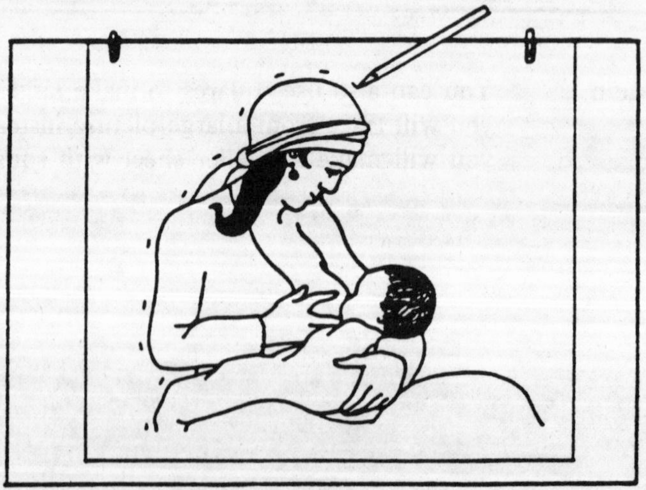

Series of images adapted from *Prenatal Nutrition and Breastfeeding*

2 At the distance you have decided on, trace *outside* the original lines of the picture until you have traced the entire outline.

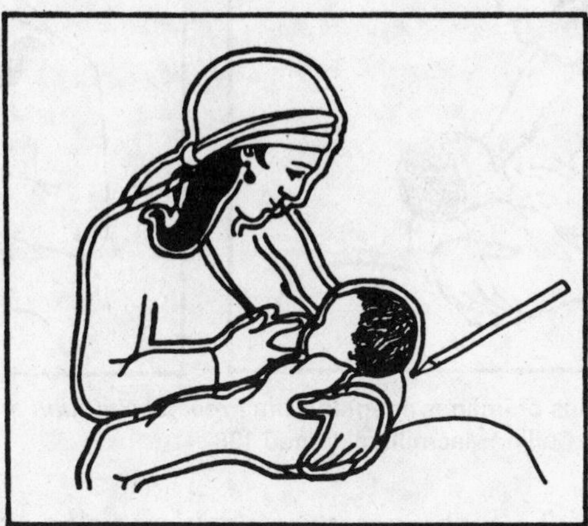

3 If your picture has detailed lines within the person or object, such as facial features, you will have to estimate where the lines should be located in relation to the outline you have already drawn. Look carefully at the original picture, estimate where the lines within the figure should go, and mark them on your thin paper.

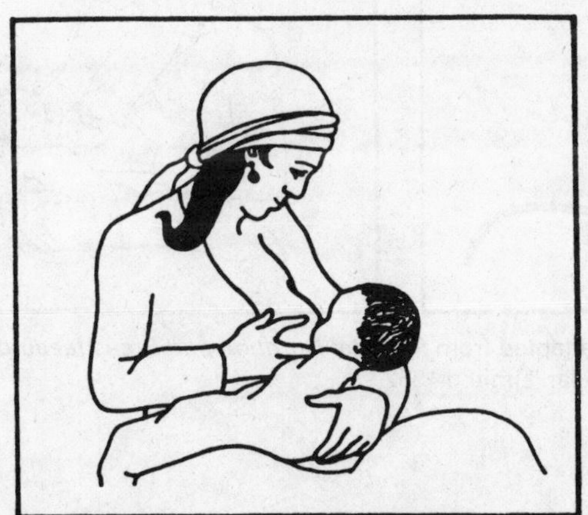

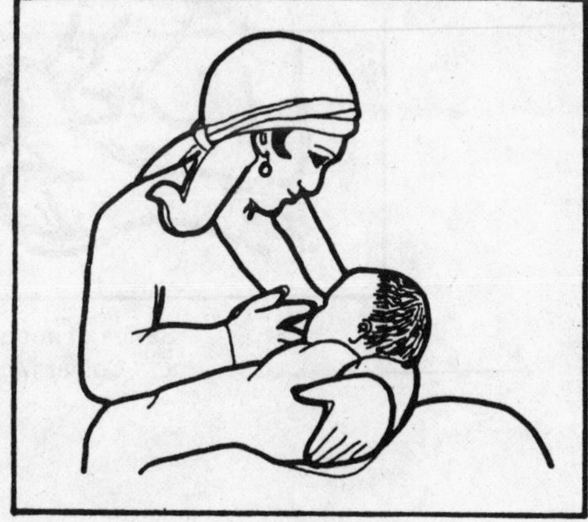

Series of images adapted from *Prenatal Nutrition and Breastfeeding*

4 Compare your larger copy to the original picture. Erase the lines that are incorrectly placed. Sketch new ones until they are correctly placed in the drawing.

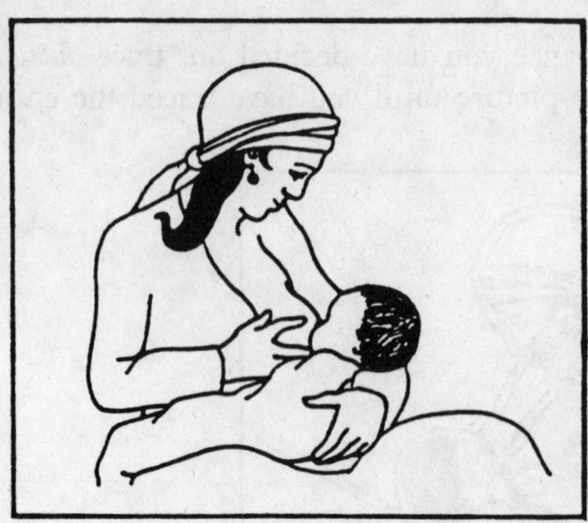

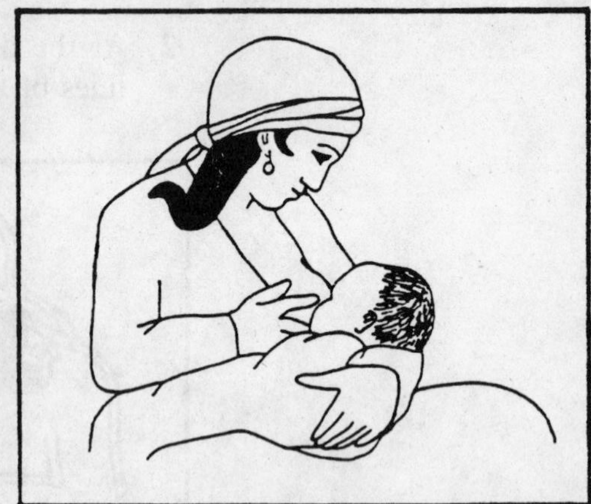

Series of images adapted from *Prenatal Nutrition and Breastfeeding*

5 *To make a picture slightly smaller*, follow steps 1–4, but trace *inside* the outline of the original picture at the distance you decide upon.

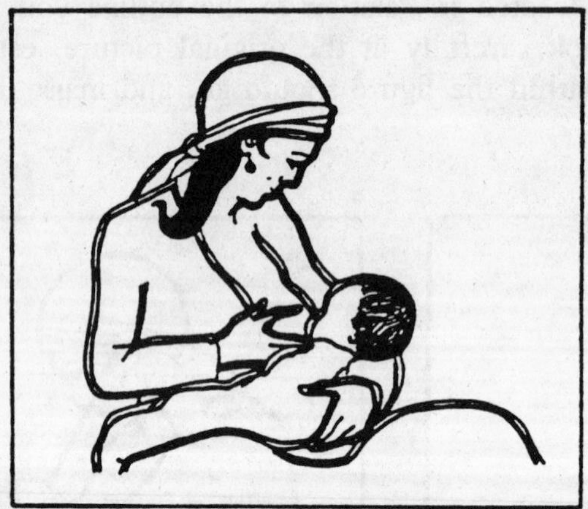

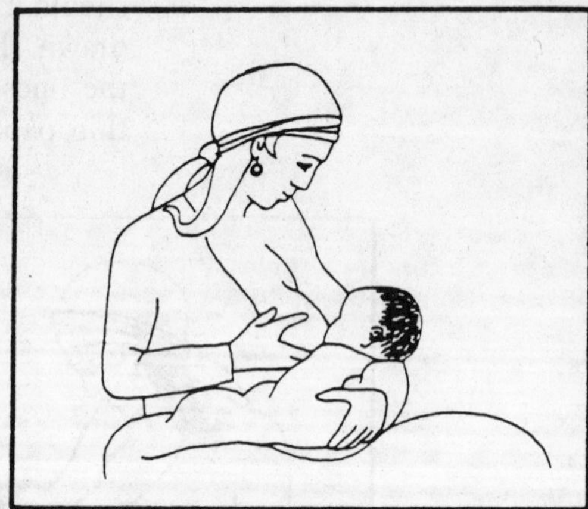

Series of images adapted from *Prenatal Nutrition and Breastfeeding*

Lettering

Objective

Learners will be able to letter words by hand or by using a lettering stencil.

Information and notes to the trainer

Visual aids sometimes have words on them to explain a picture or to label the parts of a drawing. Commercially-produced visual aids have words that are mechanically lettered. If you are making your own visual aids, there are ways you can put words on them by hand lettering or by using a lettering stencil. These activities will show your learners how to hand letter and how to use a lettering stencil.

Your learners will need to practise these 2 lettering techniques in order to make words clearly and neatly. It would be a good idea for you to practise them before conducting these activities so that you can demonstrate the techniques. Allow plenty of time for your learners to practise during the activity.

You may want to use the following information to introduce the lettering activities.

When should I use words on a visual aid?

Usually, the picture is the most important part of a visual aid. But *when a trainer cannot be present* to explain a display or poster, words on the visual aid can provide the explanation.

Some visual aids need words to *label the parts* of a picture, as in the picture below.

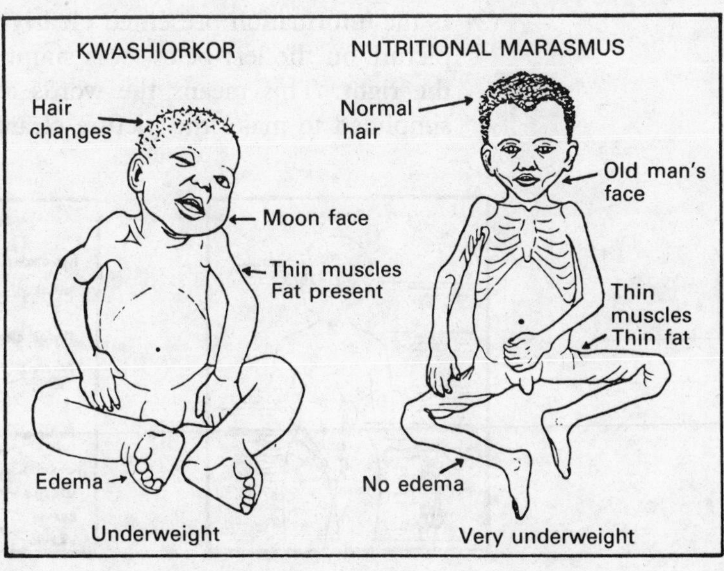

When your learners cannot read, you will want to avoid using words on your visual aids.

How should I use words on a visual aid?

Keep the *number of words* to a minimum that will still explain the picture clearly.

Use the *design questions* explained in Unit 2 to guide you. The first 3 questions are particularly helpful for lettering:

(1) Are the pictures and words **easy to see and understand?**

LETTERS

Should be:
LARGE
THICK
SIMPLE
VISIBLE

Instead of:
SMALL
THIN
COMPLEX

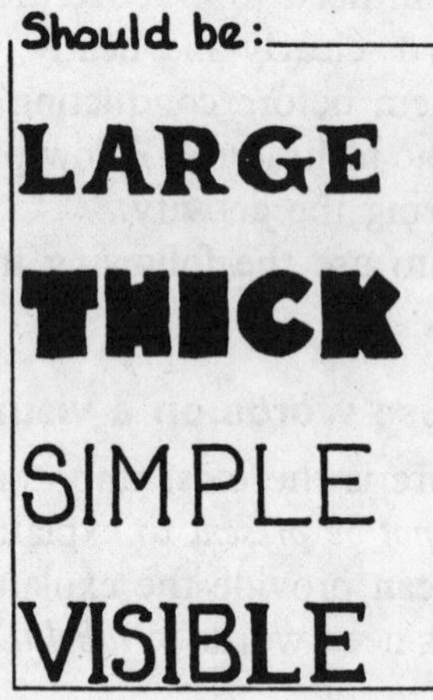

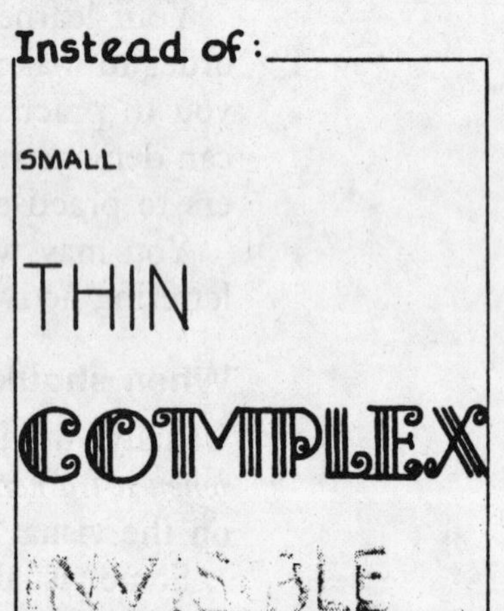

(2) Is the information presented **clearly and simply**? Notice that the picture on the left below was simplified to make the picture on the right. This means the words as well as the drawing were simplified to make the picture clearer.

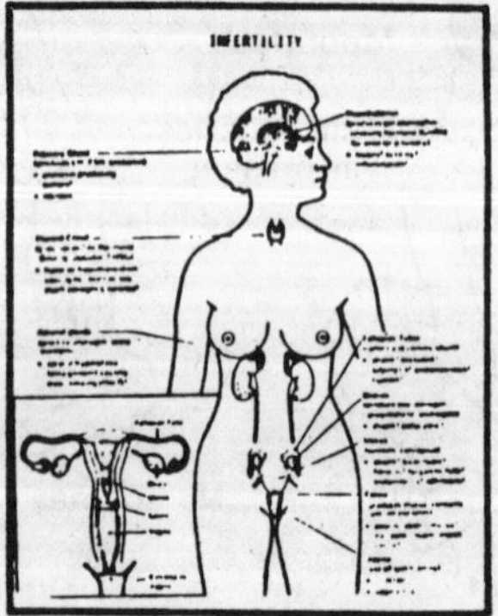

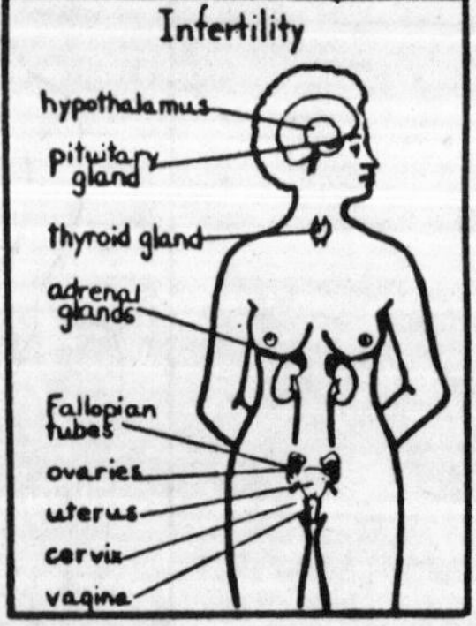

(3) Is the visual aid **well organized**? The words are part of the organization.

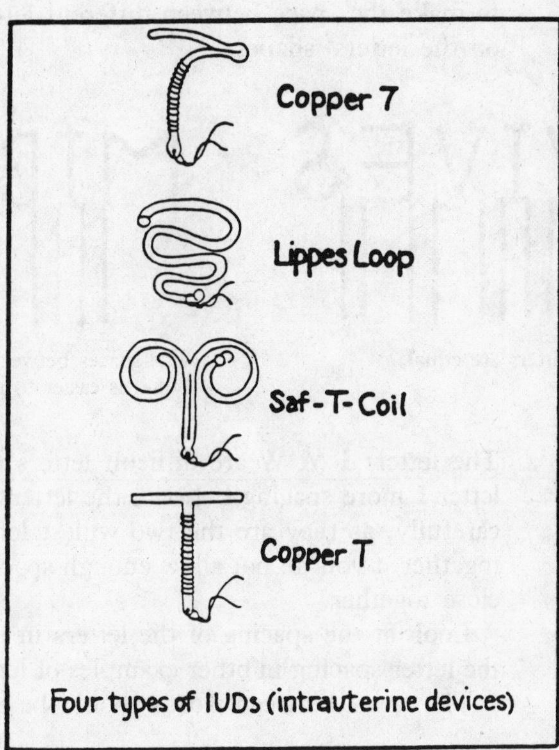

Usually, people can read a combination of *upper and lower case letters* more easily than all upper case letters. When you make a visual aid that needs to be seen from a distance and only has a few words on it, all upper case letters may be best.

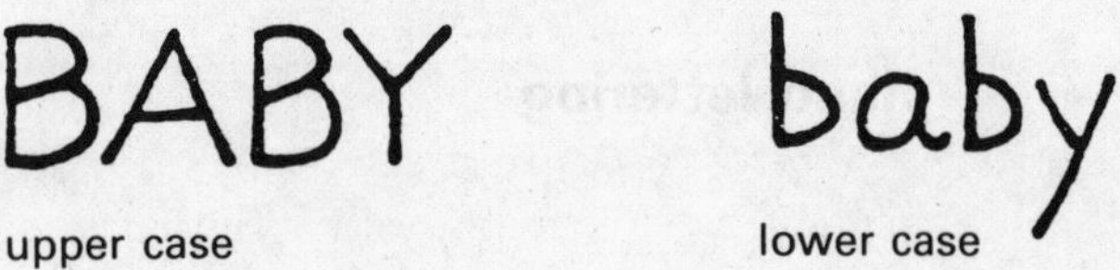

The activity on hand lettering will give your learners practice in making upper and lower case letters. The lettering stencil activity shows how to make thick upper case letters that are easy to see from a distance.

Space letters and words carefully so that the individual words and series of words are easy to read. Letters in a word should *appear* to have the same space between them. In order to do this, you will need to make the space between different letters more or less depending on the letters' shapes.

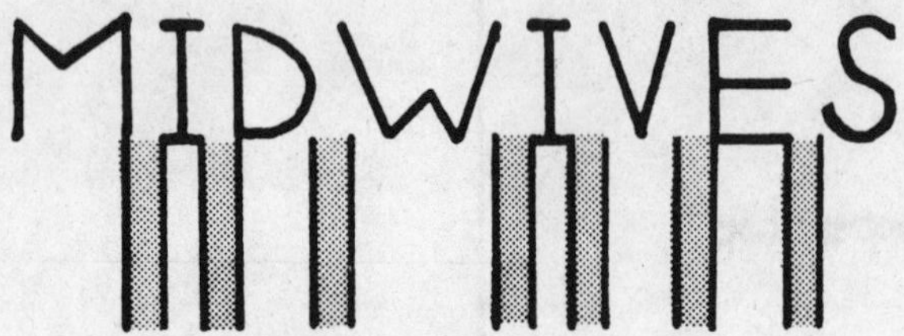

The spaces between these letters are equal, but it is hard to read.

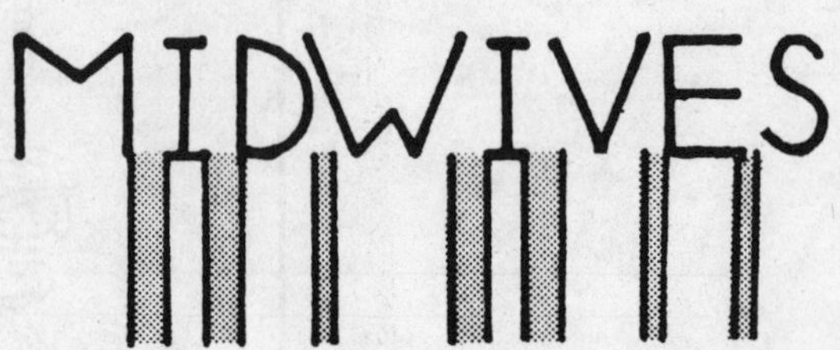

The spaces between these letters are unequal, but it is easier to read.

The letters **I M W** are difficult letters to space correctly. Give the letter **I** more spacing between the letters next to it. Place **M** and **W** carefully, as they are the two widest letters and can look squeezed together if you do not allow enough space. Space all the other letters close together.

Look at the spacing of the letters in the example above. Look at the letter spacing in other examples of lettering that are easy to read.

The space between words should be equal to about one letter.

SMALL FAMILIES CAN LIVE BETTER

Activity 1 **Hand lettering**

Time 1 hour

Objective Learners will hand letter upper and lower case letters to make words that are readable.

Materials A ruler or straight edge for each person.
Pencils and erasers.
Blank paper.

Ink, crayons, or other materials for colouring.
Printed alphabet samples (optional).
Chalkboard and chalk or large pieces of paper.
Hand printed lower case and upper case alphabets on large sheets of paper using the 4 guidelines (see pictures under steps 4 and 11 below).

Instructions

1 Draw the 4 guidelines shown below on the chalkboard or on a large piece of paper. Write the word *baby* in upper and lower case letters on the guidelines. This will show your learners how to use the guidelines.

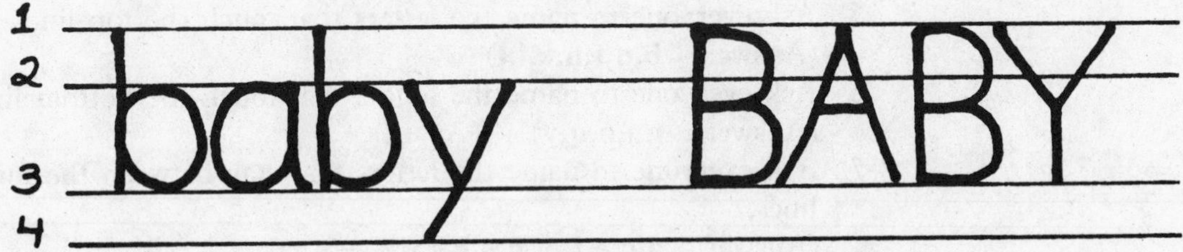

2 Point out to your learners that:
(a) the spaces between guidelines 1 and 2 and guidelines 3 and 4 are equal.
(b) the space between guidelines 2 and 3 is about twice as large as the space between guidelines 1 and 2 or guidelines 3 and 4.

3 Ask learners to use their pencils and rulers to draw 2 or 3 sets of the 4 guidelines on the blank paper.

4 Have learners write in pencil all the letters in the lower case alphabet on their guidelines. They may refer only to the sample word *baby* that you wrote on the chalkboard in lower case letters.

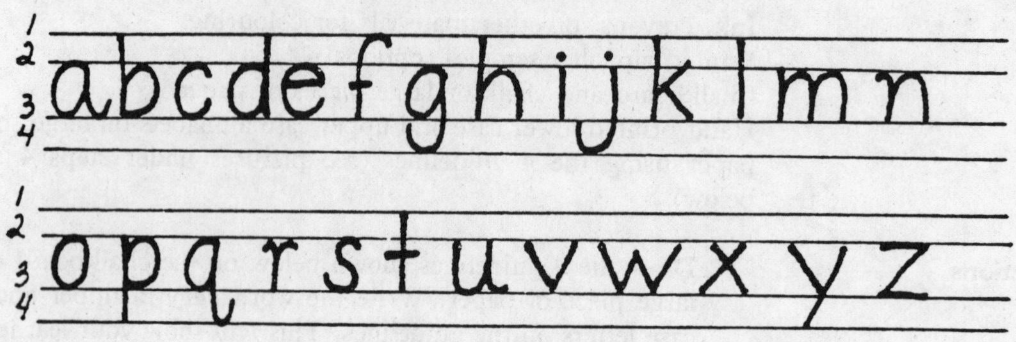

5 Ask everyone to name the letters that touch the top line. (Answer: **b,d,f,h,k,l,t**)

6 Ask everyone to name the letters that touch the bottom line. (Answer: **g,j,p,q,y**)

7 Ask everyone to name the letters that stay between the middle lines.
(Answer: **a,c,e,i,m,n,o,r,s,u,v,w,x,z**)

8 Post your large hand printed lower case alphabet on the wall and ask learners to compare it with their lower case alphabets.

9 Point out the word BABY that you wrote on the chalkboard using the 4 guidelines. Ask your learners to notice that only guidelines 1, 2, and 3 are used in upper case lettering.

10 Ask learners to draw 2 to 3 sets of the 4 guidelines on another sheet of blank paper.

11 Have learners refer to the sample word BABY on the chalkboard and write all the letters in the upper case alphabet on their guidelines.

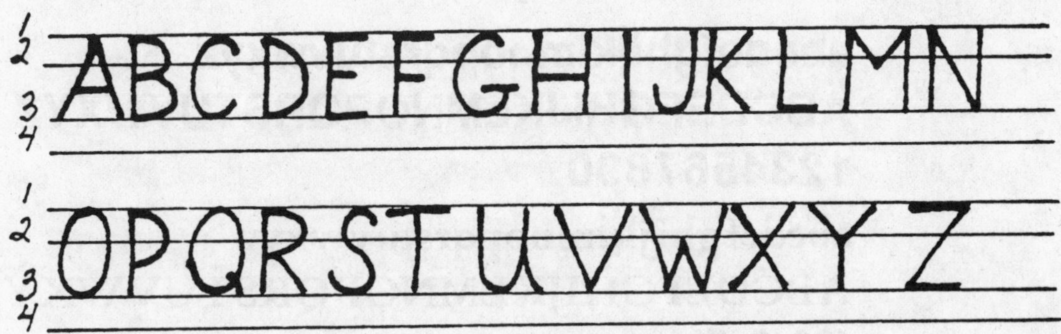

12 Post your large hand printed upper case alphabet on the wall and ask people to compare it with their alphabets.

13 Give out the materials for colouring and have learners use them to mark over their pencilled lower and upper case letters.

14 Have learners draw the 4 guidelines in pencil on a clean sheet of paper. Ask them to hand letter a word such as *pregnancy* or *infertility* in lower and in upper case letters. They can practise the suggestions you made in your introduction for letter spacing. Then tell them to use the colouring materials to mark over the pencilled letters and erase the 4 guidelines.

15 Have learners draw the 4 guidelines in pencil. Ask them to hand letter in upper and lower case letters their full name or a phrase such as 'Healthy Families Are Happy'. This will give them practice in hand lettering different kinds of letters, spacing the letters, and spacing the words.

Possible adaptations

1 You may want to give learners (or have them find) samples of alphabets such as the examples below to use as a guide for hand lettering.

abcdefghijklmnopqrstuvwxyz
ABCDEFGHIJKLMNOPQRSTUVWXYZ
1234567890

abcdefghijklmnopqrstuvwxyz
ABCDEFGHIJKLMNOPQRSTUVWXYZ
1234567890

abcdefghijklmnopqrstuvwxyz
ABCDEFGHIJKLMNOPQRSTUVWXYZ
1234567890
abcdefghijklmnopqrstuvwxyz
ABCDEFGHIJKLMNOPQRSTUVWXYZ
1234567890
abcdefghijklmnopqrstuvwxyz
ABCDEFGHIJKLMNOPQRSTUV
WXYZ
1234567890

2 You may want to give learners copies of the guidelines at the end of this activity to trace for different size letters. Tracing the guidelines will probably take less time than measuring them.

SAMPLE GUIDELINES FOR DIFFERENT SIZE LETTERS

1 ______________________________
2 ______________________________

3 ______________________________
4 ______________________________

1 ______________________________

2 ______________________________

3 ______________________________

4 ______________________________

1 ______________________________

2 ______________________________

3 ______________________________

4 ______________________________

1 ______________________________

2 ______________________________

3 ______________________________

4 ______________________________

Activity 2 **Using a stencil to make letters and words**

Time 2 hours, minimum

Objective Learners will use a stencil to make letters and words.

Materials A lettering stencil for each person in the shape of one of the lettering stencils shown at the end of this activity. You can cut these out of any heavy paper.

A copy of the alphabet guide to using lettering stencils shown at the end of this activity for each person. If it is not possible for each person to have a copy, it would be helpful to have several copies around the room for them to share. You can draw the alphabet guide on the chalkboard before your session if you cannot make copies.

A ruler or straight edge for everyone.

Pencils and erasers.

Blank paper.

Materials for colouring, such as ink or crayons.

Instructions

There are 3 different sets of letters you can make with a lettering stencil: straight letters, curved letters, and turned-over letters. Each set is a little more difficult to make than the previous one, so your learners should practise the straight letters first, then the curved letters, and last the turned-over letters. Then you can have them make words using a combination of letters.

1 *Straight letters:* **E F H I L N T K**
   (a) Use a pencil to draw a line with a ruler or straight edge.
   (b) Place the bottom of the lettering stencil just above the line so that all letters will be level.
   (c) Trace all possible lines for **E** from the stencil as shown below. Use the handout on the alphabet as a guide.

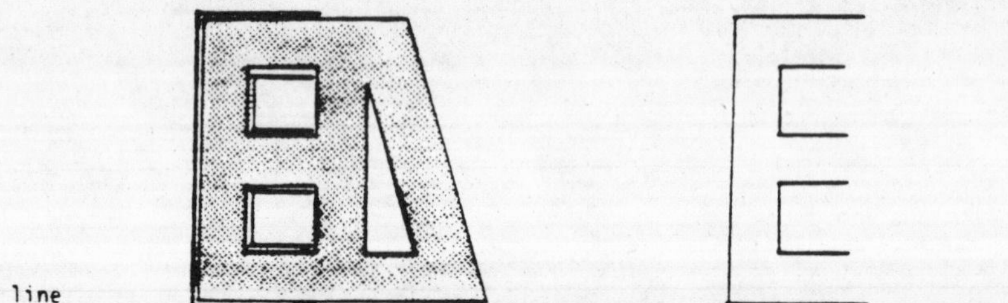

   (d) Use your straight edge to add the missing lines and fill in the letter with markers or other colouring tools as shown below.

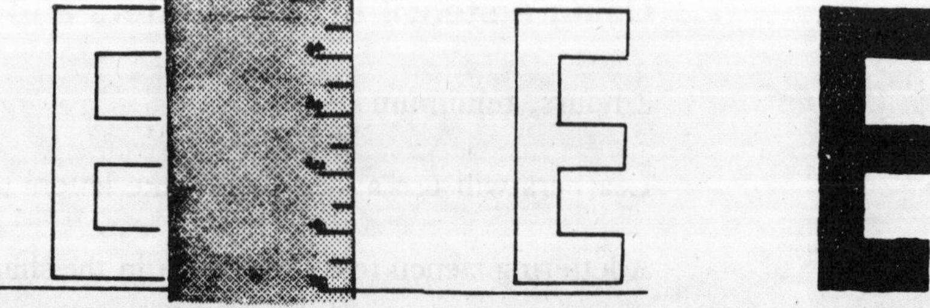

(e) Demonstrate and have your learners practise making as many other straight letters as they have time.

2 *Curved letters*: **A B C D G J O P Q R S U Y**

(a) Draw a straight line.

(b) Place the stencil just above the line.

(c) Trace the shape of the letter **C** using the stencil as shown below. Use the handout on the alphabet as a guide.

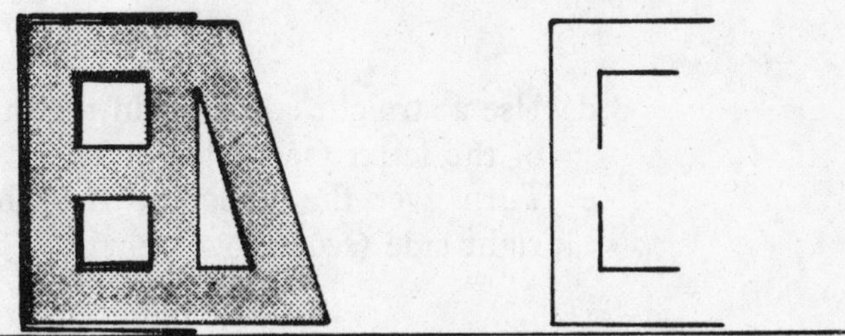

(d) Using a straight edge, add the missing lines as shown below left.

(e) Round the corners of the letters as shown below centre.

(f) Erase the unnecessary lines and fill in the letter as shown below right.

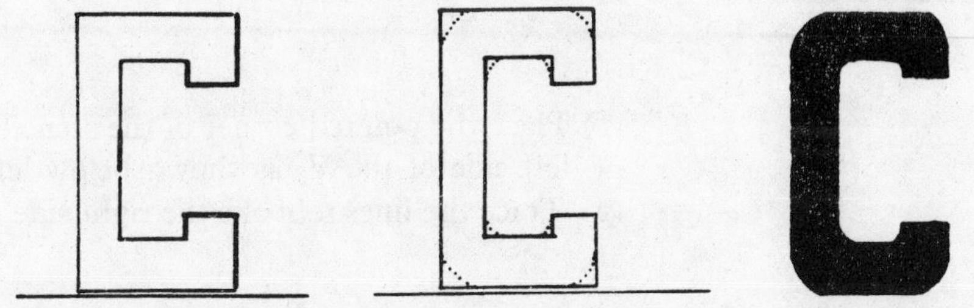

(g) Demonstrate and have your learners make as many other curved letters as they have time.

3 *Turned-over letters* (letters that require turning over the stencil to complete them): **M V W X Z**

(a) Draw a straight line.

(b) Place the stencil just above the line.

(c) Trace the left side of the letter **V** as shown on the next page.

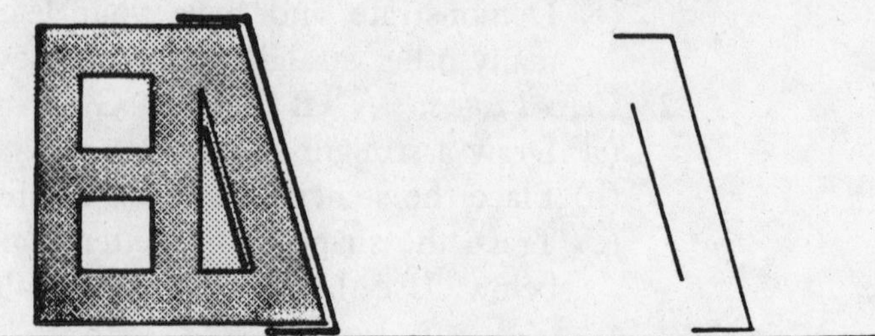

(d) Use a straight edge to add the missing lines for the left side of the letter (see below left).

(e) Turn over the stencil so that the squares are now on the right side (see below right).

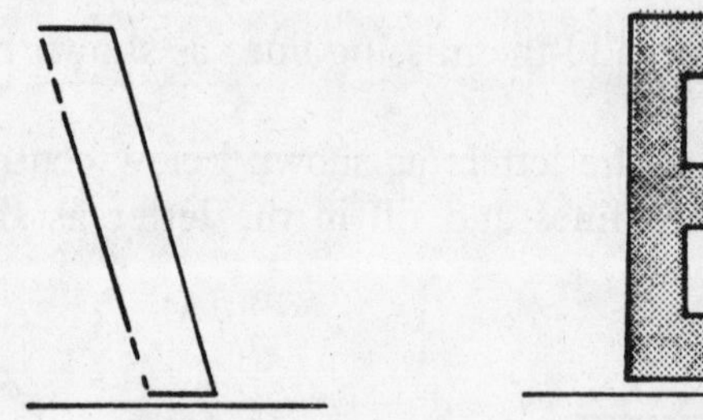

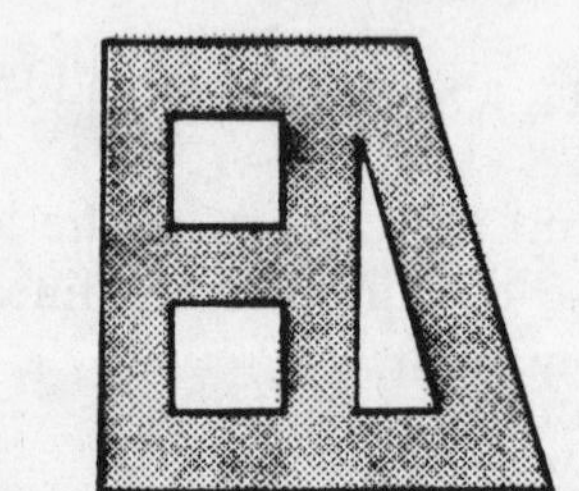

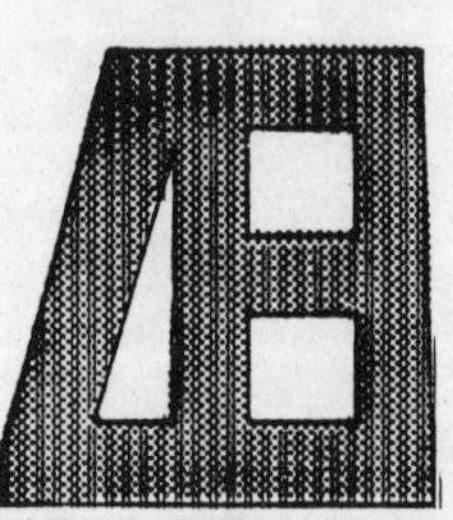

(f) Place the pointed corner of the stencil into the bottom of the left side of the **V**, as shown below left.

(g) Trace the lines to make the right side of the **V** (below right).

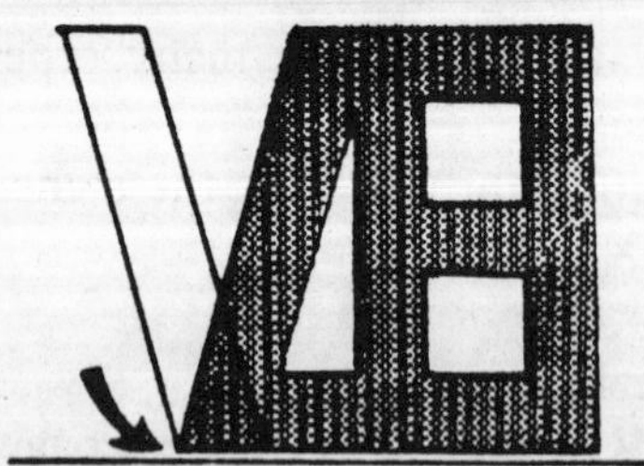

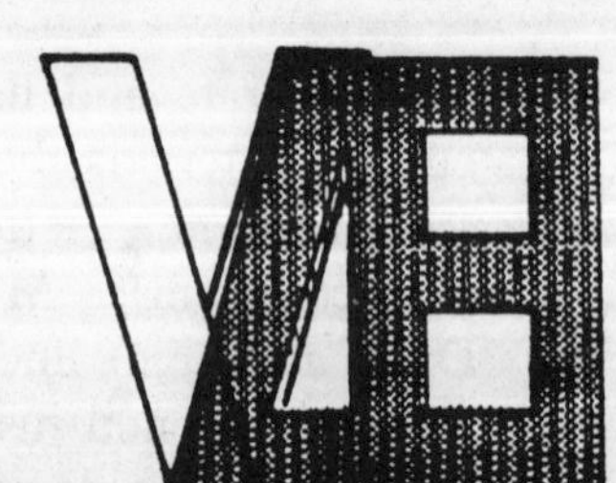

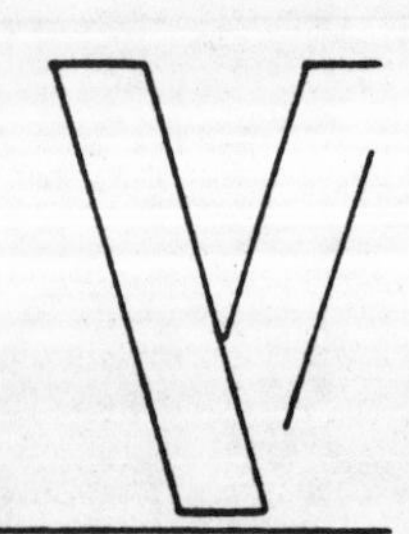

(h) Use a straight edge to add the missing lines.
(i) Erase unnecessary lines and fill in the letter.

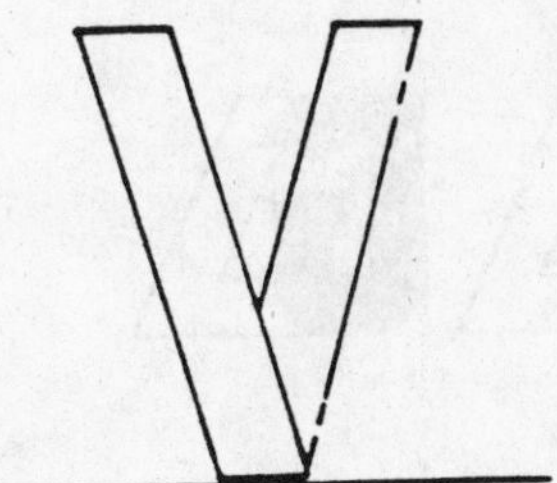

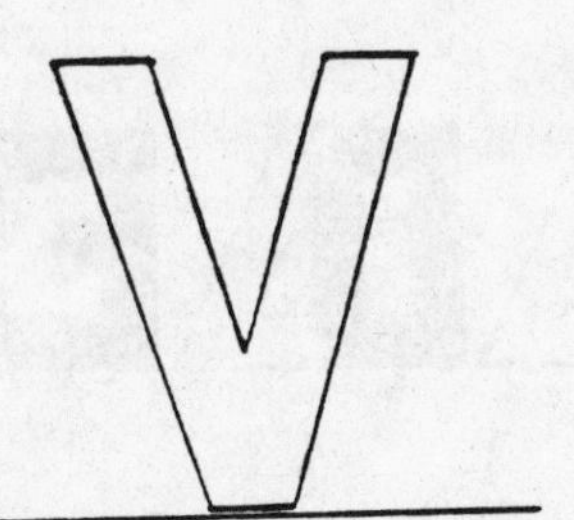

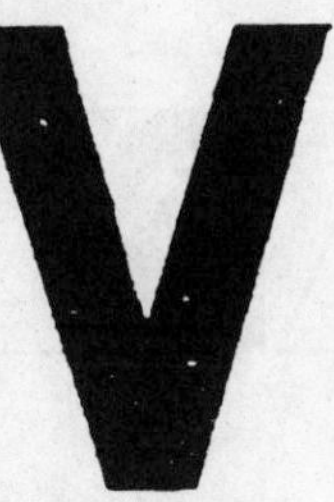

(j) Demonstrate and have your learners make as many other turned-over letters as possible. These are the most difficult letters to make using the lettering stencil.

4 *Words*

(a) Ask learners to letter a word that has different kinds of letters, such as *mother* or *family*. This will give them practice in making different letters and spacing the letters.
(b) Ask learners to letter their own first and last names, the name of their own health post or hospital, or some phrase (such as 'Birth Control Methods' or 'Small Families Can Live Better'). This will give them practice in making different kinds of letters, spacing the letters, and spacing the words.
(c) Learners can fill in the letters with colour.

LETTERING STENCILS

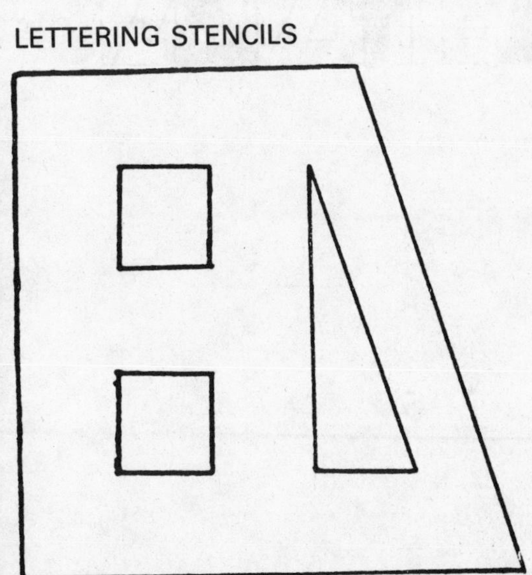

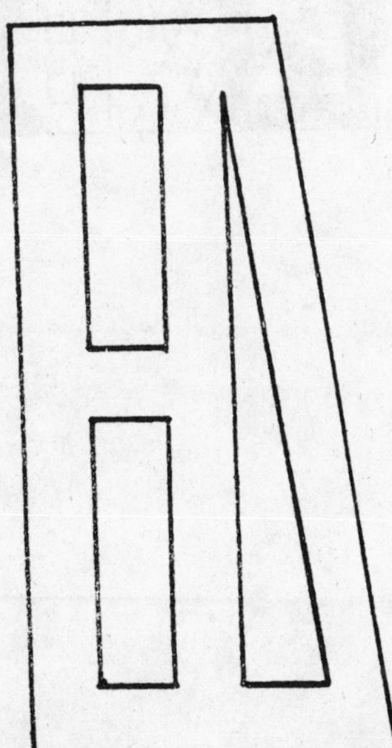

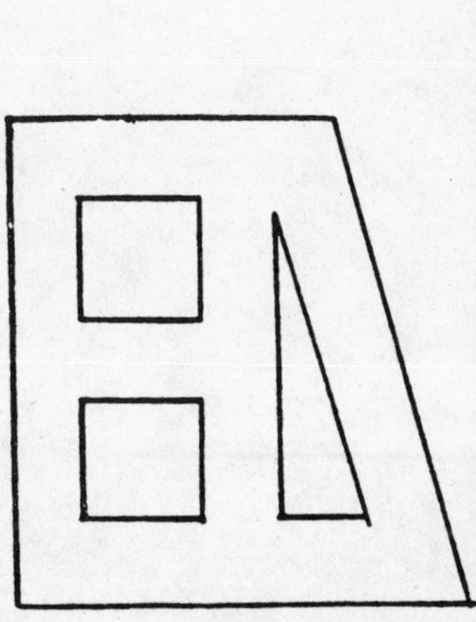

ALPHABET GUIDE TO USING LETTERING STENCILS

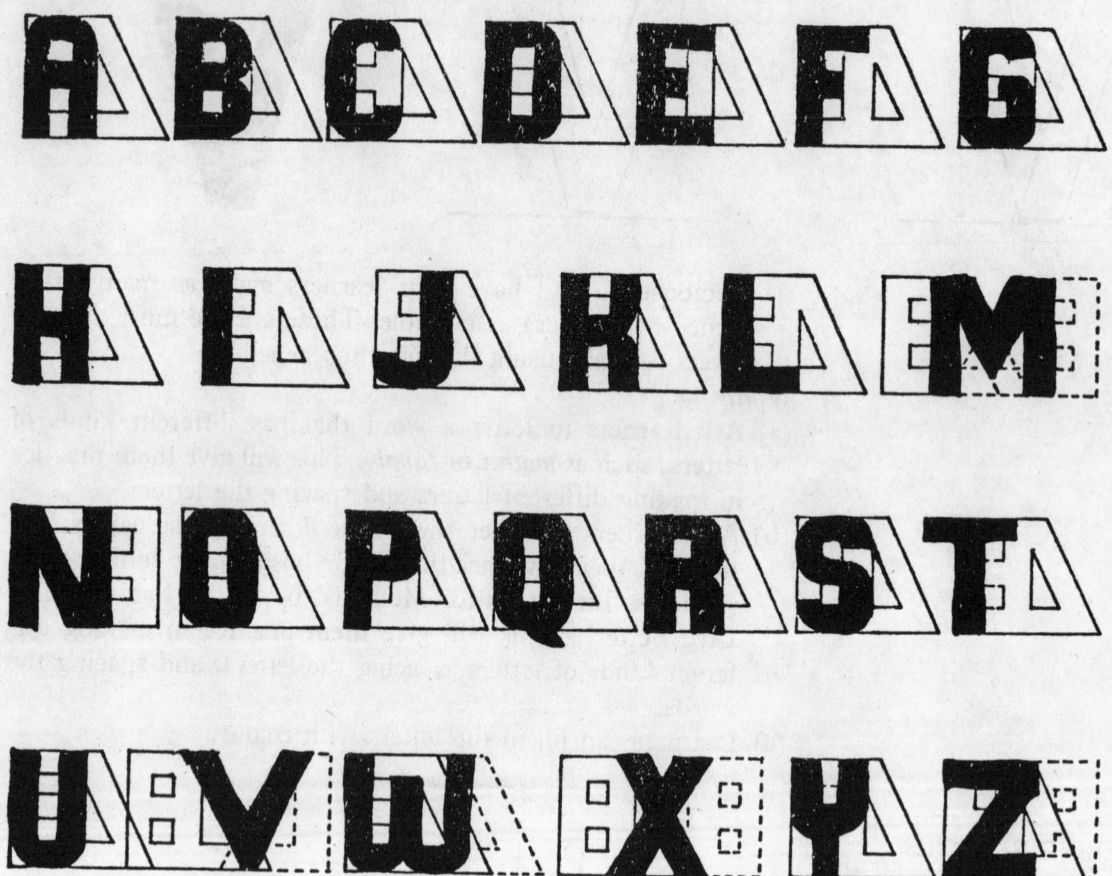

Using colour

Objectives

Learners will choose colours for a visual aid by the guidelines presented in Activity 1 and colour a visual aid with whatever materials are available for colouring.

Learners will combine colours of paints to make new colours and shades of colour. (Optional)

Information and notes to the trainer

Review comments in Unit 2 on the use of colour.

Learners need to have practice in choosing the colours for a visual aid and in using available materials for colouring. Adding colour to a visual aid makes the tracing or sketch a finished product.

Two activities are included in this section. The first, **Colouring visual aids,** gives practice in combining colours and in using colouring materials. The second activity, **Mixing colours to make new colours and shades of colour,** is especially useful where paint is available. The activity shows how to make several colours from only 5 basic colours.

Be sure you practice using whatever colouring materials are available in your area. You will need to give your learners some guidelines for using them.

Present the information that follows before learners follow the instructions in Activity 1. You will need to prepare the examples ahead of time to show everyone.

The choice of colour for a visual aid can either help a person's understanding or it can cause problems in their understanding. We have already discussed several uses of colour. Do you remember what they are? (See Unit 2).

Answers:

(a) To help make the visual aid more *readable* by showing contrast.

(b) To *direct the eye of the learner to important information.*

RASH

Dots and word 'rash' coloured red

(c) To *gain and hold the learner's attention* by making the visual aid interesting and attractive.
(Show any visual aid you think your learners will find attractive. It should be in colour.)

(d) To present the health message in a way that is *culturally appropriate* to the people who will see it by choosing colours according to their special meanings within a given community.
(Remind participants of the previous discussion on the cultural appropriateness of colour, Unit 2. Recall any examples of special uses of colour that were mentioned.)

It will be important for you to remember these uses of colour in completing this activity. Remember that colours should be chosen for a reason instead of by chance.

The choice of colour combination is especially important for the *readability* of the visual aid. Look at these examples of colour combinations. Which combination shows the most contrast?

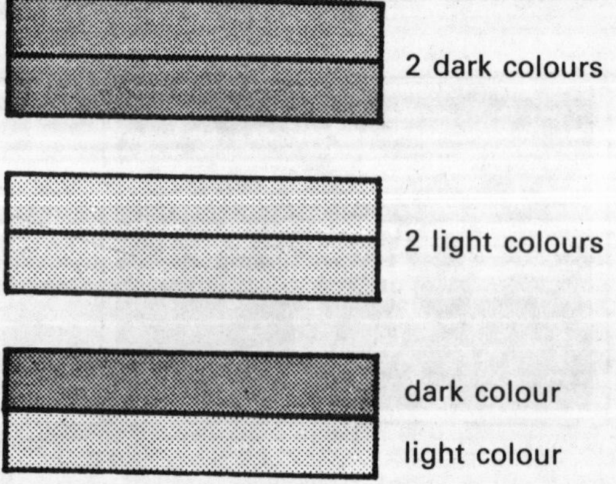

Answer: Light and dark combination. The contrast is greatly reduced when two dark colours or two light colours are side by side.

Look at these two examples. Which one is most readable?

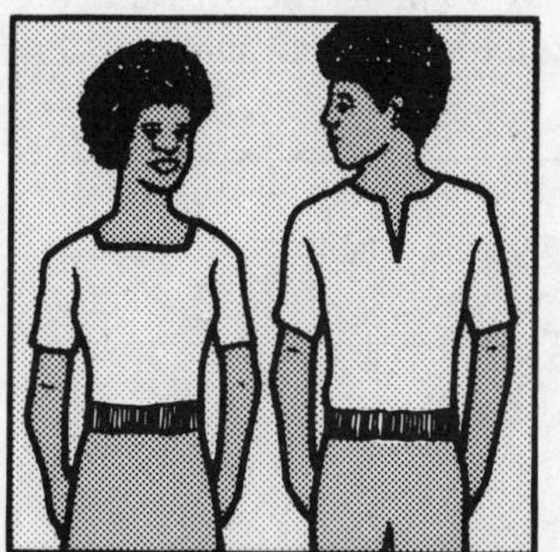

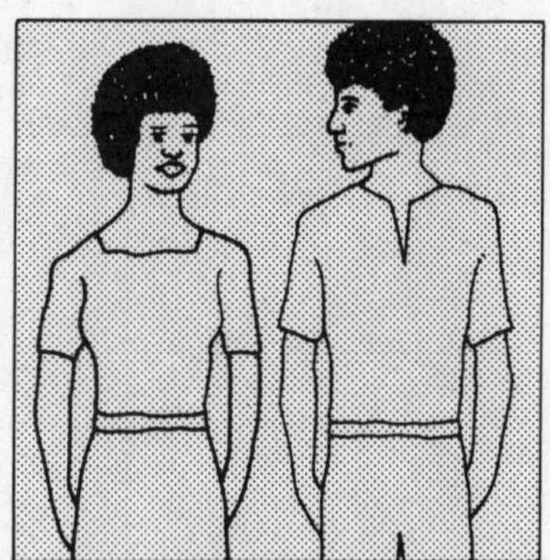

Answer: The one outlined in black because it helps to separate the different colours and to make the figures in the visual aid stand out.

You can improve readability by combining colours carefully so that each colour is easy to see and by outlining the figures in black.

Activity 1

Colouring visual aids

Time

20 minutes

Objective

Learners will colour a visual aid so that it is readable, attractive, and uses colour in the way that their intended learners do.

Materials

Visual aid for each learner to colour.
Colouring materials for each learner, such as paints and brushes, inks, crayons or coloured pencils. You can use the paints from the next activity, **Mixing colours**, if you want.
Heavy drawing paper, if paints are used.

Instructions

This activity gives practice in colouring visual aids so that they are readable, attractive, and use colour in the way that their intended learners do.

You can combine this activity with any other activity in this manual that produces a visual aid. The last visual aid in **Sketching and tracing** is used as the example. Any other drawing that has been traced or sketched will work just as well for this colouring activity.

1 Choose a visual aid from other sections of this manual to colour. You may want learners to use the last visual aid completed in the **Sketching and tracing** section.

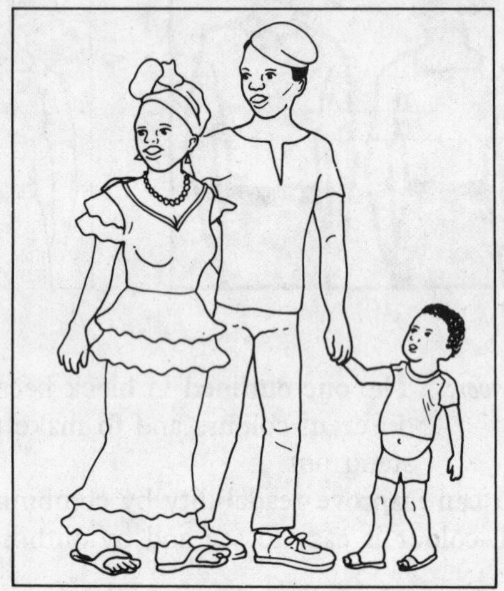

2 Ask everyone to colour the visual aid so that they can use it with their own learners. Remind them to choose the colour combinations carefully and to outline the figures in black.

3 Remind your learners to use attractive colours. They should also use colours in the way that their intended learners do.

4 Give them any special instructions for the type of colouring materials they are using.

Paints require special instructions. It is easier to allow each colour to dry before painting another colour beside it. Painting is faster if you decide ahead of time the colours for each area of the visual aid. Paint all the areas of the same colour first. For example, paint all the red that will be in the visual aid. After the first colour has dried, paint all the areas of another colour. For example, paint all the blue that will be in the visual aid.

5 Tell learners that they should be careful to stay within the lines of each area of the visual aid they are colouring.

6 When everyone has finished, display the coloured visual aids so they are easy to see. Discuss the use of colour in each: Is it

readable? Is it attractive? Are the colours used in the way their intended learners use them? Allow your learners to offer suggestions for improving the colouring of the visual aids.

Possible adaptation

Learners can find their own picture to colour or colour a drawing they have been working on during the workshop.

Activity 2 Mixing colours to make new colours and shades of colour

Time

Will vary depending on how the activity is conducted: demonstration by the trainer, small group work, or individual work.

Objective

Learners will make new colours and shades of colour by mixing the basic colours, and white and black.

Materials

Red, blue, yellow, white, and black paint.
Small containers for mixing paint.
Stirring instruments, such as thin strips of wood or bamboo.
Enlarged drawing of the colour wheel included at the end of this activity (on paper or on a chalkboard).
Colouring materials for the enlarged colour wheel (ink, crayons, paint, or coloured chalk).

Instructions

This activity can be done as a demonstration, as small group work, or as individual work, depending on the time and supplies you have available. It is a good idea to have learners do the paint combinations, either in small groups or as individual work, if it is at all possible. Remember, people learn more by doing than by just watching!

If you must demonstrate the combinations, be sure everyone can see. You might want to pass the paint around the group after each combination. See the guidelines for demonstrations included in Unit 5.

You can enlarge the colour wheel on a piece of paper or chalkboard so that everyone can see. Colour in the areas labelled on the colour wheel one at a time as you go through the activity.

The colours of paint made in this activity can be used in Activity 1, if you like.

Combining primary colours to make secondary colours

1 Display the colour wheel that you traced or enlarged with the areas for the primary colours already coloured in (red, yellow, and blue). Explain that these are basic or *primary* colours from which other colours can be made.
If possible, provide a copy of an unlabelled colour wheel for each learner (see below left) and ask them to colour in the areas in the colour wheel as you go through the activity. They can use the paints, crayons, ink, or coloured pencils.

2 Combine equal amounts of each *pair* of primary colours until you have made all the possible combinations of primary colours. (Red and yellow; red and blue; blue and yellow.)

3 Ask the learners what new colours are made for each of the combinations of primary colours. The combinations are called *secondary* colours. (See below right.)
Answers: red and yellow makes orange;
red and blue makes violet;
blue and yellow makes green.

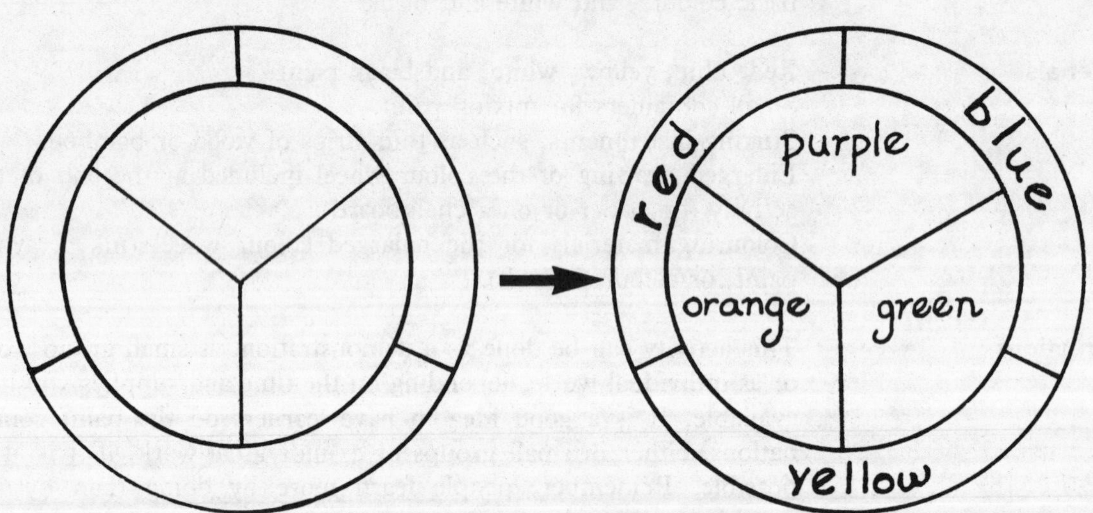

4 Colour in the areas for the 3 secondary colours on the colour wheel you have displayed. If learners have their own copies of the colour wheel, ask them to colour in the areas on their copies.

Making shades of colour by combining colours with white or black

1 Tell the participants they can make *shades* of colour by adding white or black to the colour. A *shade* is a lighter or darker version of a colour.

2 Pour a small amount of each primary and secondary colour into separate containers.
3 Add a small amount of white to each and stir. Each of the colours will become a shade lighter than they were. The more white added, the lighter the colour will become.
4 Pour a small amount of each primary and secondary colour into separate containers.
5 Add a small amount of black to each and stir. Each of the colours will become a shade darker than they were. The more black added, the darker the colour will become.

Making common colours

1 *Brown.* Shades of brown can be made in two different ways:
  (a) Mix yellow and green to make yellow-green. Add drops of red until you have made brown.
  (b) Mix yellow and orange to make yellow-orange. Add drops of black until you have made brown.
2 *Grey.* Mix white with black or equal parts of any two secondary colours.
3 Colour of *seawater*. Mix blue and green to make blue-green. Mix blue and blue-green. Add drops of either black or white until you have made the colour you want.
4 *Sky* colour. Mix a small amount of white with blue. Add a few drops of red or yellow until you have made the colour you want.

COLOUR WHEEL

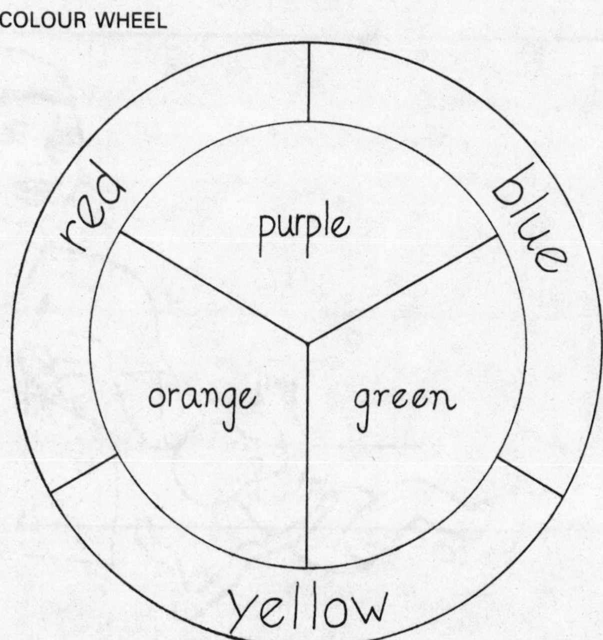

Making teaching/learning models

Objectives

This set of activities should enable learners to make simple models which:

1 can help them to discover solutions to problems on their own; and

2 can be used to demonstrate and to provide practice in a procedure or process.

Information and notes to the trainer

Models can be excellent visual aids when it is impossible to demonstrate or practise with a real object or person. They can help learners discover principles or solutions to problems. They can be used to demonstrate and practise skills.

The two activities included here give instructions for making and using two different models. Activity 1 shows how to make a 'gourd baby' for discovering the signs of dehydration in babies and small children. Activity 2 shows how to make a delivery box or 'birthing box', placenta, and cord to demonstrate and practise delivery skills.

Both of these models use low-cost, everyday types of materials. If some of the materials needed for the activities are not available in your area, use your imagination to think of other materials you can use. By using locally available materials you can make simple but effective models.

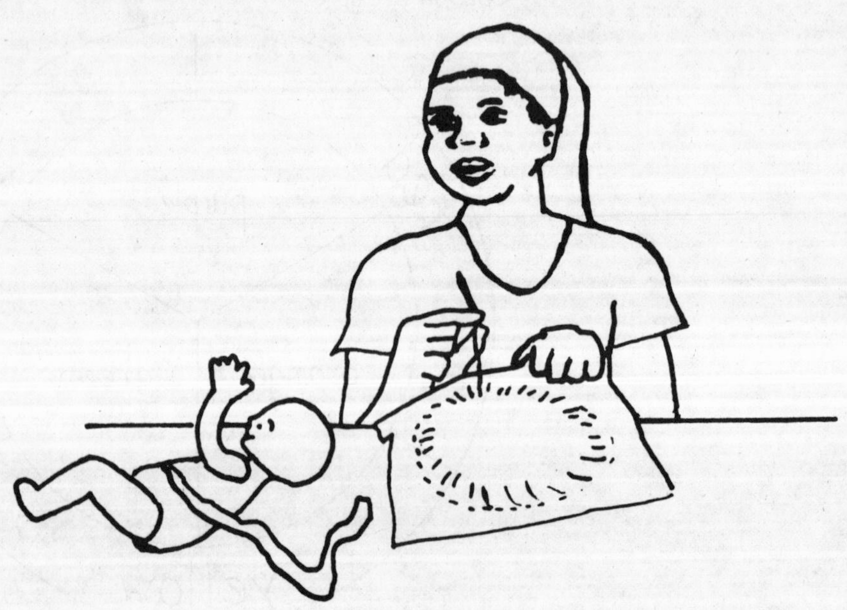

Activity 1

Making models to discover solutions to problems: a 'gourd baby' model for discovering the signs of dehydration

Time

1 hour

Objective

Learners will make a 'gourd baby' and will practise using it to discover the signs of dehydration.

Materials

Gourd, tin can, or plastic bottle.
Knife or other cutting tool.
Paint or pen.
Small piece of thin cloth cut into a square.
Water.
Sticks or corks to serve as plugs.

Instructions

Dehydration is the loss of water in the body tissues. It is a common problem among infants and children in many places. It usually results from diarrhoea.

There are many rumours and traditions throughout the world which prevent correct treatment of dehydration. In some places, people believe the brains have slipped down and caused the baby's diarrhoea. In other places, people believe they should not give anything to drink or eat to a child or baby with diarrhoea. These rumours and traditions are extremely dangerous to the health of babies and small children.

The instructions which follow will enable your learners to make a 'gourd baby'. This model allows people to figure out for themselves the signs of dehydration and the need for rehydration when a baby has diarrhoea. If gourds are not available, tin cans and plastic bottles can be used instead.

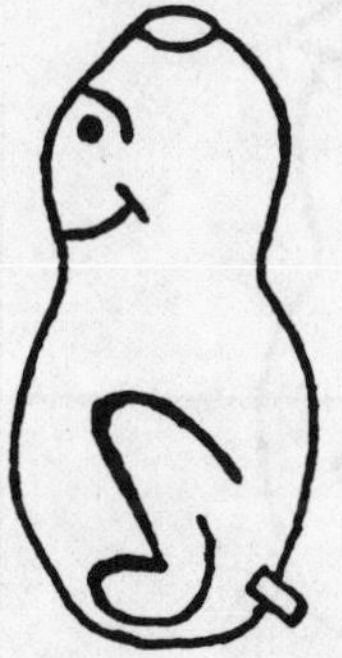

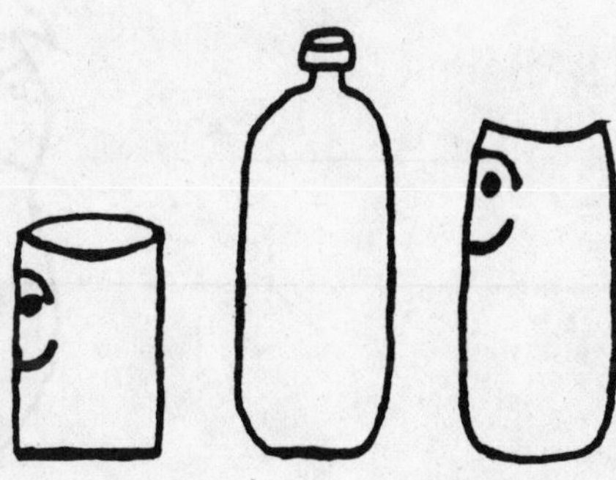

Making the gourd baby

1 Cut off the top of the gourd. Scoop out the seeds and allow the gourd to dry.
2 Make a small hole near the bottom of the gourd and plug the hole with a stick or cork.
3 Draw a mouth, eyes, eyebrows, and legs onto the gourd, as shown here.
4 Fill the gourd to the very top with water.

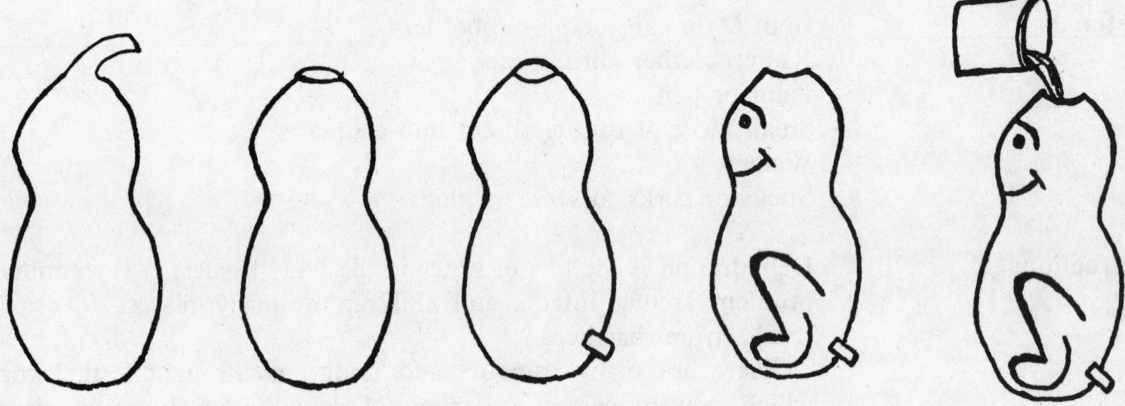

Ways to use the gourd baby to teach the signs of dehydration

Exercise 1. (See diagrams below.)

1 Cover the top of the gourd with a thin, wet piece of cloth or paper. The cloth or thin paper should be touching the water in the gourd.
2 Pull the plug and ask your learners to watch what happens to the cloth (soft spot) on the gourd baby's head. (The cloth will sink in.)

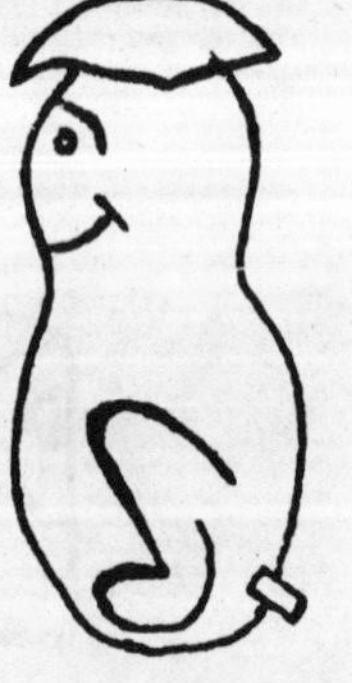

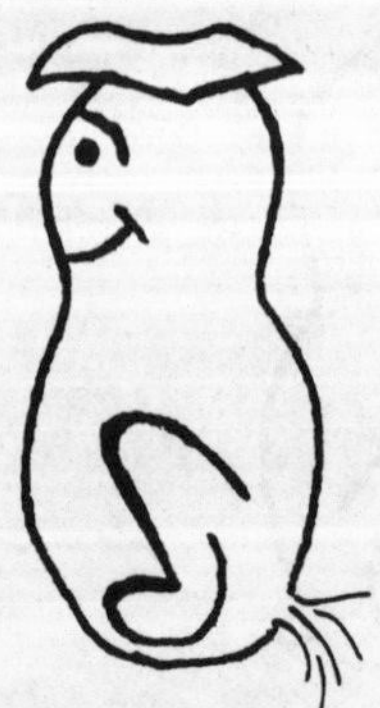

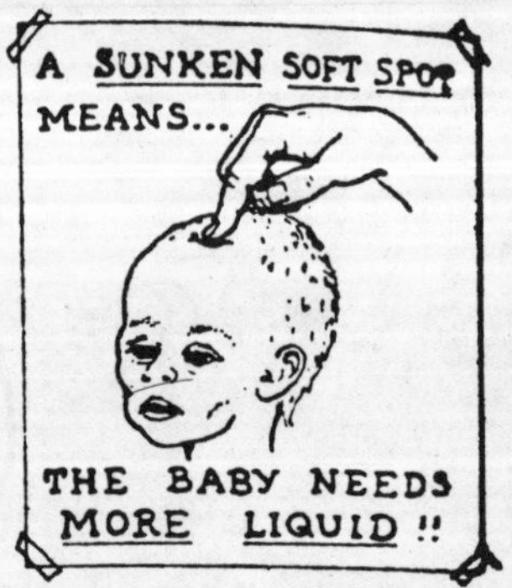

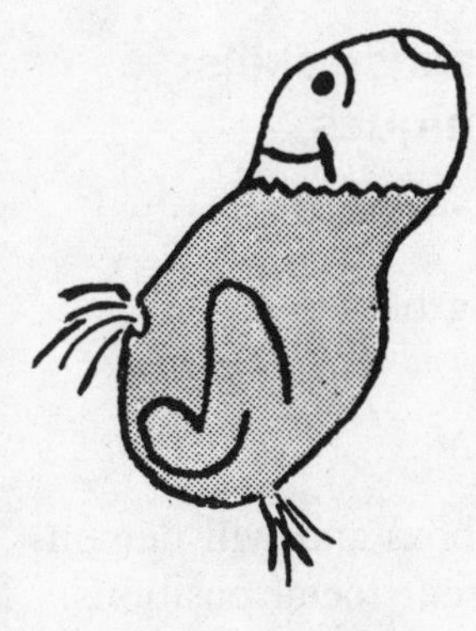

3 Ask questions, such as:
Why did the cloth sink in? (Too much water going out too quickly.)
What does the baby need to make the soft spot rise again? (More water.)

4 In this way, the group learns that one of the signs of dehydration in a baby is the sunken soft spot.

Exercise 2. (See diagrams left.)

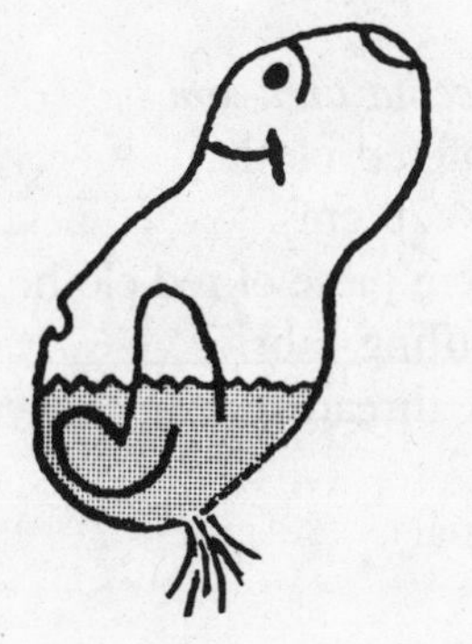

1 Make a hole in the lower front of the gourd baby (for urination) and put a plug in it.
2 Fill the gourd baby again with water.
3 Tilt the baby backwards and unplug both of the holes.

4 When the gourd baby has lost a lot of liquid, he no longer passes urine (even though the diarrheoa continues).

5 In this way, your learners discover that a child who passes little or no urine is probably dehydrated.

Exercise 3. (See diagrams below.)

1 Make a small hole in the corner of each eye.

2 Again fill the gourd baby with water.
3 When the gourd is full of water, it forms 'tears'.

4 Pull both plugs at the bottom of the gourd baby.
5 When the water level drops, tears no longer form.
6 In this way, your learners discover that if a baby does not form tears when he cries, he is probably dehydrated.

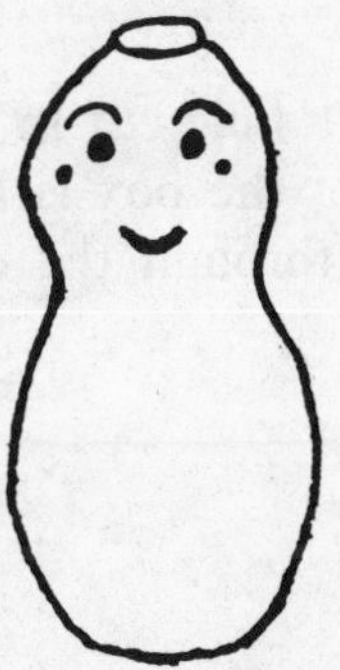

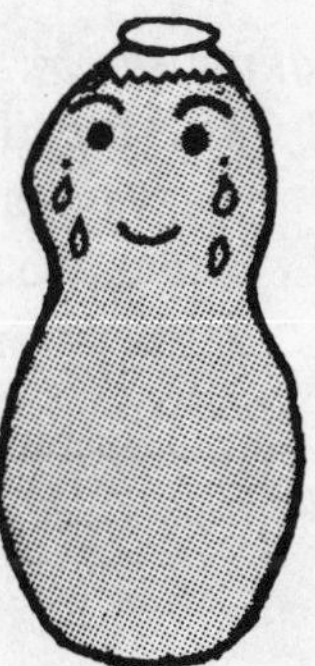

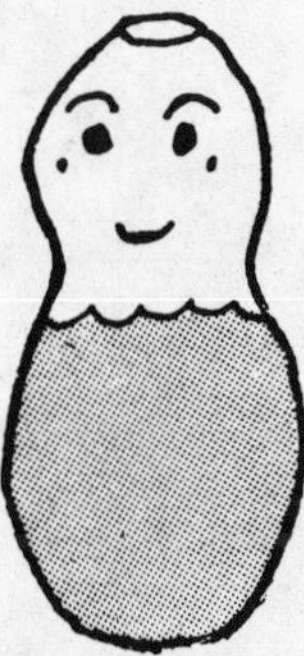

Activity 2 — Making models to demonstrate and practise skills: a birthing box to practise delivery techniques

Time

20 minutes to make the birthing box
20 minutes to make adaptations to the birthing box
50 minutes to make the placenta and cord
30 to 60 minutes to practise using the box

Objective

Learners will make a 'birthing box' (delivery box) and will demonstrate at least one delivery technique for different foetal positions.

Materials

For the birthing box
Cardboard box.
Ruler.
Pencil.
Sharp cutting tool.
Child's doll.
Paint (optional).
Tape (optional).
Elastic material (optional).

For the placenta and cord
2 squares of red cloth (20 cm × 20 cm).
65 cm × 5 cm piece of red cloth.
Padding/stuffing fabric.
Needle and thread.
Scissors.
Pins (optional).

Instructions

Midwives, nurses, and traditional birth attendants who will be responsible for assisting in deliveries need to know what to do in both usual and unusual deliveries. During their training, they will probably observe and assist in deliveries. But they may not have the opportunity to ask questions during the delivery. They also may not have the opportunity to see unusual deliveries, such as breech births.

The birthing box is a simple model which can be used to demonstrate delivery techniques. It can provide practice in the steps for assisting in a delivery. The trainer can demonstrate each step, ask and answer questions, and supervise the learners as they practise the steps.

Making the birthing box

1 The birthing box has a hole cut in one of its sides to represent the vagina. The top of the box is left open so that the trainer can move the 'baby' through the opening to demonstrate the delivery process.

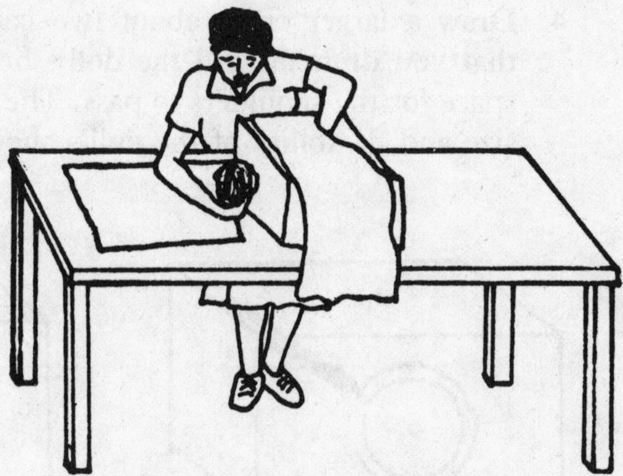

2 Use a ruler to find the centre of one of the *longer* sides of the box. Mark the spot with a pencil or pen. (This will be the centre of the vaginal opening.)

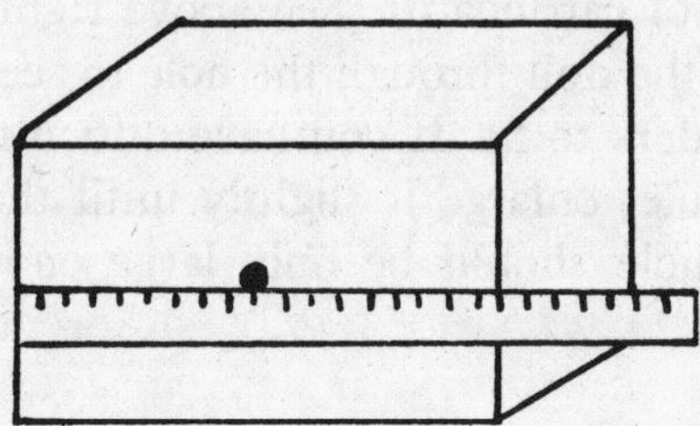

3 You will need to have a doll in order to know what size to make the hole in the box. Place the top of the doll's head against the centre of the box. Use a pencil to draw a circle on the box by drawing around the head of the doll as shown below. It is easiest to start at the top of the head and draw a half circle to the right. Return to the top of the head and draw a half circle to the left.

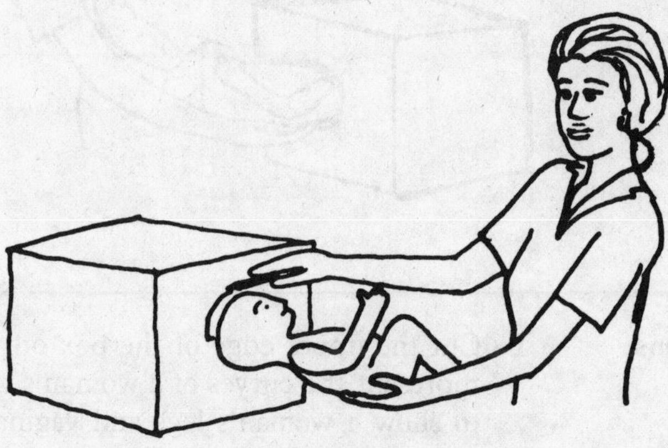

4 Draw a larger circle about two centimetres outside the circle that you drew around the doll's head. This larger hole makes space for the shoulders to pass. The exact size will vary with the size and flexibility of the doll's shoulders.

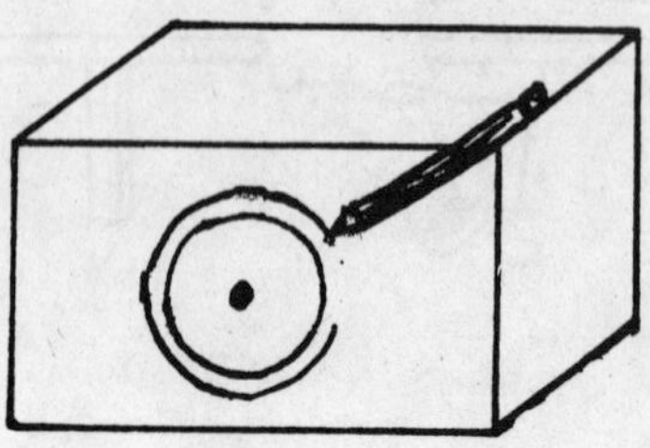

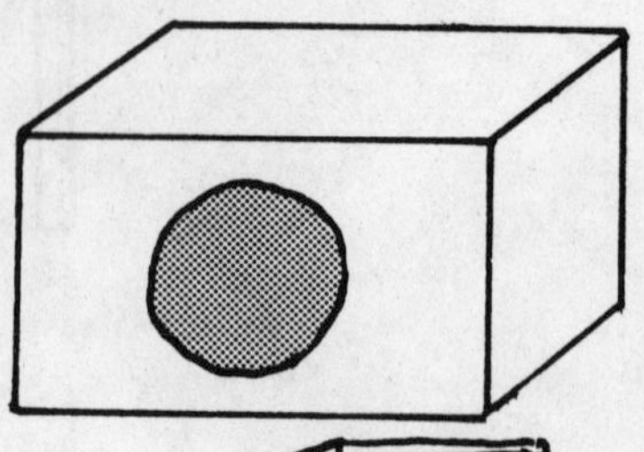

5 Carefully cut along the lines of the larger circle using a sharp cutting tool such as an old surgical knife. Remove the centre piece of cardboard. (See above right.)

6 Push the doll through the hole to see if it is large enough for the shoulders to fit. If you have difficulty pushing the doll through the hole, enlarge it slightly until the doll will pass through it. The hole should be only large enough for the doll to fit, no larger.

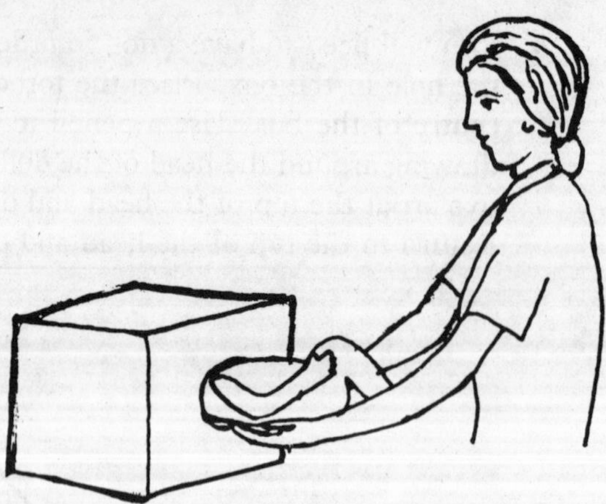

Possible adaptations

1 Cut the upper edge of the box on the side with the opening to represent the curves of a woman's legs. Paint the side of the box to show a woman's legs and vagina.

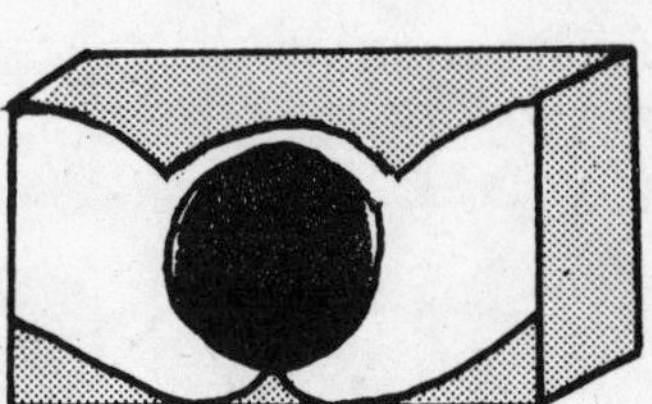

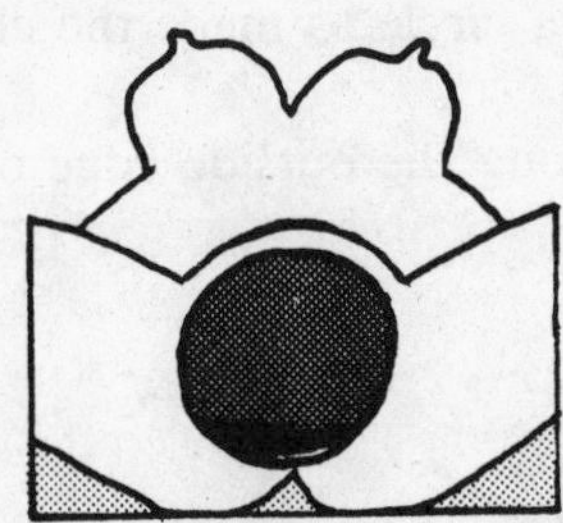

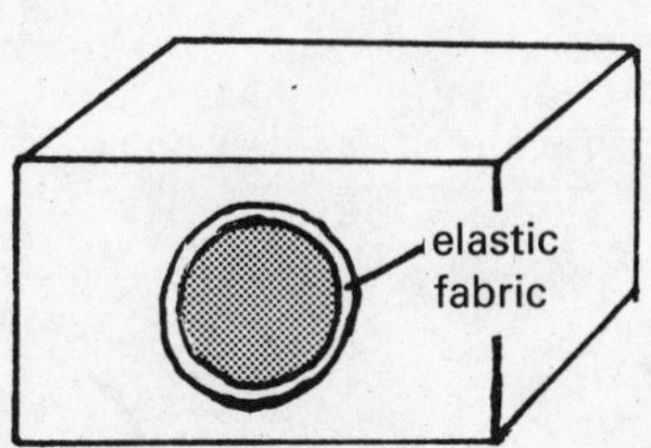

2 On the opposite side from the opening, cut the top flap of the box to look like breasts. Tape the flap in an upright position so that the breasts show above the top of the box. Then have learners practise putting the baby to the breast right after birth to prevent haemorrhage and to push out the placenta.

3 To make the opening more flexible, like the vagina, you can wrap the edge of the opening with any kind of elastic material and staple the material to the box. Some of the materials which could be used are: old nylon stockings; the fabric that goes under casts for broken bones (knit stockinette); or very wide elastic like the type sometimes used in sewing.

Instructions

Making the placenta and cord

1 Cut 2 pieces of red cloth into a 20 cm square. (It is easier to place one piece of cloth over the other and cut them at the same time. This way they are both the same size.) These pieces of cloth will make the placenta.

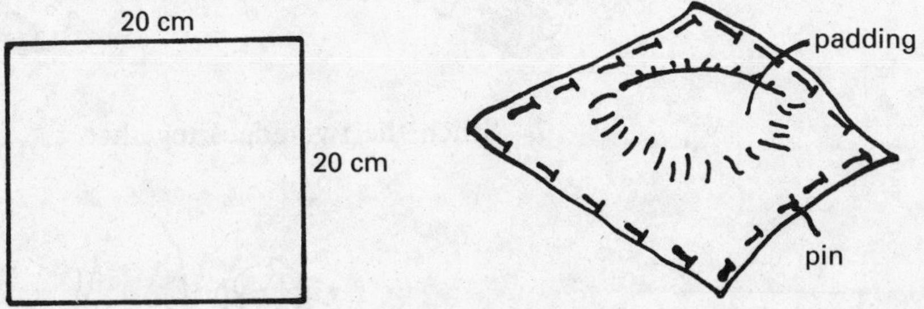

2 Place a piece of thin padding or old cloth scraps between the two squares of red cloth. Put pins around the edges of the square to hold the 2 pieces of cloth together. (If you do not have pins, loosely stitch the pieces of cloth together around the edges.)

3 Stitch a circle to make the cloth placenta shape.

4 Cut along the outside edge of the stitched circle.

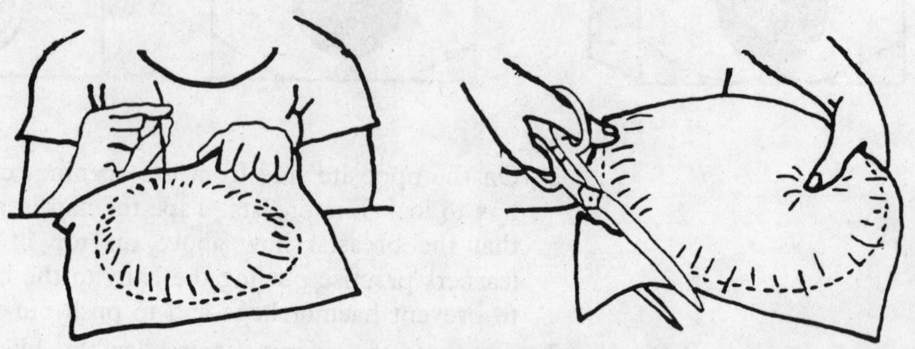

5 Cut a piece of red cloth (like that used for the placenta) to a 65 cm by 5 cm size. This piece of cloth will be the umbilical cord.

6 Fold one of the long edges of the cloth over to meet the other edge.

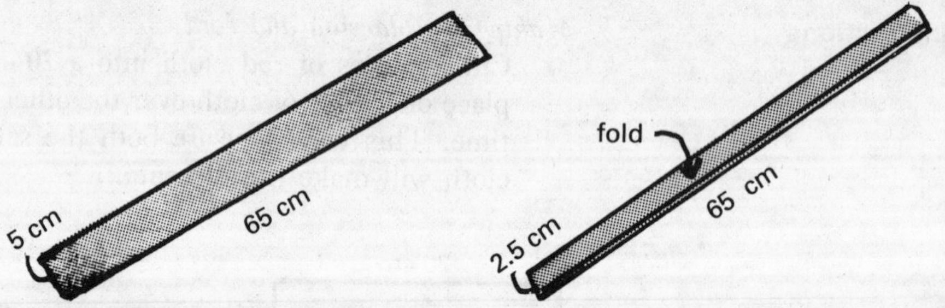

7 Stitch the two edges together.

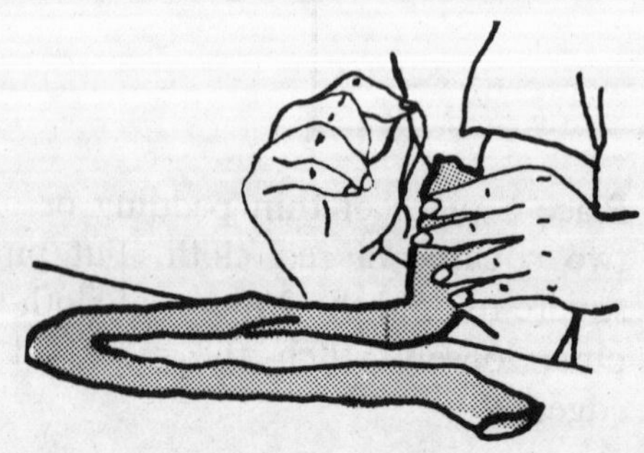

8 If you would like, you can turn the stitched cloth inside out so that the stitches are inside the cord.
9 Sew the cord securely to the centre of the placenta and loosely to the doll where the navel would be.

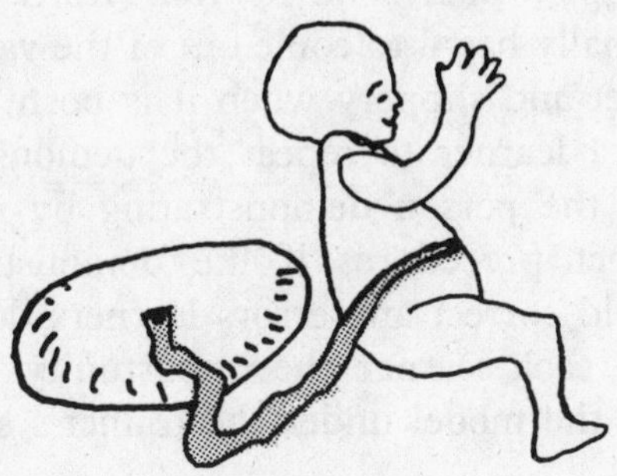

You will want to cut the cord during the demonstration, so you may want to make several cords or sew the cloth back together after cutting it.

Instructions

Using the birthing box

1 Place the birthing box on top of a table. Leave space on the table in front of the box for 'catching' the baby as it comes out of the box.
2 Demonstrate any of the following delivery techniques:
(a) Usual delivery (head presented first – see below left)
(b) Unusual deliveries:
(1) Buttocks presented first (breech – see below centre)
(2) Foot or arm presented first (see below right)

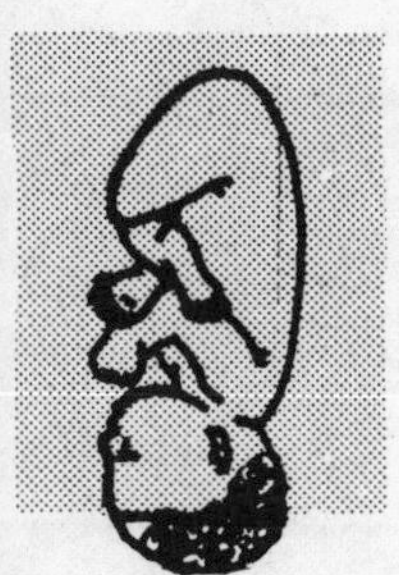

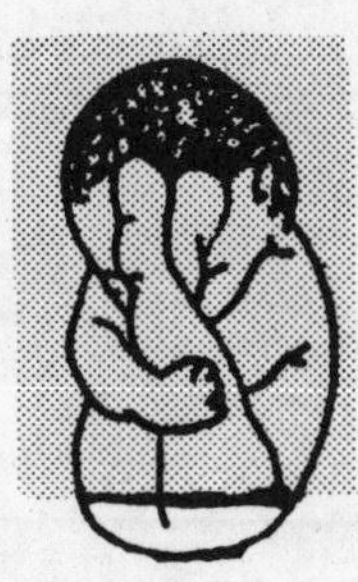

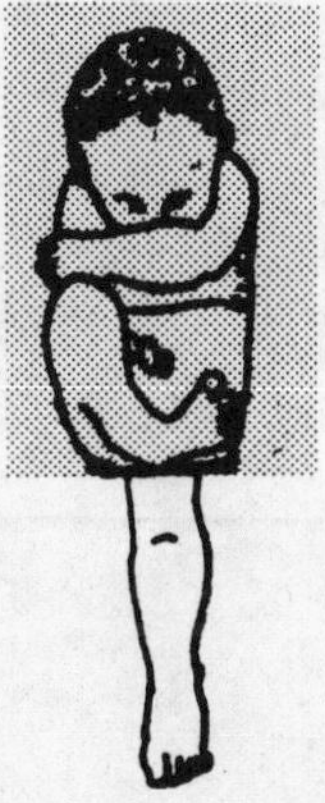

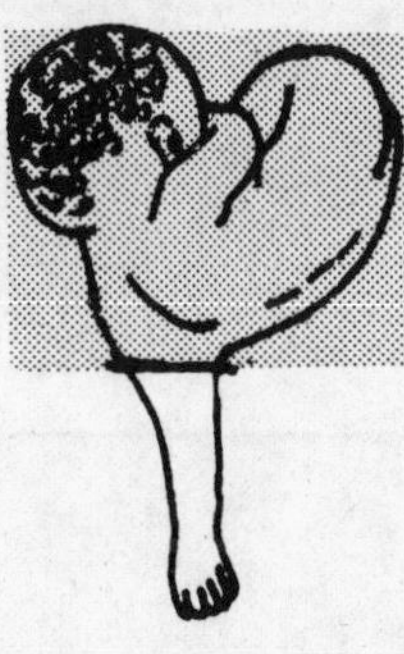

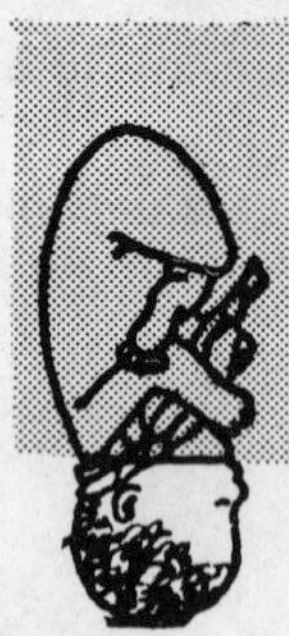

(3) Cord wrapped around the baby's neck (see left)

3 For each demonstration, do one step at a time, explaining what you are doing. Give learners the opportunity to ask questions as you go through the steps. Explain the differences between a real delivery and the practice delivery using the model. (For example, point out to your learners when the blood would normally begin to come out of the vagina. Explain that the baby is wet and slippery when it is born.)

4 Ask a learner to repeat the demonstration. Ask the others to help the person demonstrating by recalling the steps and the correct procedures if the demonstrator forgets. The trainer should correct any errors learners do not see.

5 Give each learner the opportunity to practise the procedures with the model under the trainer's supervision.

Evaluation

1 Ask your learners the following questions:
(a) How was the use of the model helpful to you in learning to perform a new procedure?
(b) Did the model make it difficult for you to learn the new procedure? If so, how?

2 Ask yourself the following questions:
(a) Did the model help me to teach my learners what I wanted them to be able to do? How many were able to perform the procedure correctly after the demonstration and practice?
(b) Did I use the model as well as I might have? How could I improve my use of the model?
(c) Was the model easy to use? Will it last for many activities?

Making rope and pole displays

Objective

These activities should enable learners to construct 1 or 2 different types of portable displays.

Information and notes to the trainer

Displays can be very helpful to trainers or health educators. They can attract attention or provide information to other people when the trainer or health educator cannot be present. See Unit 2 for an example of using a display.

These activities will show your learners how to construct 2 different kinds of display. Both displays are easy to make and portable.

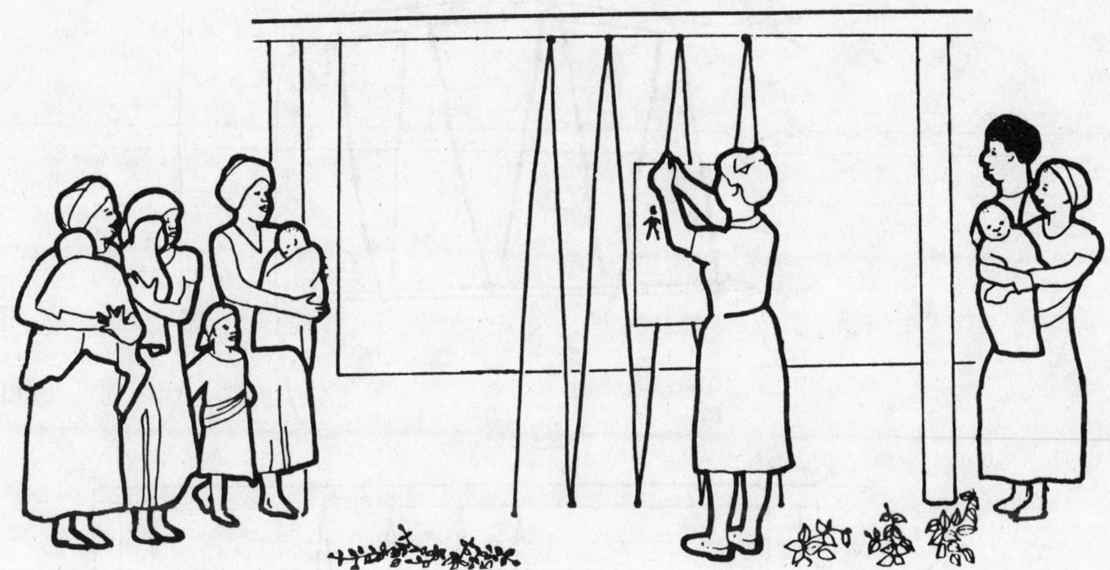

Activity 1

Making a rope display

Time

30 minutes

Materials

Rope or heavy string.
Pole(s).
Small hooks or nails (optional).
Pictures, posters, real objects (to be displayed).

Instructions

1 Choose a location for the display. It can be under a tree, inside a building, beside a building, outside in the open, or any place where it will be seen by the people you want to teach.

2 Your location will determine how you construct the rope display.

(a) If you have chosen to place the display under a tree, you can use a tree branch to loop the rope over. Put a pole in the bottom of the rope loops to hold them in place, as shown in the picture below.

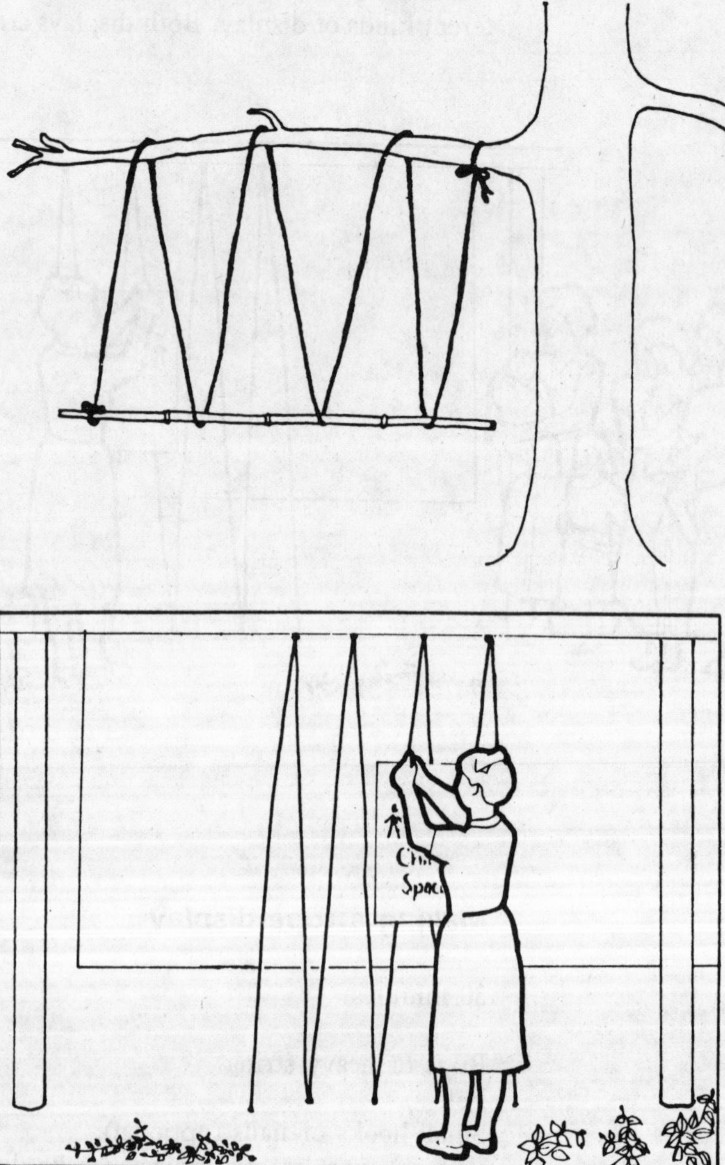

(b) If you put the display beside a building, you can attach the rope loops to the roof overhang using small hooks or nails. Insert a pole in the bottom of the rope loops. Or attach the bottom of the rope loops to the ground using nails or sticks. In the example in Unit 2, Mrs Goko used long nails (see previous page).

(c) If you put the display inside a building, you can attach the rope loops to the ceiling and the floor using nails or small hooks (see below).

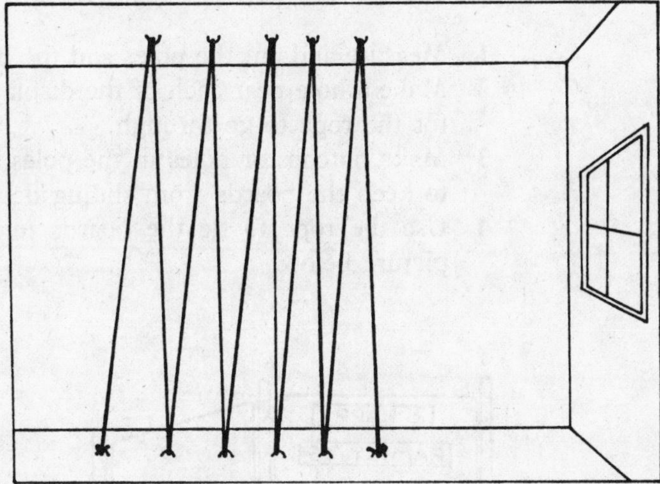

3 You can attach pictures, real objects, posters, or other materials to the ropes with pins or string.

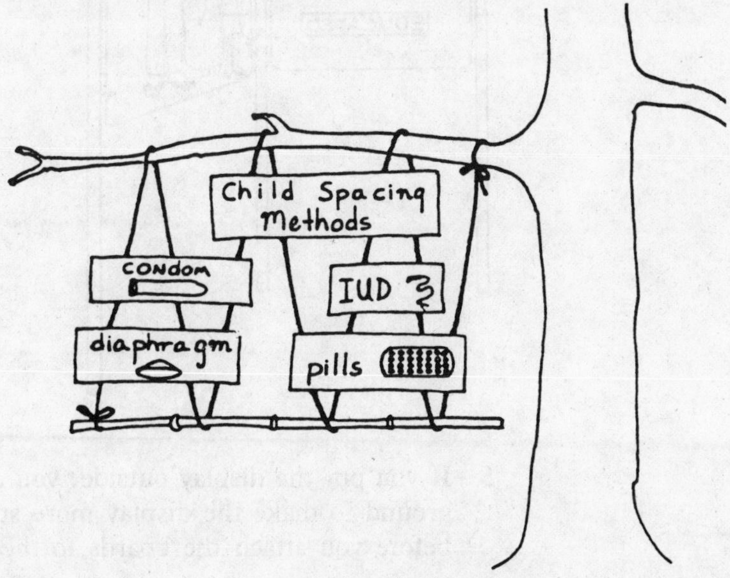

Activity 2

Making a pole display

Time

1 hour

Materials

Hand saw.
Measuring tape (optional).
3 poles, about 3–4 cm. in diameter.
2 pieces of thin, lightweight plywood, wallboard, or pegboard.
Rope, heavy string, or wire.

Instructions

1 Measure and cut the poles and the boards to the size you want.
2 Make a hole near each of the display board corners big enough for the rope to go through.
3 Make notches or holes in the poles where the rope will be tied to keep the boards from sliding down.
4 Use the rope to tie the boards to the poles as shown in the picture below.

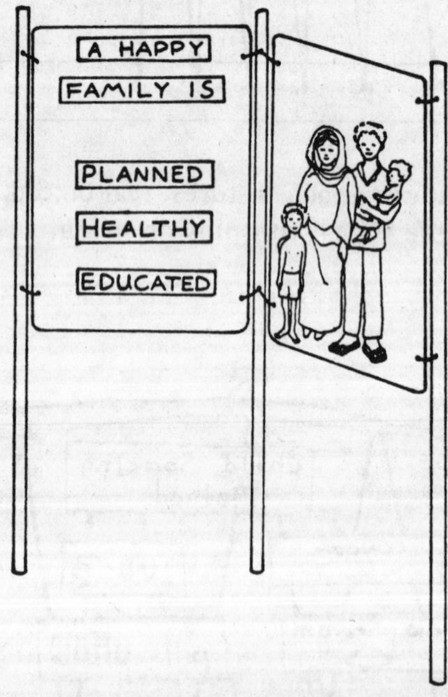

5 If you put the display outside, you can push the poles into the ground to make the display more stable. It is easier to do this before you attach the boards to the poles. Make sure the dis-

tance between the poles is the same as the width of the display boards.

6 If you put the display inside a building, it should stand up without any other support as long as the poles are *not* placed in a straight line.

7 You can attach pictures, real objects, posters, or other materials to the display boards with tape or small nails. Or you can paint your visual aid directly on the display boards if you want it to last a long time.

Possible adaptations

1 You can make a larger display by adding more poles and more display panels.

2 You can use different materials for the display panels, such as cloth or woven mats. If you use cloth or mats, be sure the poles are pushed into the ground to make the display sturdy.

Making your own supplies: paste, chalk, modelling dough and paint

Objective

Learners will make one or more of the supplies included in this set of activities by using locally available ingredients.

Information and notes to the trainer

Sometimes, especially in rural areas, it is impossible to find some basic supplies for making visual aids. Recipes for paste, chalk, modelling dough and paint are included here. It is a good idea for you to experiment with the recipes before introducing them to your learners. You may have to find other ingredients to use which are more available in your area.

The paste and paint can be used for many purposes in making visual aids. The chalk can be used not only on chalkboards, but also on a board painted with a dark, flat paint or on a board covered with oil cloth. The modelling dough can be used for making models. For example, the gourd baby included in the section on **Making models** can be made from modelling dough. You can also make a small model of a village out of modelling dough to show where latrines must be placed in relation to the houses and water supply.

Evaluation

You can assess the value of these activities in two ways:

1 Can learners make useable supplies from the recipes or from other ingredients which you suggested?
2 Do learners make their own needed supplies when they return to their home areas?

Activity 1

How to make starch paste

Time

10 minutes for flour paste; 1½ hours for rice paste

Objective

Learners will make starch paste from one of the recipes listed below or from other ingredients which you suggest.

Materials

Flour Paste
Wheat, millet, or cassava flour.
(Note: corn flour will not make useful paste. The flour must be sticky when wet.)
Water.
Flour sieve.

Rice paste
1 part rice.
3 parts water.

Instructions

Making flour paste

1. Remove all lumps in the flour by sifting it through a flour sieve.
2. Add water, a little at a time, and stir mixture until the flour is wet. The mixture should be a smooth paste.
3. Store paste in a closed container.

Possible adaptations

1. You can cook the flour and water mixture over low heat while stirring it constantly. Allow to cool before using.
2. You can add insecticide to the flour in areas where insects are a problem. Be sure to store the paste out of reach of children who sometimes eat paste!

Instructions

Making rice paste

1. Cook rice in water as you usually do until rice is moist and sticky. Do not allow rice to become dry. (Brown rice does not work well for making paste.)
2. Drain off any excess water and let rice cool.
3. Put a small amount of cool, sticky rice on the surface to be pasted.
4. With your finger, smooth the rice onto the paper and press out any lumps.
5. Press the other paper to be pasted on top of the rice paste.
6. Store remaining paste in a closed container.

Activity 2

How to make chalk

Time

15–30 minutes of preparation time on different days. The mixture must sit for two nights. So total time before you have finished chalk is 3 days.

Objective

Learners will make chalk from the recipe listed below or from other ingredients which you suggest.

Materials

1 part chalky soil (or other soil that can be used to make a mark).
4 parts water.
Bucket and shovel.
Bag made of muslin or other coarse, porous cloth.
Bamboo (optional).
Dye (optional).

Instructions

1. Shovel some chalky-looking soil into a bucket. Leave room for 4 times as much water as soil.
   You can use any soil found in your area which can be used for marking.
2. Add 4 times as much water as soil. Stir very hard. Crumble large pieces with your hand so that the soil is completely mixed with the water. Do not worry about any rocks or pebbles in the mixture.
3. Allow the soil to sit overnight in the bucket.
4. The next day, carefully pour the water off the top of the soil and water mixture.
5. Pour the top layer of silt from the mixture. The silt is usually several inches thick. This layer will be the chalk.
6. Put the 'chalk' into a bag made of muslin or other coarse, porous cloth. Squeeze as much water out of the bag as you can. Let it drip until the chalk feels like dough or clay. (This will take several hours to one day.)
7. The next day, the chalk will look like clay or bread dough.
8. Roll the chalk into long pieces that look like snakes. Thicker chalk will not break as easily as thin chalk.
9. Cut the chalk to the desired lengths. Let it dry.
10. Try out the chalk by marking on a flat, hard surface. If the soil is the right kind, you have chalk.

Possible adaptations

1. If you want coloured chalk, add any dyes you have to the layer of chalk you have taken from the top of the bucket (step 6).
2. If you want, you can use bamboo stalks as moulds for the chalk. Just split the bamboo stalks and press the chalk into the hollow middle.

Activity 3 **How to make modelling dough and papier mâché**

Time Will depend on recipe used.

Objective Learners will make modelling dough or papier mâché from one of the recipes listed below.

Materials See each recipe listed below.

Instructions

Recipe 1: Modelling dough
Materials:
Equal amounts of wheat, millet, or cassava flour and salt.
Small amount of water.

1. Mix the flour and salt.
2. Add enough water so that the flour and salt mixture feels like bread dough (elastic and not sticky).
3. Knead like bread dough.
4. Store in a closed container.

Recipe 2: Papier mâché
Materials:
Newspapers.
Starch paste. (You can use the flour paste recipe.)

1. Shred newspapers into long, thin pieces.
2. Mix the newspapers with starch paste.
3. Knead the mixture like bread dough.
4. Store in a closed container.

Possible adaptations If you want to have coloured modelling dough or papier mâché, add a dye in the desired colour to the mixture before it is a dough. For example, in Recipe 1, add the dye when you add the water. (You will not need as much water if you add a liquid dye.)

Activity 4 **How to make paint**

Time 30 minutes

Objective Learners will make paint from the recipe listed below or from other ingredients which you suggest.

Materials

60 ml cornstarch (¼ cup).
Small amount of water.
460 ml boiling water (2 cups).
30 ml soap flakes (⅛ cup).
Colouring (dye).

Instructions

This recipe makes good paint for posters.

1 Boil water.
2 Mix the cornstarch with a small amount of water until wet.
3 Stir the wet cornstarch into the boiling water.
4 Bring to boil again, stirring continuously. (Mixture may be a little lumpy.)
5 Remove from heat and stir in the soap flakes.
6 Add the colouring.
7 Store in a closed container.

Unit 5
Using Visual Aids in a Training or Health Education Session

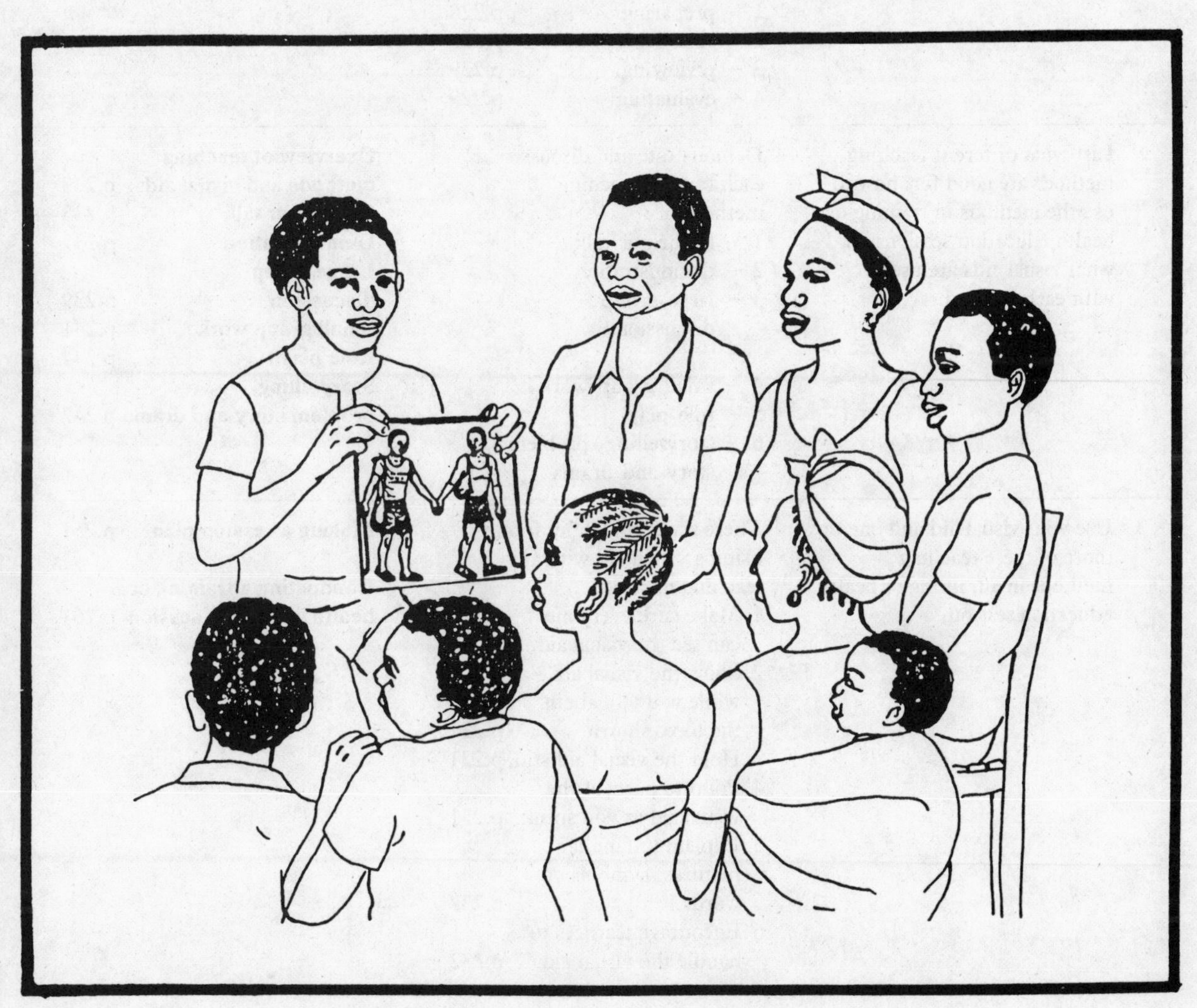

Now your learners know when to use visual aids and how to decide what kind is best. They have planned and made their own visual aids. Unit 5 explores how to use those visual aids effectively with different teaching methods. Using this unit you can guide learners in a review of teaching methods including lecture, demonstration, role play, large group discussion, and small group work as well as storytelling, problem stories and drama. The activities in this unit ask your learners to apply the information and skills they have learned in all the units of the manual. You can use this unit to teach how to plan and how to evaluate a training or health education session. You may want to duplicate parts of this unit also for your learners to use.

Unit 5: Using visual aids in a training or health education session

Objective	Information	Activities
1 Demonstrate several different teaching methods and how to use visual aids with each.	There are 4 parts in a training or health education session, no matter what teaching methods you use. 1 – preparing p.228 2 – conducting p.229 3 – reviewing p.229 4 – evaluating p.229	
2 List what different teaching methods are good for, how to use the methods in training or health education sessions, and what visual aids are useful with each method.	Demonstrate and discuss each kind of teaching method: 1 – lecture or talk 2 – demonstration 3 – large group discussion 4 – small group work 5 – role play 6 – storytelling, problem story and drama	**Overview of teaching methods and visual aids:** p.233 **Lecture or talk** p.235 **Demonstration** p.237 **Large group discussion** p.239 **Small group work** p.241 **Role play** p.244 **Storytelling, problem story and drama** p.247
3 Use your visual aid and one or more of these teaching methods in a training or health education session.	There are 6 guidelines for using a visual aid with any teaching method: 1 Make sure everyone can see the visual aid. p.230 2 Show the visual aid while you talk about the topic shown. p.231 3 Hold the visual aid still. p.231 4 Point to parts of the visual aid as you speak. p.231 5 Explain unfamiliar pictures, symbols or words. p.232 6 Encourage learners to handle the visual aid. p.232	**Making a session plan** p.251 **Conducting a training or health education session** p.261

Evaluation:
At the end of the **Overview** activity, look at learners' lists on the teaching methods. Is much discussion necessary to add other points from the guidelines included in the manual? Do learners understand the importance of using different teaching methods?

Evaluate the learners' lesson plans with each person individually. More specific evaluation ideas are included with Activity 2, **Making a session plan.**

In Activity 3, **Conducting a training or health education session,** you can evaluate the learners' skills in carrying out their lesson plans by using the observation form. You can tell how well all of your learners understand this unit by looking at their evaluations of each other on the observation forms.

Parts of a training or health education session using any teaching method.

The first thing to do when planning a session is to answer the 7 teaching questions. As mentioned in Unit 2, it is important to think about the first 4 teaching questions (1 What is the problem? 2 Who are my learners? 3 What do I want them to be able to do? 4 Where will the instruction take place?) when deciding what kind of teaching method or methods to use. Combining different methods and using visual aids is usually more effective and interesting to your learners.

After you have decided what teaching methods and visual aids will be best, you must then think about *how to use* the methods and visual aids in the actual training or health education session.

An effective session has 4 parts, no matter what teaching method you use. These four parts are:

1 preparing,
2 conducting,
3 reviewing, and
4 evaluating.

Write these 4 headings on the chalkboard. Ask learners to tell you briefly what kinds of things come under each heading. Use the following information as a guideline as you lead the discussion.

1 *Preparing*

Preparing can mean getting any of the following things ready:

- the classroom or place of training
- the trainer
- the learners

Anything the trainer or learners do before the part of the session which involves new information is called preparing.

The first thing you need to do to prepare is to answer the 7 teaching questions.

See the section in Unit 2 on **Choosing visual aids to fit teaching situations.**

You need to collect all the visual aids you will use before the session. It is helpful to stack these in the order in which you will use them.

You should also practise with the visual aids before the session. This is part of preparing yourself.

Sometimes it is a good idea to tell your learners what they will be able to do as a result of participating in this activity. Sometimes it is also necessary to give learners background information, to help them get the most out of the activity. It is helpful to remind your learners of information and skills they already know which will help them learn the new information more quickly. This is all part of preparing your learners.

2 *Conducting*

In this part of the session your learners either receive or discover for themselves the new information or skills. You will need to conduct the session differently depending on what method you are using, but there are some things about conducting a training session which are true for most methods:

- Be sure that all learners can see you and any visual aids you use and that everyone can hear well.
- Relate the activity to experiences and interests of your learners.
- Try to keep learners actively involved.
- Encourage questions.
- Watch your learners' reactions and listen carefully to their questions and answers. Make changes in the activity if necessary.

3 *Reviewing*

You and your learners then look at what they have learned, and try to summarize it and apply it to other things they know already.

During this part of the session, it is good for both the trainer and the learners to do the following things:

- Summarize what was learned from the activity.
- Relate the new information or skills to what learners already know.
- Decide how the new information can help them in their daily lives or in their work.

4 *Evaluating*

A good trainer is always evaluating, both during and after the session.

A good trainer knows how to improve the effectiveness of the training session by asking these kinds of questions:

- Can my learners do what the objective says they should be able to do?
- What are the learners' suggestions concerning how to improve the session?
- How can I make the session better next time?

Within all 4 parts of the session, a good trainer sets up situations which require learners to *do* something. This may be to discuss how things relate, to solve a problem, to identify and discuss feelings, or to make something.

Keep in mind that people learn and remember more if they learn by *doing*. A trainer can combine teaching methods and use visual aids to keep the session interesting and to make sure learners are actively involved in learning.

Using visual aids with teaching methods

When you combine visual aids with teaching methods in preparing, conducting, reviewing, and evaluating a session, remember that the way that you use the visual aid also affects learning and remembering.

The best designed visual aid is effective only when you use it well. The following guidelines apply to using visual aids with any teaching method.

You may want to review Unit 2, particularly the 7 teaching questions and the 6 design considerations. Explain that the guidelines for using visual aids are based on these questions and considerations.

1 *Make sure everyone can see the visual aid.*

- Is it large enough for the whole group to see?
- Are you standing in front of the visual aid?
- Is anything blocking the view of anyone?

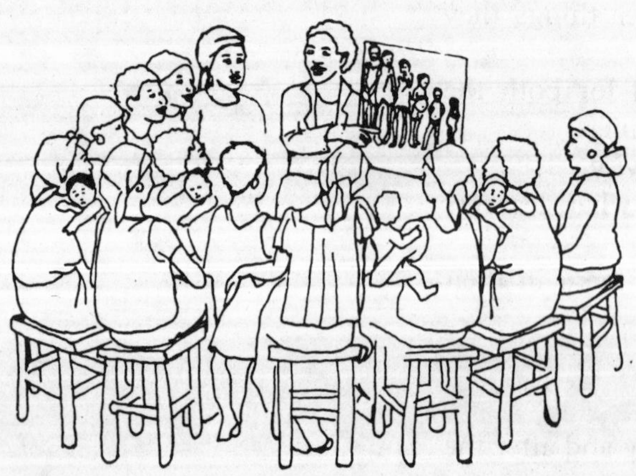

Demonstrate this guideline by asking someone at the back of the room if they can see a visual aid that you hold up. Hold it so it can be seen. Then stand in front of it as you talk and ask the learners how that has affected their learning.

Guidelines 1–3 are based on the design consideration, 'Words and pictures should be easy to see and understand' and the teaching question, 'Who are my learners?' (How many people).

2 Show the visual aid while you are talking about the topic it illustrates.

- Show it long enough for everyone to look at it.
- Put it aside when you finish talking about the topic.

Demonstrate use of this guideline as you describe it. Give a good and a bad example as you did for 1. Do the same for the other guidelines.

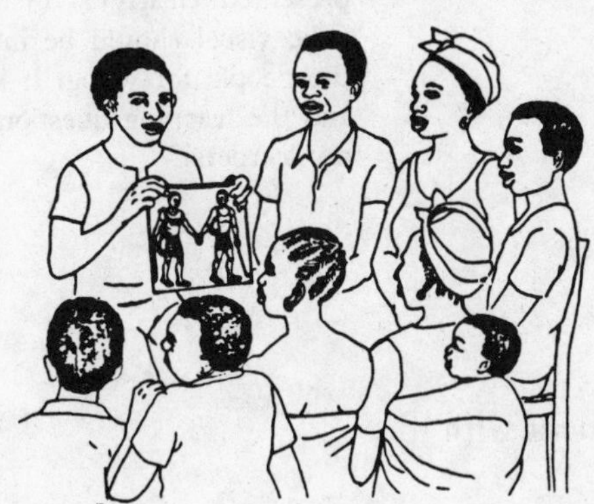

3 Hold the visual aid still or tape it to the wall. Moving it around can confuse or distract the people looking at it.

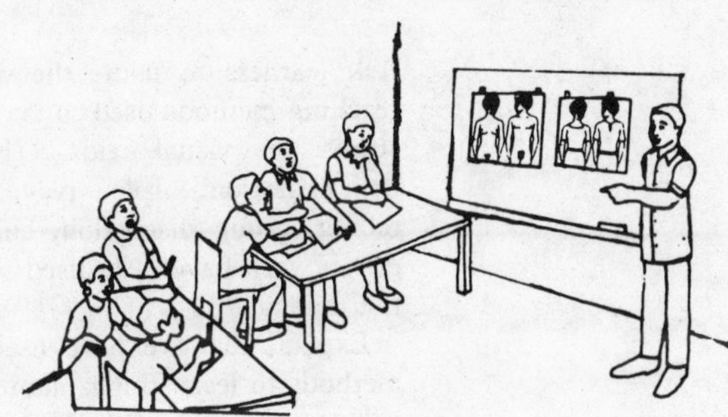

4 Point to parts of the visual aid as you talk about them.

The fourth guideline is based on the design consideration, 'The viewer's attention should be directed to important information.'

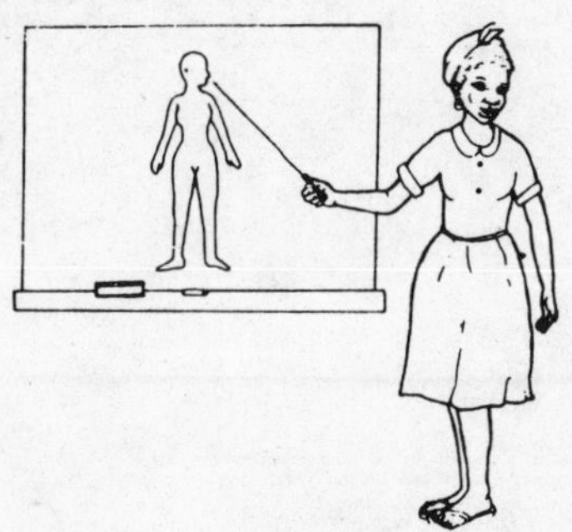

5 Explain any picture or symbols or words that may be unfamiliar. This is very important with people who are not used to learning from pictures.

This is based on the design considerations, 'The information should be presented clearly and simply', and 'The visual should be interesting to the people for whom it is intended' and the teaching question, 'Who are my learners?'

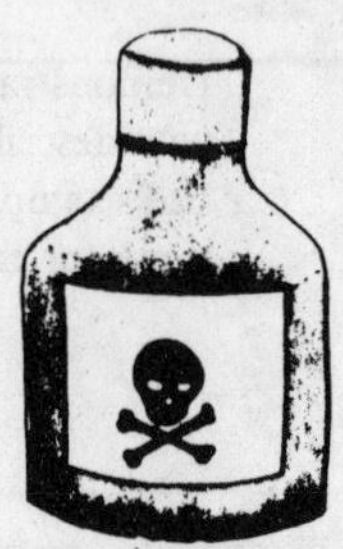

6 Encourage your learners to handle and experiment with your visual aids and to make their own.

- Pass them around during discussion.
- Put them on display.
- Make up activities in which the learners make and use visual aids.

Ask learners to name the different teaching methods used so far in their study of visual aids. (Lecture, demonstration, role play, story-telling, group discussion, and small group work have been used so far in the manual.)

Explain that we have used these methods to learn things about visual aids, but now let us look at them as teaching methods.

Do Activity 1. The instructions and adaptations will help you fit this activity to your own teaching needs.

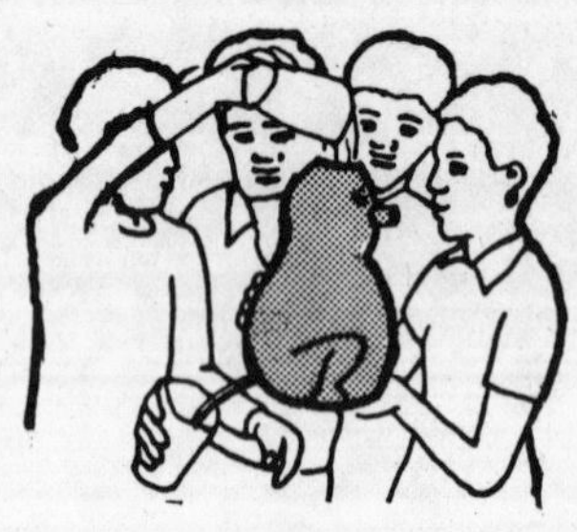

Activity 1 — Overview of teaching methods and visual aids

Time

This will depend on how many methods you want to include in the activity. Allow 10 minutes for each example session, about 20–30 minutes for small group work, and 15 minutes per group for group presentations.

Objectives

Learners will demonstrate several different teaching methods and how to use visual aids with each.

Learners will discuss and make up the following list for each teaching method you choose to include in this activity:
(1) Definition.
(2) What kinds of things the method is good for.
(3) Guidelines for using the method in each of the four parts of a session.
(4) Suggested visual aids to use with the method.

Materials

Copies of the pages on **Lecture or talk** for each person, (if possible).
Copies of the case studies you plan to use.
Large sheets of paper and markers or pens for each small group.

Instructions

1 Information on several different teaching methods is included in the following pages. Some of the methods may be more useful to your learners than others. Pick the ones which will be most useful. You may also think of other teaching methods to use with visual aids. If so, you can make up your own guidelines for the method and include them in this activity.

2 Choose several learners to help you with this activity. Ask them ahead of time to prepare short example sessions for each method you include in the activity.
More detailed suggestions on how to do this are included at the beginning of the description of each teaching method.

3 Demonstrate one of the methods for your whole group of learners. **Lecture or talk** is good for this. You can use the example given or choose your own example. The important thing is that you show your learners how to use this method well. Use visual aids, ask questions, and encourage discussion.
Most participants will probably have had practice in using lectures or talks. If you want to motivate them to use other methods, you can demonstrate a method other than lecture. A participant could be asked to show the lecture or talk method.

4 After your short talk, go to the chalkboard and help the group decide on a definition of the method. Then help them make the

list of what kinds of things the method is good for, guidelines for using it, and kinds of visual aids to use with it.

Encourage questions and discussion. Be sure your learners understand what each of these headings means.

5 If possible, make a copy of the pages on **Lecture or talk** for each person. If you can make these copies, distribute them now. Explain that these are only suggestions and possible answers. Your learners may or may not have thought of everything on these pages. Point out that the pages are meant to give them some ideas for using this teaching method. If an idea on their list is not on this list, it does not necessarily mean that the idea is not good. You must listen carefully and decide that yourself.

6 One by one, ask the learners who are helping you to give the short example sessions they have prepared, continuing until they have demonstrated all the methods you chose.

7 Have people divide into small groups. Ask each group to work on a different method. Each group is to define and make up its own list for that method, just as it did for your lecture or talk.

8 Go from group to group to answer questions. Be sure that all groups are accomplishing their task. Ask people to raise their hands if they need your help.

9 When the time is up, ask each small group to have one person present the group's list. Ask this person to post the list on the chalkboard or on the wall so everyone can see it.

As each person finishes presenting the group list, you may want to add ideas mentioned in these guidelines which were left off the group list.

It will be best if you can arrange to record the group lists with these additions. Have them copied and distributed to each person later. If you cannot do this, be sure everyone copies the lists. These will be valuable notes for them for their own teaching.

10 At the end of each presentation, lead a large group discussion. You may want to ask learners such questions as these:

- 'How many of you have used this teaching method?' 'How successful has it been for you?' 'Do your learners stay interested?' 'Do they learn what you want them to?'
- 'Have any of your previous teachers or trainers used this method to teach a session you were in?' 'How did you like it?'
- 'Can you think of any situations in your own work when you can use this teaching method?'

11 At the end of the activity, ask:

- 'Was this activity helpful for you?' 'Why or why not?' 'What improvements would you suggest?'

Possible adaptations

The approach used in the activity takes more time than either of the following adaptations, but the advantage is that everyone sees a demonstration of each method. These demonstrations will make the discussion after group presentations more meaningful. If you do not have time to do the activity as it is written, you can try one of the adaptations below.

1 Ask people to give short example sessions using different methods. After each session, lead a large group discussion about the use of the method.
Help learners develop the list as explained in step 4 of the activity. Then go on to another method.
This approach takes less time than the one described in the activity, but it may become boring if you want to include more than two or three different methods. There is less chance for all people to participate in a large group discussion.

2 If you have very little time, you can simply present the lists which are included here. You can do this as a lecture or make copies of the pages for each person.
Lead a large group discussion on each method and then go straight to the next activity.
This approach is quickest, but least effective. Your learners will remember less because they have not done anything with the teaching methods. They also have not seen examples of these methods to help remember them.

Lecture or talk

Note to the trainer

Present part of the section of Unit 2 on **Adapting an existing visual aid.** Give learners a good example of effective use of the lecture method. (Show the pictures as you talk, and ask questions.)

Ask your learners to describe the method, and suggest what things it is useful for. Have them suggest some guidelines for using the method. Write their suggestions on the chalkboard.

Use the guidelines given here to add ideas they do not mention.

The guidelines for each method given here have been tried many times all over the world, and they seem to work well. Your learners may also have good ideas to add.

Continue the discussion until your learners have agreed on a set of guidelines for using the lecture method.

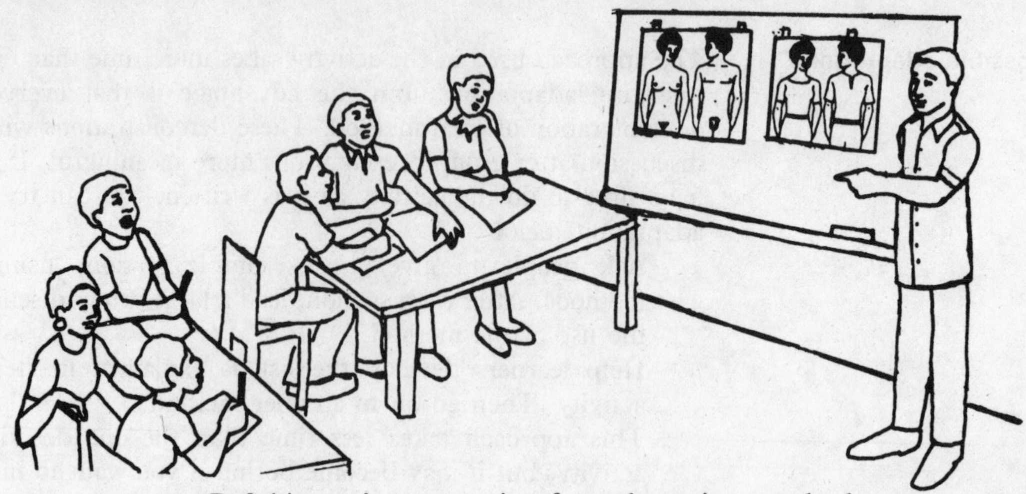

Definition: A presentation from the trainer to the learners.

What a lecture or talk is good for:

- presenting an overview of a topic or introducing a topic to be used as a basis for discussion
- reporting experiences to others
- reviewing or summarizing
- inspiring or motivating others
- hearing from resource persons

Guidelines for using lecture:

1 Preparing
   - Arrange chairs and visual aids in the room or wherever the training will take place.
   - Practise using the visual aids.
   - Let learners know what they will be able to do as a result of this training session.
   - Give learners background information, if necessary.

2 Conducting
   - Make the lecture interesting by relating it to experiences and interests of your learners. Try to adapt the information so that all your learners will be interested in it.
   - Present new information one idea at a time, in a sensible order.
   - Show how new information relates to information learners already know.
   - Ask questions at different points during the lecture. If learners do not understand, stop and have a discussion, or modify the lecture.
   - Encourage learners to discuss the information after the lecture.

3 Reviewing
- Have learners discuss what was learned and how it relates to what they already know.
- Lead discussion of ways learners can use what they have learned.
- Summarize the main things learned and how they can be used.

4 Evaluating
- Find out if learners can do what your objective says they should be able to do. You can do this by asking questions, assigning a project or activity, or giving a short test.
- Ask learners to tell you what was good and what can be better about the session.
- Modify the session based on this information.

Suggested visual aids:
- display (Example: Mrs Goko in Unit 2.)
- picture series (Example: Mrs Ebrahim in Unit 2.)
- flipbook
- flannelboard
- models, real objects
- chalkboard

Demonstration

Note to the trainer

Ask someone to prepare and present the birthing box demonstration from Unit 4. Make a copy of the instructions for using the box (Unit 4) for this person ahead of time. Have a birthing box ready for the person to use.

Have the session leader demonstrate how to use the birthing box. After the demonstration, return to step 6 in the **Overview** instructions on page 234.

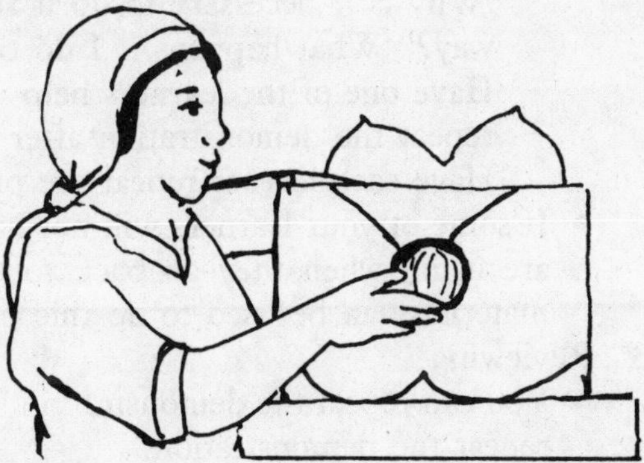

Definition: Trainer, learner, or resource person shows others how to do something.

What a demonstration is good for:

- showing exactly what needs to be done and in what order, also how much time it takes to do it
- showing procedures and processes which are hard to describe
- encouraging interest in the topic

Guidelines for using demonstration:

1 Preparing

- Collect the equipment and materials you will need. Arrange them so that everyone can see them and you can reach them easily. Use the same equipment and materials your learners will be using at their jobs or in their community or homes.
- Be sure everyone can see you and whatever visual aids you will use. Also be sure that everyone can hear well.
- Give an overview of the entire demonstration at the beginning. Use a picture, model, or real object to show what the finished product will be.
- Write the main steps on the chalkboard or show a picture series of the steps before beginning. If you do not have a chalkboard or large piece of paper on which you can write the main steps, then at least tell your learners the main steps.
- It is useful to give learners a list of materials necessary for doing the procedure.

2 Conducting

- Keep the demonstration simple and short.
- Show only one procedure at a time.
- Involve your learners in the demonstration. There are several ways to do this. Here are a few ideas:

  Ask learners questions such as, 'What should I do next?' 'Why is it necessary to do it this way instead of another way?' 'What happens if I do this the other way?'

  Have one of the learners help with the demonstration, or repeat the demonstration after you have finished.

  Have each learner repeat the procedure while you watch.
- If some of your learners will not have the same materials you are using when they go back to their jobs, ask what other materials can be used to do this procedure.

3 Reviewing

- You can repeat the demonstration, or have one of the learners repeat the demonstration.

- Have learners discuss the procedure and how it applies to their work.
- Have learners put a picture series of the steps in the correct order.
- Help learners relate this demonstration to things they already know.

4 Evaluating

- Can the learners repeat the demonstration correctly?
- Do your learners ask questions that show they understand the procedure?
  Do they seem to understand why to do the procedure and when to do it?

Suggested visual aids:

- models
- picture series showing the procedure or process
- real objects

Large group discussion

Note to the trainer

Ask one of your learners to prepare and present a large group discussion. Ask the person to use a visual aid as the basis of discussion. Make a copy of the pages in Unit 1 which explain how to use visual aids as the basis for discussion. Give these pages to the person ahead of time to prepare to lead the discussion.

After this presentation, return to step 6 of the instructions in the **Overview** on page 234.

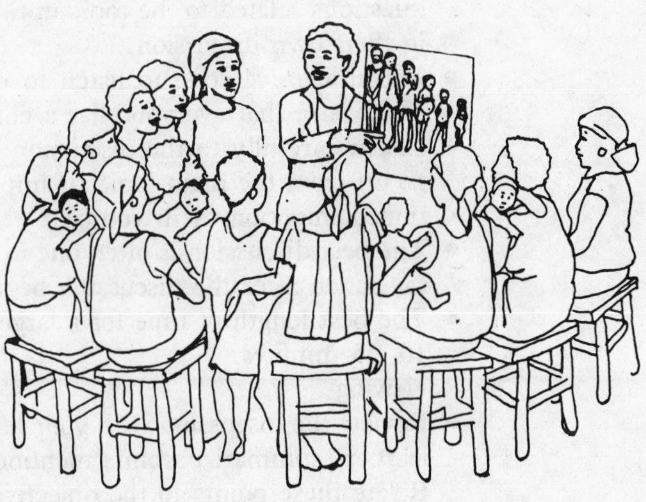

Definition: A whole group of learners discusses a given topic or problem, or shares opinions and experiences.

What a large group discussion is good for:

- exploring a topic of interest to the whole group
- discussing new goals and directions for the group
- bringing out ideas and experiences after a presentation or a small group discussion

Guidelines for using large group discussion:

1 Preparing
- Collect the visual aids you will use to begin the discussion.
- Practise using the visual aids if this is necessary.
- Decide on the objective for the discussion.
- Prepare some open questions you can ask to start the discussion.
- It is useful to have an informal setting where learners can see each other. For this reason, some trainers have participants sit in a circle or square.

2 Conducting
- Use the visual aid, if you want to base your discussion on it.
- Ask an open question. When someone responds, comment on the response, or ask others to comment. You might ask other open questions, such as, 'What do you think about that?' or, 'What has your experience been?'
- If you are using real objects or models, you can have learners pass these around so that everyone can look at them more closely during the discussion.
- Encourage others to add their comments. Keep asking open questions related to the topic until your learners are involved in their own discussion.
- Encourage everyone to listen to the person who is talking. Make sure that everyone has a chance to talk.
- Listen carefully to the discussion. Do not let the discussion go off from the main topic. If important points are not mentioned, mention them yourself.
- The best discussion is often one in which the trainer does not say much after the discussion begins.
- The best length of time for a large group discussion is about 10–15 minutes.

3 Reviewing
- Review the discussion with your learners. Summarize or have learners summarize points mentioned during the discussion. Relate these points to the objective of the discussion.

4 Evaluating

- Watch learners during the discussion to be sure that they remain interested, and not bored and restless.
- Ask learners how well they think the objective of the discussion was accomplished.
- How well do you feel the objective of the discussion was met?

Suggested visual aids:

- models or real objects
- posters
- flannelboard
- picture series
- display or exhibit

Small group work

Note to the trainer

Ask one of your learners to lead a session using this method. Suggest that the person begin by showing the entire group a visual aid which is *not* appropriate for them to use in their teaching. You may want to find the visual aid yourself, or you can ask the session leader to find one. It will be helpful to review the sections in Unit 2 on the 6 design considerations, and then find a visual aid which you know needs to be adapted.

Have the session leader show the visual aid and explain that people are to divide into small groups. Each small group will choose a leader and a recorder. Each group will have 5 minutes to list as many things they can think of which need to be changed to make the visual aid more useful to them.

The learners divide into groups of 4–6 people. They have 5 minutes to do their group work.

The session leader then calls everyone together again and leads a brief large group discussion. If you have time, it would be good for all small group leaders to present their lists and use the visual aid to explain their comments. The large group can discuss each suggestion as it is made.

Have the session leader summarize the discussion, and repeat what everyone agrees needs to be changed in the visual aid.

After this demonstration of small group work, return to step 6 of the instructions in the **Overview** on page 234.

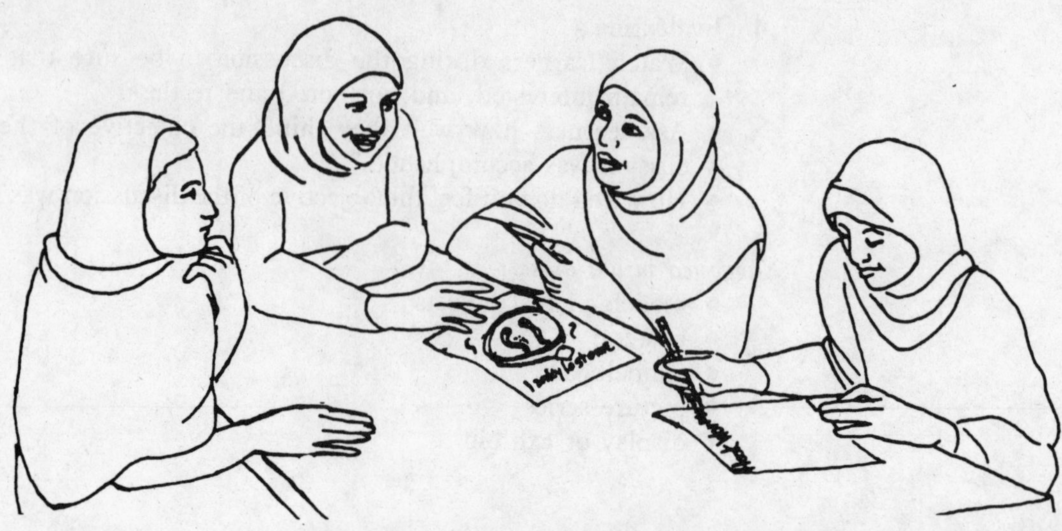

Definition: The trainer divides a large class into smaller groups of 6 or less. The small groups have a short time to discuss a topic or solve a problem.

What small group work is good for:

- Encourages individual thinking and participation.
- Provides a fast way to solve problems. Individual participants produce many ideas in a short period of time.
- Gets a discussion started after you have introduced a topic or issue to be discussed.
- Helps keep learners interested when used in the middle of lectures or large group discussions.
- People are often more comfortable and will talk more easily with a small group of their peers rather than in a large group with a trainer.

Guidelines for using small group work:

1 Preparing

- Collect any real objects or other visual aids you want to use as the basis for discussion or problem-solving. Visual aids can be very useful for this purpose.
- Practise using these, if necessary.
- Decide on an objective for the small group work. Think about combining the small group work with another method. Do you want to have a large group discussion afterward? Do you want the small groups to report or present their work to the whole group? Or do you want to do both and have the group presentations followed by a large group discussion?

Decide these things as you plan what you want the small group to do.

2 Conducting

- Present the problem or topic you have chosen as the basis for small group work.
- Explain what the small groups are to do. Have participants divide into equal-sized groups.

  There are several ways to divide into groups. Choose the way which seems most comfortable for your participants:

  (a) Participants choose their own groups.

  (b) Group according to seating.

  (c) Have participants count off 1–7 or as many groups as you want. Each eighth person becomes a 1 until everyone has a number. Then ask the people with like numbers to group together.

  (d) Have cards with numbers or pictures on them. Everyone picks a card. People with like cards form a group.
- The trainer chooses or the group chooses one person to be the leader and another to be the recorder. It is good to give groups a time limit for this if they are doing it, so that everyone can get on with the activity. 2 minutes is usually enough.
- Have available any reference or resource materials you want the groups to use. If you are having the groups discuss a topic or problem which involves real objects or other visual aids, you can have participants pass these around so that everyone can look at them more closely during the discussion.
- Giving the groups too little time is usually better than giving them too much. Depending on the topic and what you ask the groups to do, 5–20 minutes is usually enough for people to think of several ideas but still have more to talk about. Set a time when everyone will meet again as a large group.

3 Reviewing

- Meet again as a large group. Have each group summarize its discussions and ideas. To save time and avoid repetition, you may want to have people raise their hands when one of their ideas is mentioned.
- Conduct a large group discussion. Help learners summarize what they learned.

4 Evaluating

- Go from group to group to be sure that everyone is participating in the discussion. Sometimes one or two people will dominate a group. In this case, try to involve others in the group by asking what they think.

- Watch learners to see if they remain interested, or are becoming bored or tired.
- How well did the small groups meet the objective you set? Can the learners do what you wanted them to be able to do as a result of this work?
- Was the topic or problem useful or does it need to be changed if you use it again? Was anyone confused?
- Ask people what was good about this session and what could have been better.

Suggested visual aids:

- real objects
- models
- picture series
- posters
- flannelboards
- displays or exhibits (Groups can take turns examining the display.)

Role play

Note to the trainer

Ask a small group of your learners to prepare and present a role play. You can ask them to repeat the role play from Unit 3, Activity 3, **How to pre-test visual aids: a role play.** Or you can use the guidelines below and make up another situation and other role descriptions. Be sure that the role play requires participants to use visual aids. Give the people who will be presenting the role play copies of the situation and role descriptions ahead of time so they can prepare.

After the role play, return to step 6 of the instructions in the **Overview** on page 234.

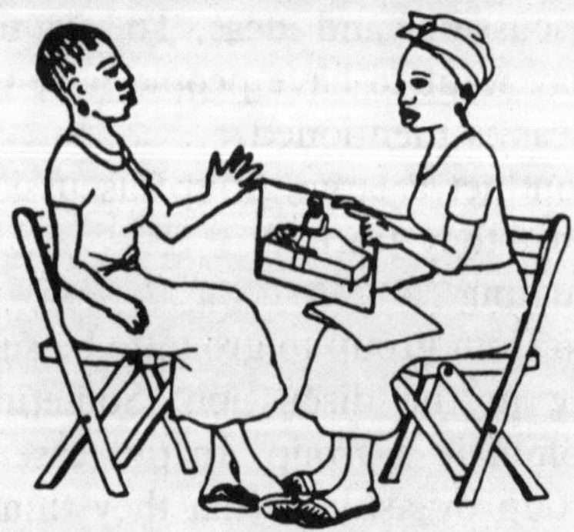

Definition: A short, spontaneous play. A role play is not rehearsed or written. Learners receive a problem situation and a short description of characters. They take the role of the characters and make up their own lines. Role play is often used to show the emotional reactions of people involved in the situation. It is also often used to practise interacting with other people.

What role play is good for:

- Helps learners see that other people have similar problems.
- Helps people look at personal problems in a more impersonal manner.
- Shows different ways of handling a problem situation.
- Provides a safe way of expressing emotional feelings and working out conflicts between people.
- Provides a basis for discussion.
- Gets learners actively involved.
- Gets the whole group working together.
- Identifies the attitudes of different people in the group.
- Studies problems in personal relationships and group behaviour. Also helps participants gain insight into their own behaviour and feelings.

Guidelines for using role play:

1 Preparing

- Choose a problem situation which is:
  (a) related to your objectives
  (b) interesting to your learners
  (c) suitable for acting
- Collect all the props and real objects you will need for the session. (Props and real objects make the role play more realistic.)
- Plan some questions you can ask during the review discussion.
- Describe the characters and roles to your learners.
- Choose 2 or 3 learners to act as the characters in the role play.
- Encourage the people who are acting to let themselves feel and act like the characters they are supposed to be.
- Ask the other learners to choose one of these characters. Then ask them to compare their feelings and reactions with those of the person acting out that character in the role play.

2 Conducting

- Be sure that everyone can see and hear well enough to follow the role play.
- Watch carefully to see if the actors are raising issues which

are appropriate to the main problem. It is a good idea to take notes during the role play. Then refer to your notes during the discussion which follows.

- Watch everyone else during the role play to see if they are still interested, or are becoming bored and restless.
- Stop the role play when you feel the actors have shown the feelings and ideas which are important in the problem situation, or when the other learners become bored and restless.
- Thank the actors for their help and good work.

3 Reviewing

- Ask the actors and other learners to discuss their feelings.
- Ask questions you have prepared.
- Ask learners what they discovered by doing this activity.
- Ask learners how this related to what they already know, and how this information can help them in their daily lives or in their jobs.

4 Evaluating

- Ask your learners if this was a valuable activity for them. Why or why not?
- Listen to the comments during discussion. Do people have a better understanding of personal feelings and values which are part of this problem situation?
- Ask how the role play can be improved next time.

Suggested visual aids:

- real objects to make the scene more realistic (Tables, chairs, brooms, and other such things.)
- costumes or clothes appropriate to the role the person is playing
- posters or signs (Perhaps a sign above a doorway saying, 'Welcome to your health clinic'.)
- props (Examples: baby dolls, cardboard animals, and other such things. See also the section on **Storytelling, problem story and drama**. Basins or tubs are useful for making the sound of someone knocking on a door. It is not necessary to have real walls and doors if you make the sound as the actor knocks.)

Storytelling, problem story and drama

Note to the trainer

Decide which variation of this teaching method you will include in the activity. Four variations on this method are listed below. Ask one or more learners to prepare and present 'The Story of Fatu and Musu'. For more information on open and closed questions, see the information section of Unit 3 on pre-testing visual aids.

Try to incorporate local traditional stories and characters in other stories or dramas that you use. You also may want to use songs or poetry as a part of these activities. You or your learners can make up new words to familiar songs.

Storytelling

You can ask one person or a small group of people to present the storytelling method. One person can present the storytelling method by telling the story of Fatu and Musu and showing the picture series. The person can make up some questions about the story ahead of time. Following the story, the person can lead a discussion of what the listeners learned from the story.

Drama

You may want to ask a small group to present storytelling, by acting out the story of Fatu and Musu instead of showing the pictures. Encourage them to use real objects, costumes, and scenery to make the story more realistic. They also must make up some open questions ahead of time, and lead a discussion at the end of the performance.

Problem story

You can ask someone to present the problem story method. 'The Story of Fatu and Musu' becomes a problem story if you stop after picture 4, where the two men disagree on the best way to have a large family. The person preparing the presentation can make up some open questions ahead of time. Because the problem is not resolved in a problem story, the questions need to be different from the kind used after a finished story. The questions used with a problem story must encourage listeners to discuss different possible solutions to the problem, and their advantages and disadvantages.

Problem drama

You may want to have a small group present the problem story by acting it out. The group can make up the questions and have one person lead the discussion afterward.

After the demonstration of this teaching method, return to step 6 of the instructions in the **Overview** on page 234.

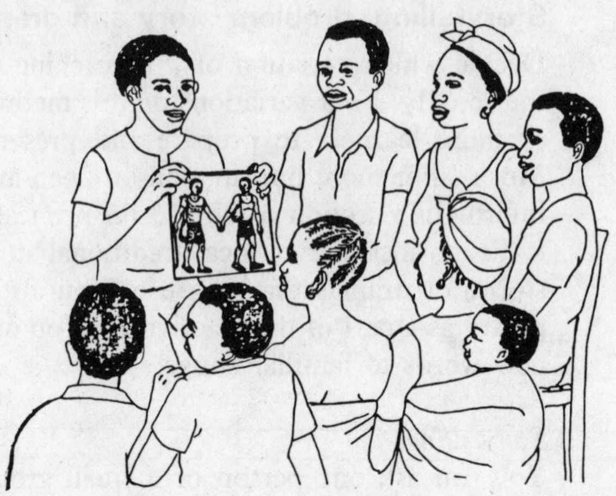

Definitions

Story telling: The trainer or health educator tells a story based on what he wants the learners to be able to do. The story is usually about a person or persons who solve their problem when they gain new knowledge and change the way they do some things. The trainer prepares questions to ask, and uses them to lead a discussion after the story.

Problem story: The trainer tells enough of the story to present the problem situation, but stops with the end of the story unfinished. The trainer then asks very open questions to encourage learners to discuss different ways to solve this problem and advantages and disadvantages of each solution.

Drama: Trainers, health workers, or villagers can act out either stories or problem stories, prepare questions, and lead a discussion afterwards.

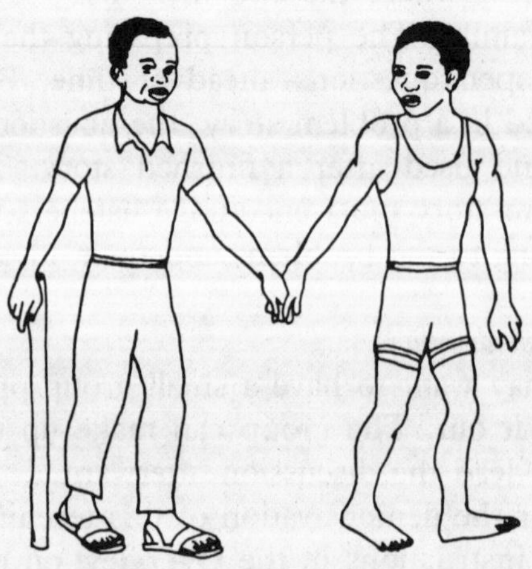

What they are good for:

- Community teaching.
- Including many local details, and so being more interesting to local people. The story is about people like them, who have problems like their own.
- Exploring a problem important to the learners.
- Showing people a better way to do things without having their feelings criticized.
- Encouraging local people to think about and discuss community problems.
- Allowing people to discover possible solutions to the problem for themselves.
- If you present the story as a drama, you can make it very interesting and entertaining. Have local people act parts in the drama. Ask them to help you adapt the story to that particular village. Use colourful objects and costumes if you are presenting it to the whole village. Your actors may be able to help you add humorous touches to the story.
- Health stories are a good way to reach many people indirectly. A person does not have to have much medical knowledge to tell a health story. Even school children can share health stories with their families.

Guidelines for using storytelling:

1 Preparing

- Decide what you want your learners to be able to do. For example, you may decide that there are 5 things you want mothers to do to improve infant nutrition:
  (1) Breast-feed as long as possible.
  (2) Start feeding groundnut porridge at 4 months.
  (3) Start giving bean cakes and other soft foods at one year.
  (4) Give at least 5 feedings a day.
  (5) Do not become pregnant again for at least 2 years.
- Make up a story which tells about a local mother or mothers whose children develop malnutrition because one or more of these things was not done. The mothers learn to do some of these 5 things, and their children become healthy.
- Prepare some questions to ask at the end of the story.
- Help the large group evaluate the performance of each group. You may want to repeat the best drama for a public performance.
- Memorize the story. Have actors memorize their parts if you are doing a drama.
- If you are using visual aids, be sure that you pre-test them

(see Unit 3). You may want to use a picture series or flip-book, as in the example of Mrs Ebrahim in Unit 2.

- If you are doing a drama, prepare simple props or scenery. Decide what clothing actors will wear. Collect the real props and objects you will use, such as baby dolls, beds, chairs, farming tools, or medical equipment.

2 Conducting

- Tell your learners the story using the visual aids, or act out the story, using the props and objects you have prepared.
- At the end of the story, ask the questions you have prepared. Lead discussion on what people have learned from listening to the story.
- Lead discussion on how the story applies to the local community.

3 Reviewing

- Divide your learners into small groups of 4 or 5 people. Each person tells the story to other members of the small group.
- Each group decides how it would act out the story and practises acting it out.
- Each group presents its drama to the large group.

4 Evaluating

- The answers to your questions after the story should show whether learners understood the story in the way you wanted them to.
- As a homework assignment, have each person make up a story and questions around a main idea which you assign. Have each person tell his or her story to the group the next day. Do the stories show that they understand how to use this teaching method?

Suggested visual aids:

- picture series
- flipbook
- flannelboard
- props (Examples: baby dolls, beds, chairs, cardboard chickens to pay the midwife, radios made from boxes.)
- real objects (Examples: scales for weighing babies, syringes, wash basins.)
- clothing or costumes (These can often be both descriptive and humorous. Examples: a rich man can wear a suit with money coming out of the pockets.)

Activity 2 Making a session plan

Time

Time required to complete a session plan will vary among individuals. Time for meeting with individuals will depend on the number of learners. Allow 20 minutes for explanations, 1–2 hours for developing the plan, and 10 minutes individual meeting time for each learner.

Objective

Learners will make up a lesson plan they can use in their work, using one or more of the methods described in this unit.

Materials

Each person should have:
The answers to the 7 teaching questions and the visual aid he or she made in Unit 3, Activity 5, **Making your own visual aid**, or see possible adaptation to this activity.
Copies of the guidelines for using each method, developed by the large group agreed upon in Activity 1. Copies of planning form (if you intend to use it).
Pencils and paper.

Instructions

1 If possible, copy the guidelines for using each teaching method from the chalkboard and duplicate them for each person. If this is not possible, be sure that everyone copies the different guidelines from the chalkboard. Ask them to use their notes in all of these activities.

2 Ask learners to work individually. Ask them to look again at the teaching method they chose when they were making their visual aid. Do they still think it is the best choice? Tell them they can change their choice, if they think another method would be better.

3 Ask learners to use their answers to the 7 teaching questions to plan a session they can use in their work. You may also want to suggest that they use the form included with this activity for planning a session.
Be sure to explain to your participants that they should use the same information they used to plan their visual aid. They have already worked with this topic in Unit 3, Activity 5, **Making your own visual aid.** This will help them as they are making out a lesson plan and developing the session.

4 If you use the form included in this activity for planning a session, be sure to present the example to your learners. The form used in the example that follows is one kind of form. It is useful for planning both long and short sessions. You may have

a different form that you will want to use here instead. A form will help your learners organize their planning.

The length of the session you require your learners to plan depends on how much time you have available for this activity. Planning a 20-minute session will give everyone a chance to put several different teaching methods and visual aids into the session. Remember when you assign the length of the session that it is very important that each participant has time to conduct at least part of this session.

5 As people finish their session plan, meet with each person individually to review and evaluate the lesson plan. Have the person revise the plan if necessary.

Some people will finish and be waiting to see you. These people can review each other's work while they are waiting.

6 When you have approved a person's session plan, suggest that they plan how they will do each of the four parts of the session.

7 Meet with learners individually again when they finish developing their sessions. Review their work, explain anything that is unclear, and ask people to revise their plans if necessary.

It is best to have individuals present their entire session. But if you do not have time for this, help each person choose a 10-minute section of their plan to conduct for the large group. (See Activity 3).

Possible adaptations

1 If you have not had time for learners to make their own visual aids, they can use visual aids which you bring. This will mean that they also do not have answers to the 7 teaching questions for a situation in their own work.

In this case, ask people to choose one of the available visual aids and think of a situation in their own work in which they can use it. Then have them answer the 7 teaching questions for that situation. You may have to help them with the 7 teaching questions to be sure that their topic can be taught in the time you have assigned.

Allow about 30 extra minutes for the activity if you do this adaptation.

Planning a session

Information and notes to the trainer

Your learners must be familiar with the 7 teaching questions to be comfortable doing this activity. Remind them of the story of Mrs Ebrahim in Unit 2. Review Mrs Ebrahim's answers to the 7 teaching questions.

Explain that this is how Mrs Ebrahim used her answers to the 7 teaching questions to actually plan the session she conducted for the women at the well. You can write these things on the chalkboard as you tell the story.

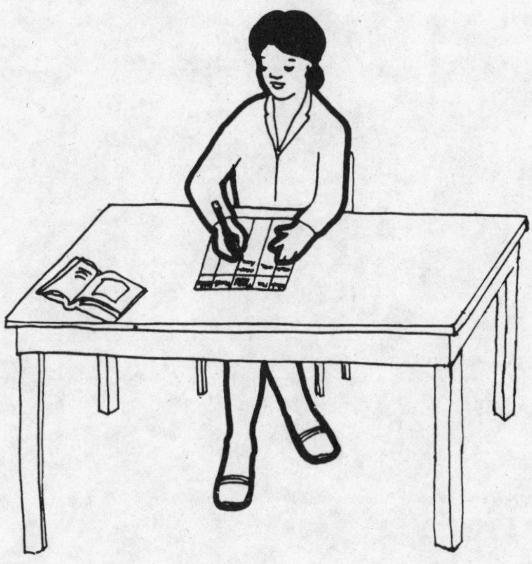

Mrs Ebrahim plans a health education talk

After Mrs Ebrahim finished answering the seven teaching questions shown below, she began planning the session.

1 **What** is the **problem**?
Kwashiorkor is a widespread problem in the community.

2 **Who** are my learners?
Women in the community who are not regular clients at the clinic. Many do not know about the clinic services. Many are not literate.

3 **What** do I want them to be able to **do**?
Name at least 3 high protein foods to feed children as a way to treat and prevent kwashiorkor.

4 **Where** and for **how long** will the instruction take place?
At the well for 15 minutes.

5 What **teaching methods** will I use?
Storytelling and discussion.

6 What **visual aids** will I use?
A picture series on kwashiorkor. Real food examples.

7 How will I know how **effective** the training was?
Comments and questions from the women that show they understand during the session.
The women can name at least 3 high protein foods, when shown pictures of them.
More women come to the cooking demonstrations at the clinic.

Mrs Ebrahim began filling in the chart shown below to plan her session. She wondered how much time the women would have to spend talking with her at the well. They will not be expecting her, and she will be talking with them in the middle of their work day. Mrs Ebrahim decided that she would make the session about 15 minutes long. In the first column of her chart she wrote:

KWASHIORKOR

Time	Objectives	Content	Method	Materials	Evaluation
15 minutes					

In the column titled Objectives, Mrs Ebrahim wrote her answer to teaching question number three: What do I want them to be able to do?

KWASHIORKOR

Time	Objectives	Content	Method	Materials	Evaluation
15 minutes	Mothers will name at least 3 high protein foods to feed children as a way to treat and prevent kwashiorkor.				

Mrs Ebrahim then decided what information the mothers must know to be able to accomplish the objective. She wrote in the Content column:

KWASHIORKOR

Time	Objectives	Content	Method	Materials	Evaluation
15 minutes	Mothers will name at least 3 high protein foods to feed children as a way to treat and prevent kwashiorkor.	1. Kwashiorkor is caused by not eating enough protein. 2. Some local foods which are good sources of protein are: - cous-cous porridge - meat broth - dried beans - groundnuts 3. The clinic gives demonstration sessions every week on how to cook nutritious and high protein foods.			

Mrs Ebrahim looked at her plan. She had already decided to use storytelling and discussion as her teaching methods. Now she needed to decide which method to use to teach which part of the information.

She decided to write a story which would include all three of the main points. She thought it would be useful for the women to discuss what local foods were a good source of protein. In this way, Mrs Ebrahim could be sure that they understood the story. She also knew that she needed to mention in the closing discussion that the clinic had cooking demonstrations every week. So she put 'discussion' beside the second and third content points as a teaching method.

KWASHIORKOR

Time	Objectives	Content	Method	Materials	Evaluation
15 minutes	Mothers will name at least 3 high protein foods to feed children as a way to treat and prevent kwashiorkor.	1. Kwashiorkor is caused by not eating enough protein.	story telling		
		2. Some local foods which are good sources of protein are: - cous-cous porridge - meat broth - dried beans - groundnuts	story telling and discussion		
		3. The clinic gives demonstration sessions every week on how to cook nutritious and high protein foods.	story telling		

In the Materials column, Mrs Ebrahim wrote what visual aids she wanted to use to teach each of the 3 main points. Since she was planning to use the picture series to teach all 3 points, she only wrote 'picture series' once.

KWASHIORKOR

Time	Objectives	Content	Method	Materials	Evaluation
15 minutes	Mothers will name at least 3 high protein foods to feed children as a way to treat and prevent Kwashiorkor.	1. Kwashiorkor is caused by not eating enough protein.	story telling	picture series to go with story	
		2. Some local foods which are good sources of protein are: - cous-cous porridge - meat broth - dried beans - groundnuts	story telling and discussion	real food examples	
		3. The clinic gives demonstration sessions every week on how to cook nutritious and high protein foods.	story telling		

In the Evaluation column, she wrote the things that she planned to do to find out how effective the session was.

KWASHIORKOR

Time	Objectives	Content	Method	Materials	Evaluation
15 minutes	Mothers will name at least 3 high protein foods to feed children as a way to treat and prevent Kwashiorkor.	1. Kwashiorkor is caused by not eating enough protein.	story telling	picture series to go with story	1. Do the women ask questions and make comments which show they understand?
		2. Some local foods which are good sources of protein are: - cous-cous porridge - meat broth - dried beans - groundnuts	story telling and discussion	real food examples	2. When shown pictures or examples of high protein foods, can the mothers name at least 3?
		3. The clinic gives demonstration sessions every week on how to cook nutritious and high protein foods.	story telling		3. Do more women come to the cooking demonstrations at the clinic?

Mrs Ebrahim's final session plan looked like this:

KWASHIORKOR

Time	Objectives	Content	Method	Materials	Evaluation
15 minutes	Mothers will name at least 3 high protein foods to feed children as a way to treat and prevent kwashiorkor.	1. Kwashiorkar is caused by not eating enough protein.	story telling	picture series to go with story	1. Do the women ask questions and make comments which show they understand?
		2. Some local foods which are good sources of protein are: - cous-cous porridge - meat broth - dried beans - groundnuts	story telling and discussion	real food examples	2. When shown pictures or examples of high protein foods, can the mothers name at least 3?
		3. The clinic gives demonstration sessions every week on how to cook nutritious and high protein foods.	story telling		3. Do more women come to the cooking demonstrations at the clinic?

Activity 3

Conducting a training or health education session

Time

Allow 15 minutes for each person

Objective

Each learner will lead a 10-minute training session, based on a session plan from Activity 2, **Making a session plan,** using a visual aid.

Materials

Copies of the guidelines for using each teaching method, from Activity 1 of this unit.
Copies of the observation form as on page 262, if possible.
The visual aids used for Activity 2, **Making a session plan.**
Paper and pencil for each person.

Instructions

1 Explain that learners will evaluate each other's sessions. They may refer to the guidelines for that method, if they wish.
You may also want to have them use the observation form included with this activity. If you cannot duplicate the form, you can write the headings on the chalkboard, and explain how you want them to evaluate each other.

2 One at a time, have each person conduct the training session planned in Activity 2. If you only have time for learners to conduct part of their sessions, then ask each person to conduct the 10-minute section you helped them choose in Activity 2.
Each person should begin by telling the group about their learners and the objective of the session. If the person is presenting only part of the planned session, ask them to describe what will be done before and after this section of the session.

3 After each session, have learners pass their observation comments to the front. Collect these and label them with the person's name who gave the session.

4 Use these comments later to help you evaluate the person's session. Then give them back so the learners can see how others reacted to their session.

5 After everyone has led a session, have a large group discussion. Ask learners if this was a valuable exercise for them. Why or why not? What did they learn about using different teaching methods and visual aids? How will they apply what they have learned?

Observation Form

Part of session	Things that were good about the session	Things that need improving	Suggestions and comments
1 Preparing			
2 Conducting			
3 Reviewing			
4 Evaluating			

Resource Pictures

The Resource Pictures are large versions of the picture series in Units 2 and 3 on the 7 teaching questions and menstruation. The training ideas in those units suggest ways to use the resource pictures to present information in a way that involves your learners. You will find more specific instructions at the beginning of each set of pictures.

The 7 teaching questions

Suggestions for using the picture series on the 7 teaching questions

Show the pictures as you tell the story. You may want to make copies to tape on a wall or chalkboard. Arrange them in a way that is familiar to your learners. Below are two possible ways to do this. The bottom arrangement is for people who read Arabic (from right to left). Note that steps 6 and 7 each have two pictures.

To avoid confusion you can place the two pictures together in one of the ways shown below.

You may want to leave the pictures in the manual or copy them to make into a flipbook as in Unit 2, Activity 5.

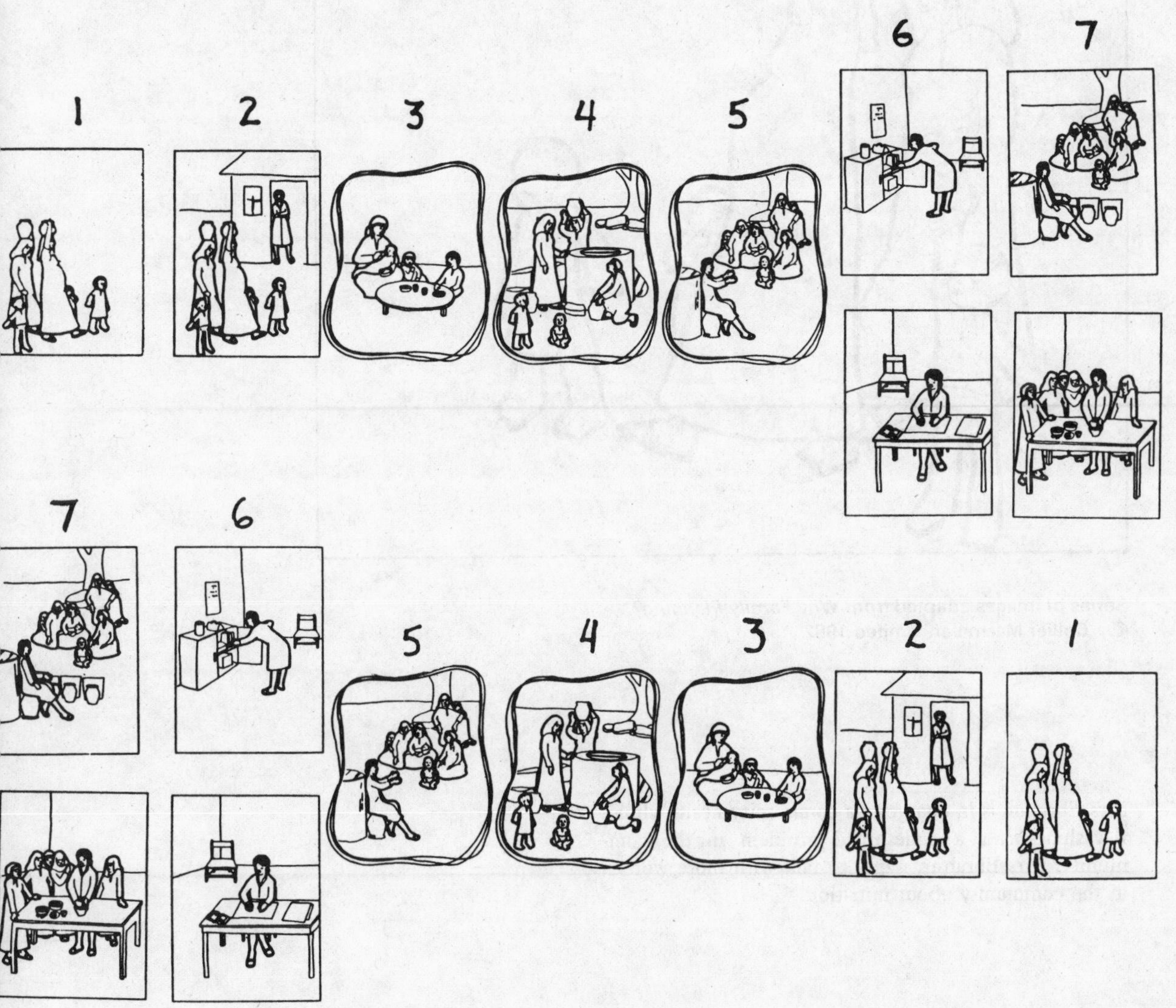

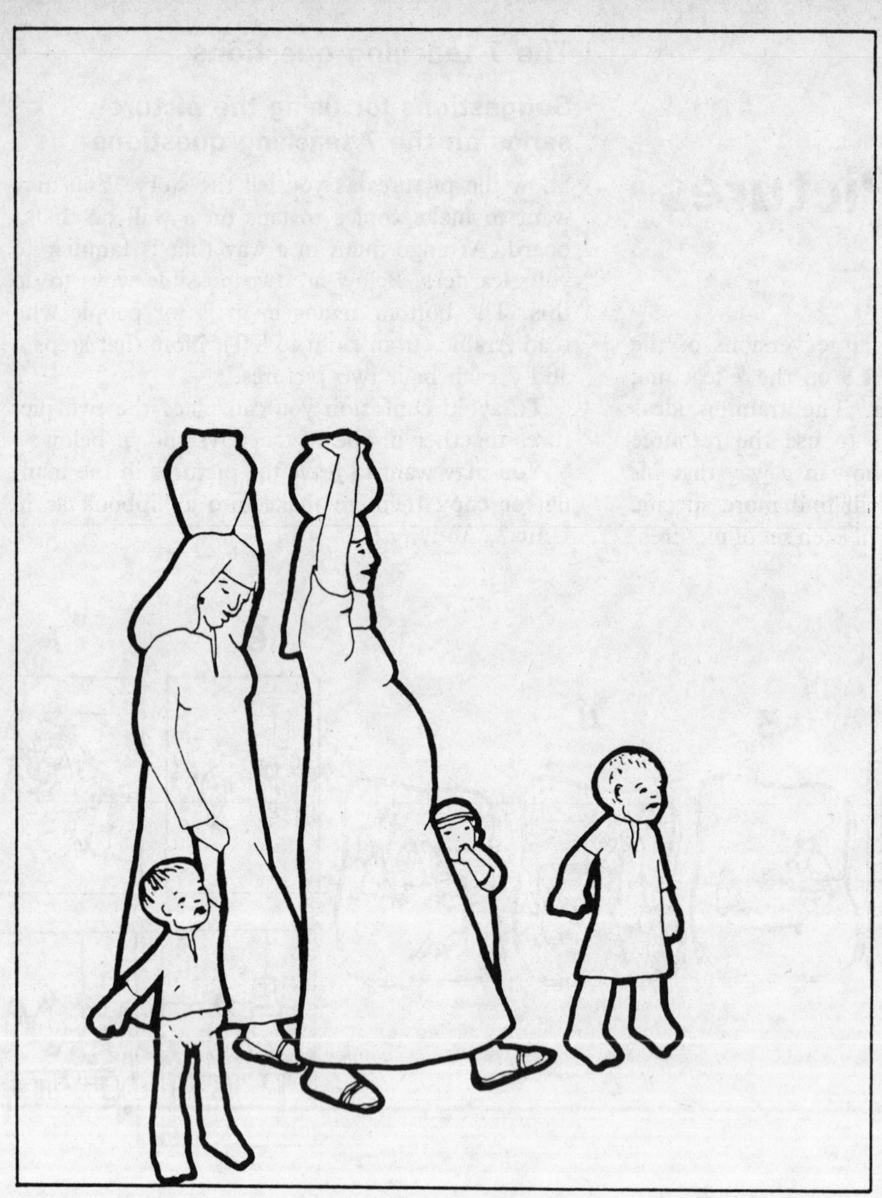

Mrs Ebrahim is in charge of a community health clinic. Kwashiorkor is a widespread problem in the community. Mrs Ebrahim wants to talk with more women in the community about nutrition.

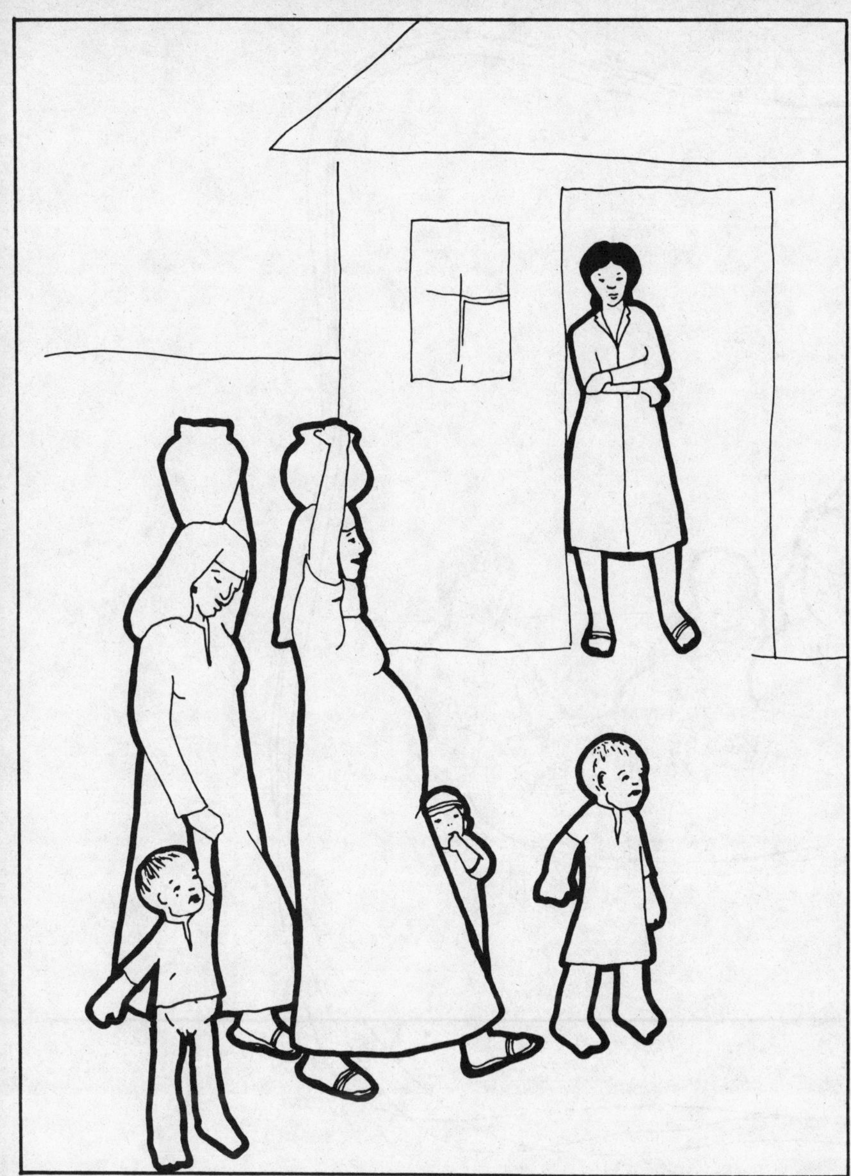

Series of images adapted from *Why Family Planning*?

She wants to talk with women who are not regular clients at the clinic. Many of the women do not come to the clinic because they do not know about the services it provides. Many of the women in the community are not literate.

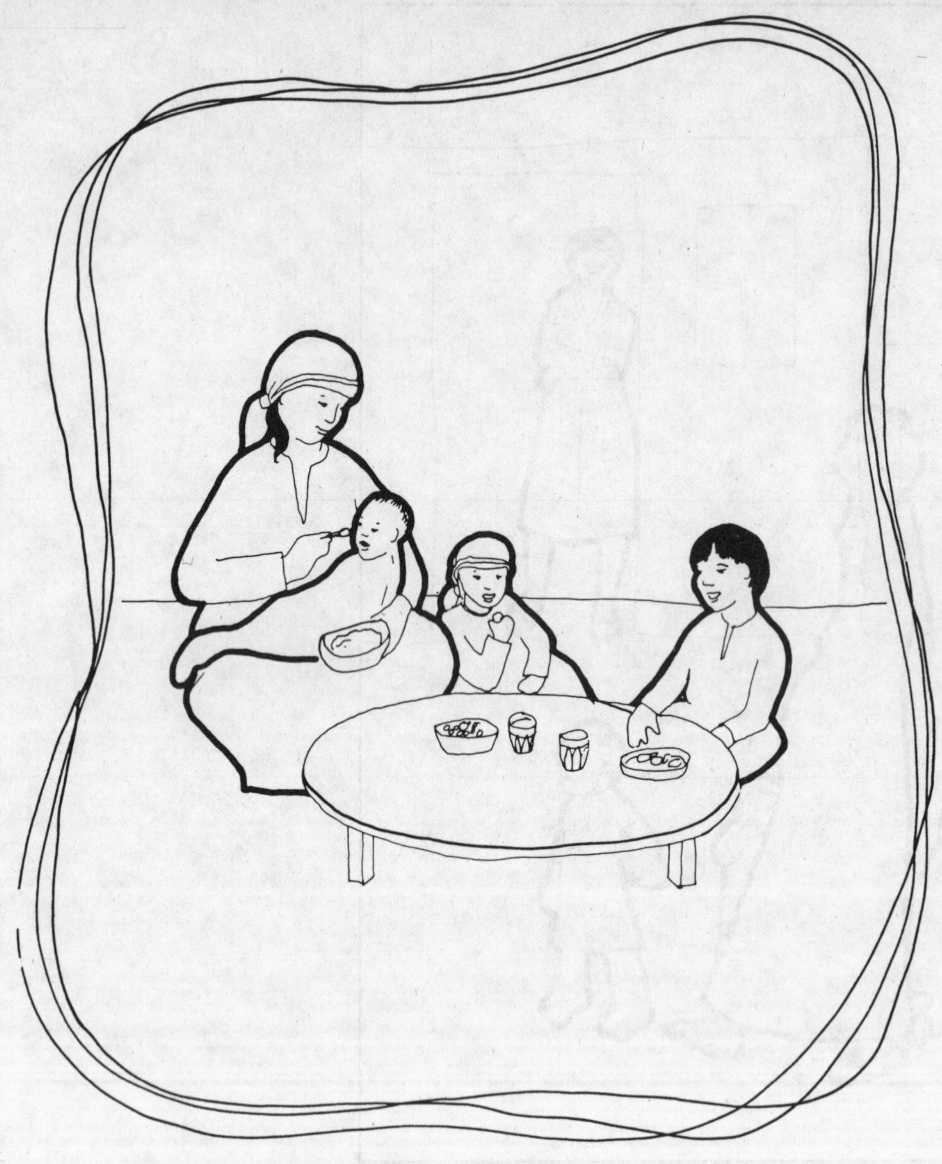

Series of images adapted from *Why Family Planning?*

Mrs Ebrahim wants the women to know that kwashiorkor is caused by not enough protein in the child's diet. She wants the women to feed their children more high protein foods.

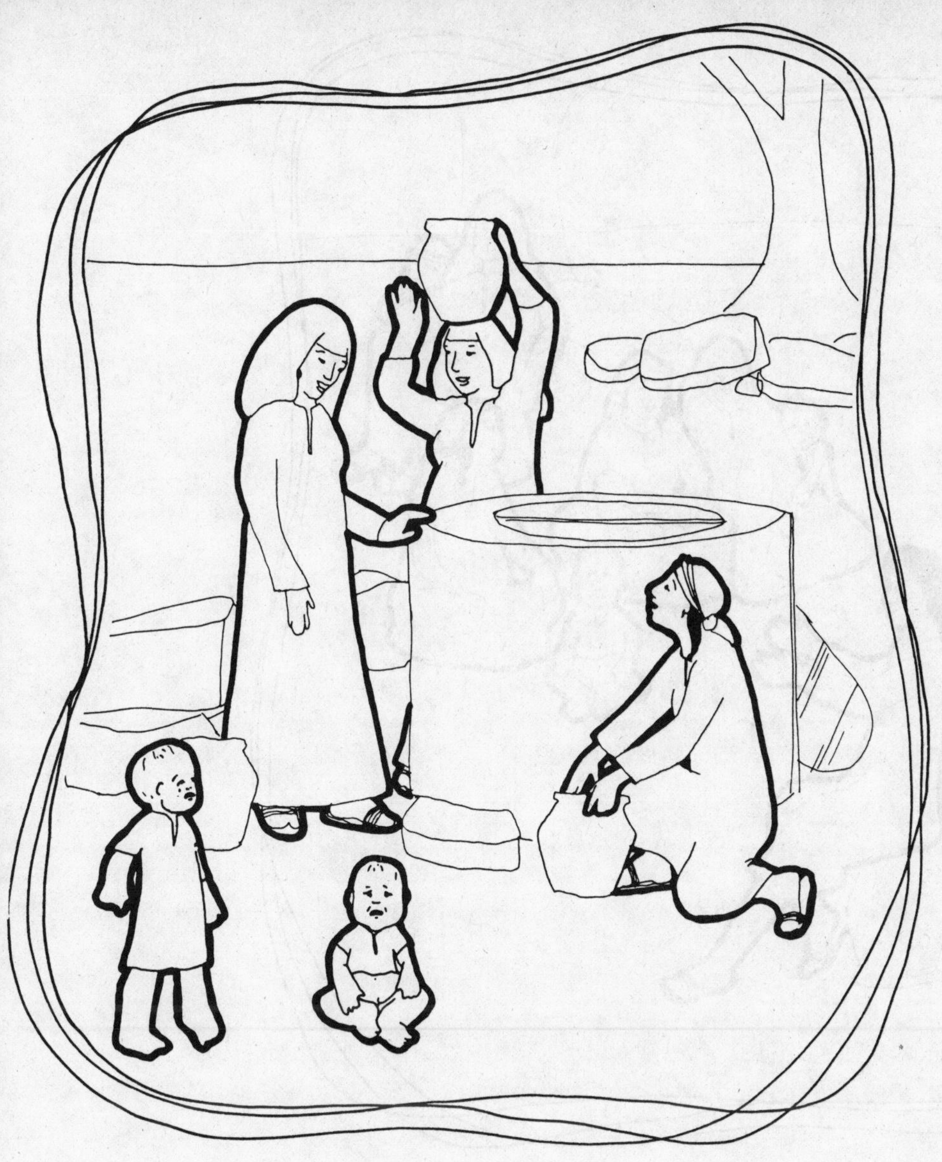

Series of images adapted from *Why Family Planning*?

Mrs Ebrahim decides that the well is a good place to meet with the women, while they are drawing water. The women will be busy and will not be expecting her. So she must have something with her which will get and hold their attention and interest them. They have little time to listen to her, so she decides to spend ten minutes talking with them.

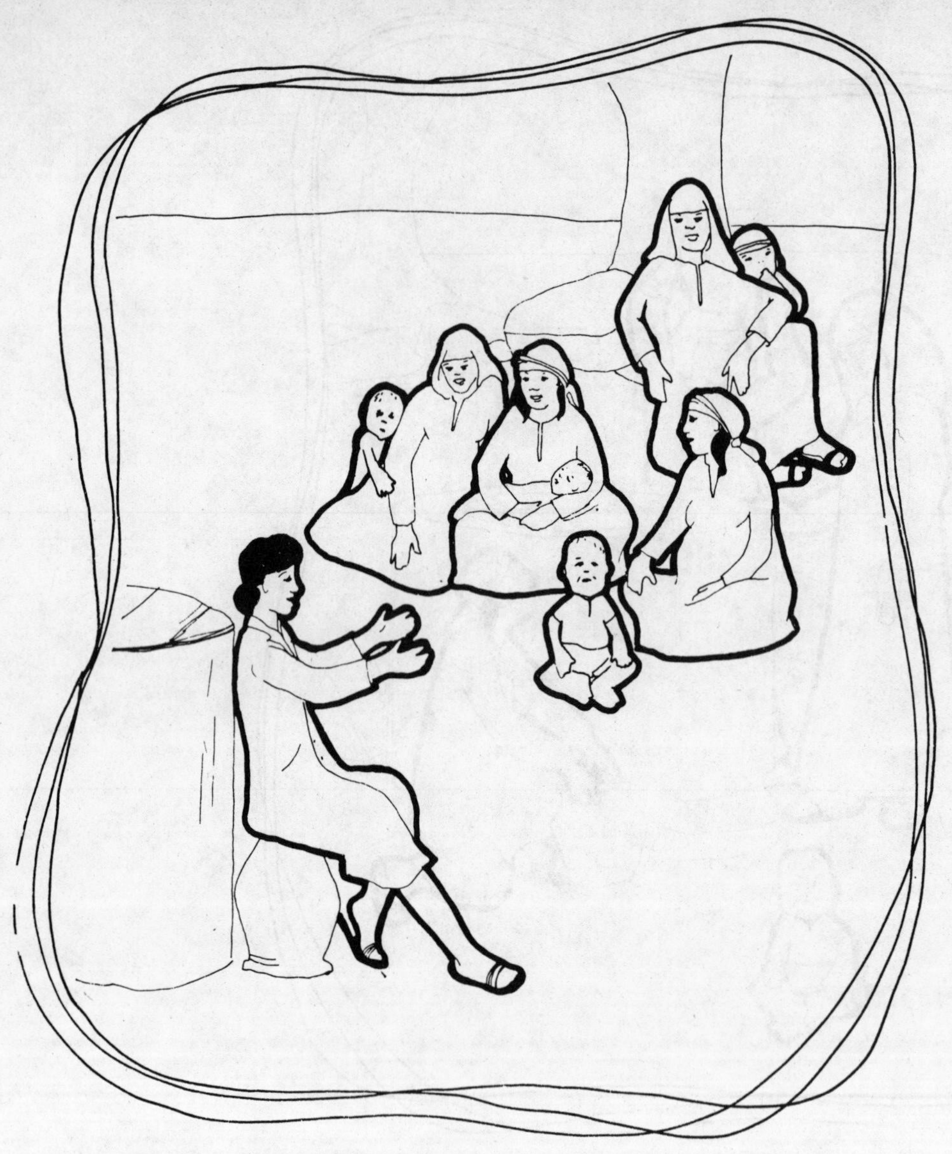

Series of images adapted from *Why Family Planning*?

Mrs Ebrahim has noticed that the women often tell stories to each other when they are at the well. She thinks the women would be interested in hearing a health story. She plans to tell a story about a mother whose child gets kwashiorkor.

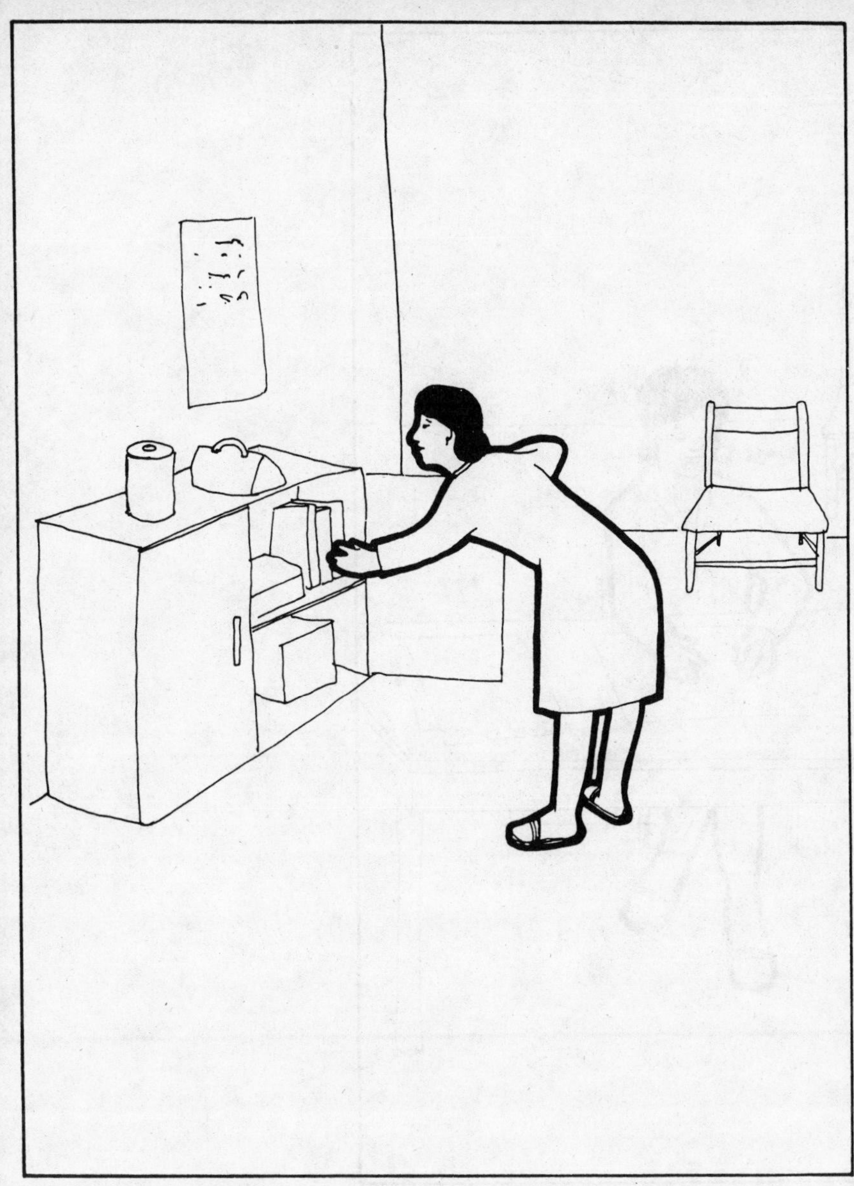

Series of images adapted from *Why Family Planning*?

Mrs Ebrahim wonders what kind of visual aid she can use. Mrs Ebrahim then wonders if she has any flipbooks or pictures in the clinic which would be useful for this meeting. She looks through her cabinet to see what she has. She does not find anything.

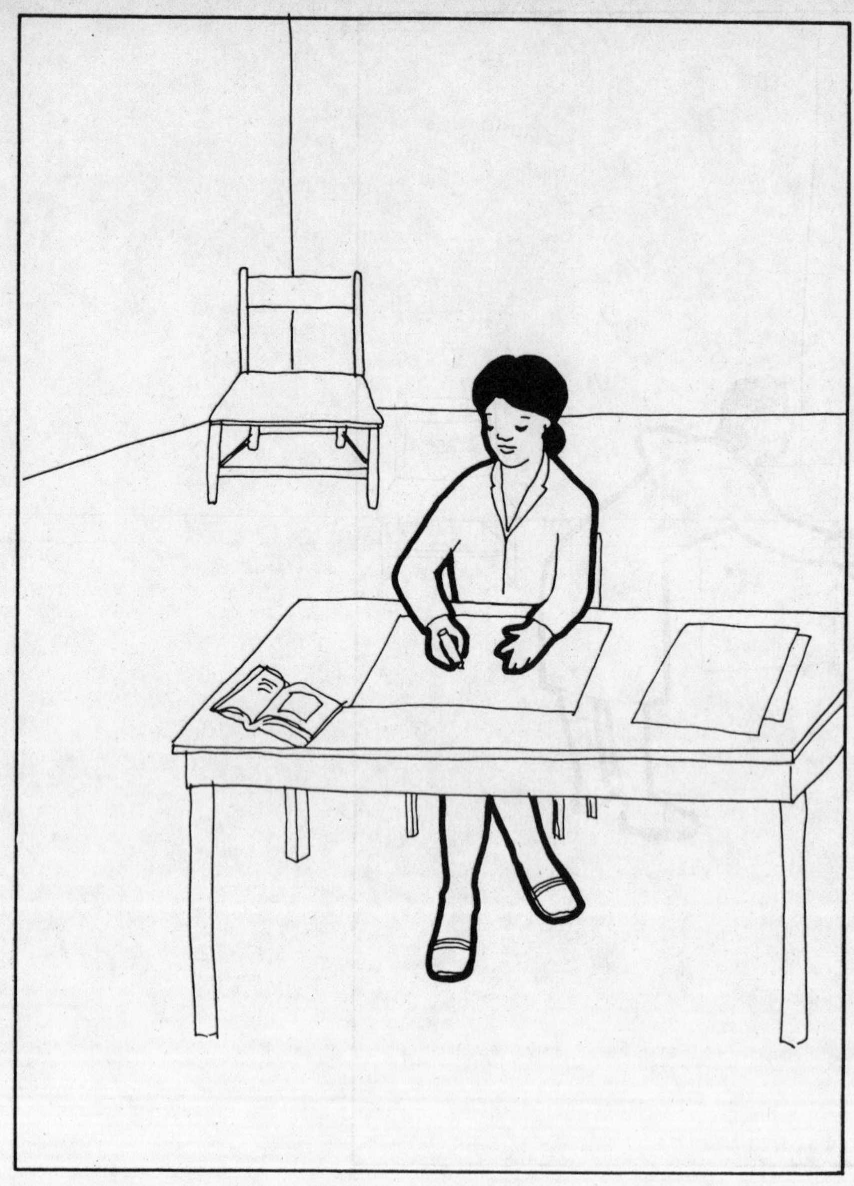

Series of images adapted from *Why Family Planning*?

Mrs Ebrahim knows that she can use a series of pictures of kwashiorkor again and again in her work. She decides to take the time to make her own picture series on kwashiorkor.

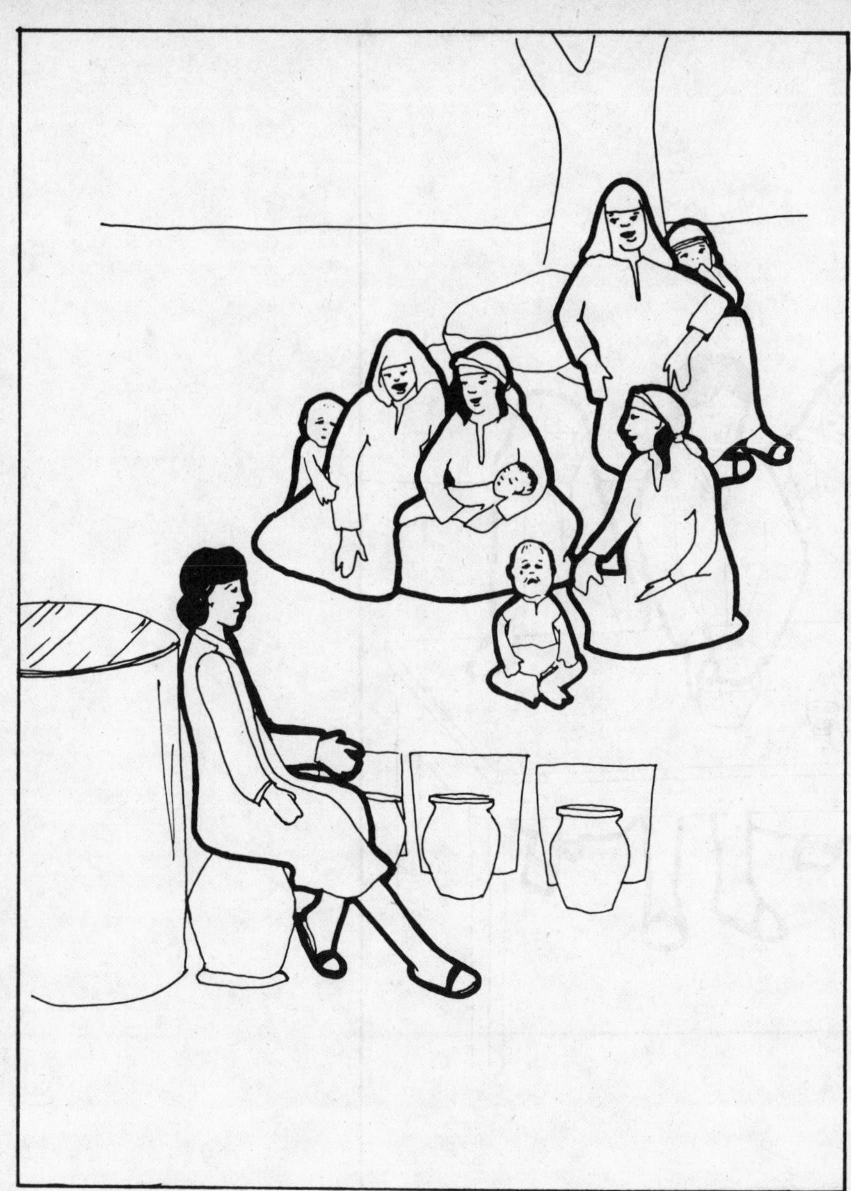

Series of images adapted from *Why Family Planning*?

Mrs Ebrahim notices the reactions of the women during her talk with them. The women seem interested. They ask questions. Mrs Ebrahim can tell from their questions that they understand the information in the story.

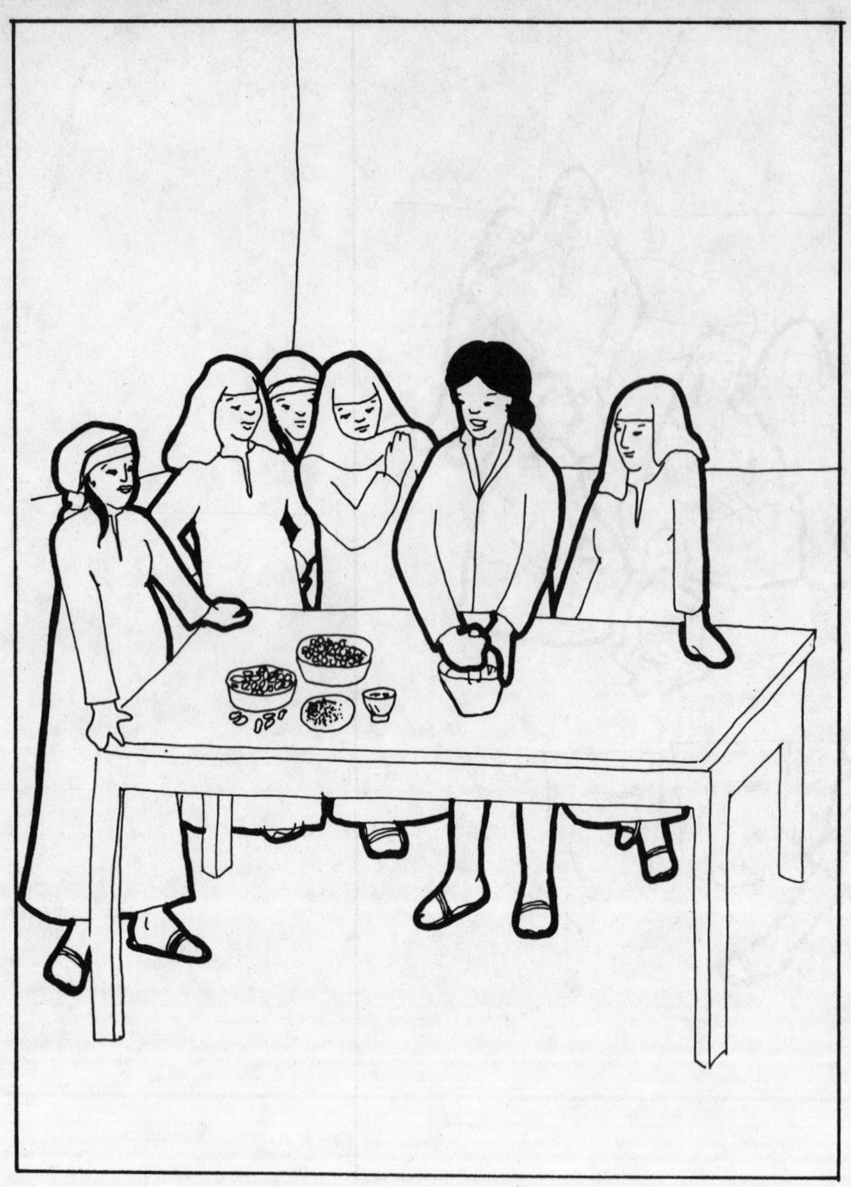

Series of images adapted from *Why Family Planning*?

Mrs Ebrahim can also tell that the talk was effective if she sees more women coming to the nutrition sessions at the clinic.

Menstruation

A guide to use

Problem:
Nurse aides have difficulty explaining the menstrual cycle to their clients.

Who:
15 nurse aides.

What:
The nurse aides will be able to explain the changes in the ovaries and the lining of the uterus that occur during the menstrual cycle.

Where and how long:
In a room at the district health centre, for 30 minutes.

Teaching methods:
Group discussion and lecture; then have 1 or 2 learners explain the menstrual cycle using the visual aids.

Visual aids:
A chalkboard, flannelboard, or wall; a wire pointer and several large paper or cloth figures:

1 a front view of the female body;
2 a small picture of the female reproductive organs;
3 three large pictures of the female reproductive organs showing three phases of the menstrual cycle;
4 the words, **Ovulation** and **Menstruation**.

How to know effectiveness: Nurse aides will use the visual aids to accurately explain the changes in the ovaries and lining of the uterus during the menstrual cycle.

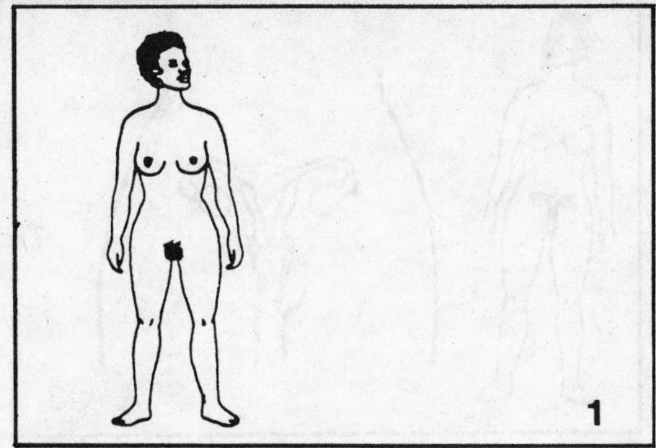

Story

Menstruation is the regular bleeding in women during the years when they can bear children.
How to use:
Tape a large picture of a woman to the chalkboard, flannelboard or wall.

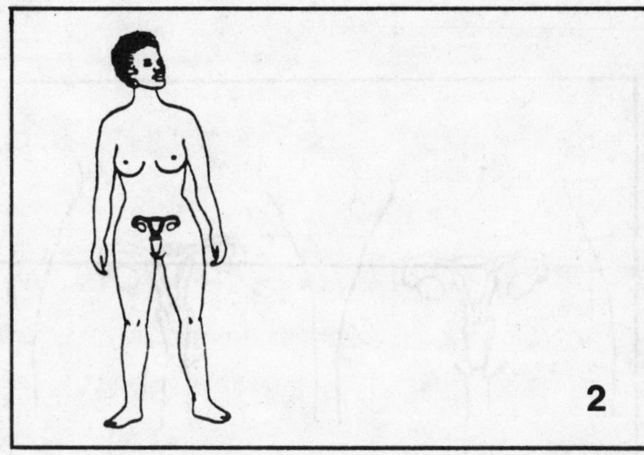

This bleeding is the shedding of the thick lining of the uterus that takes place each month.
How to use:
Tape or pin a paper or cloth uterus to the picture.

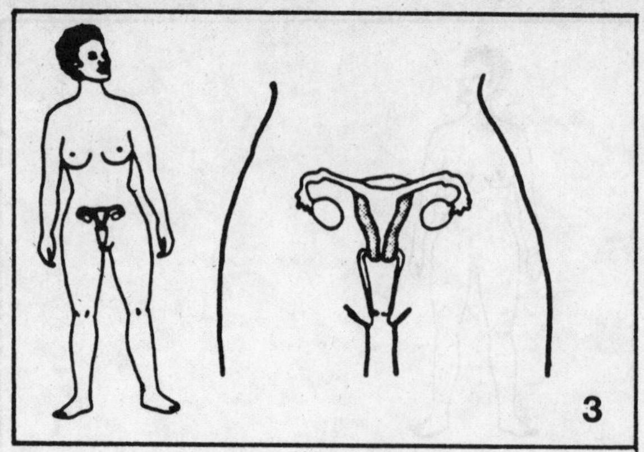

This shows where a woman's reproductive organs, including the uterus and ovaries, are located inside her body. On the right is an enlargement of this area of her body, so you can see the reproductive organs better.

How to use:

Tape a larger picture of the uterus and ovaries beside the picture of the woman. Point to the areas of the picture as they are being discussed.

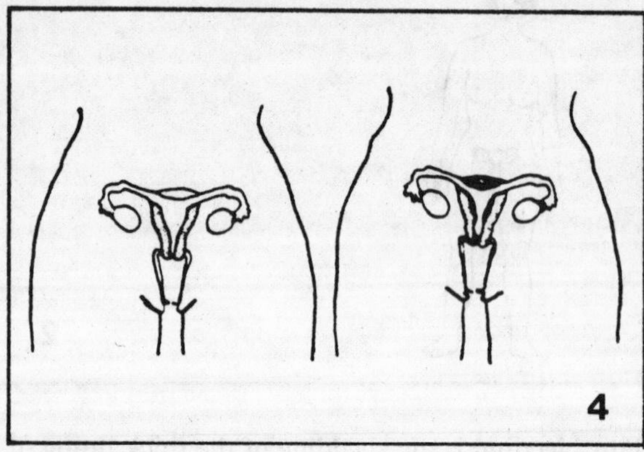

Every month the lining of the uterus thickens, preparing to receive a fertilized egg that could grow into a baby.

How to use:

Remove the picture of the woman. Tape a picture of the uterus with a thick lining beside the other picture.

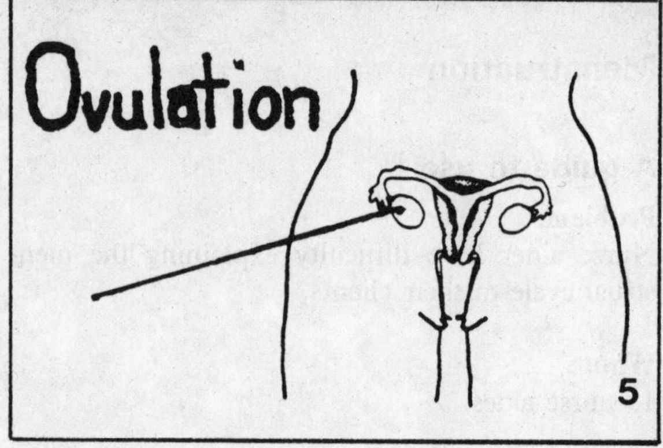

When an egg matures it leaves the ovary. This is called ovulation. Then the egg moves slowly through the fallopian tube, taking about 6 days to reach the uterus.

How to use:

Remove the picture that shows the thin lining. Write **Ovulation** on the chalkboard. Move the egg on the wire from the ovaries through the fallopian tubes.

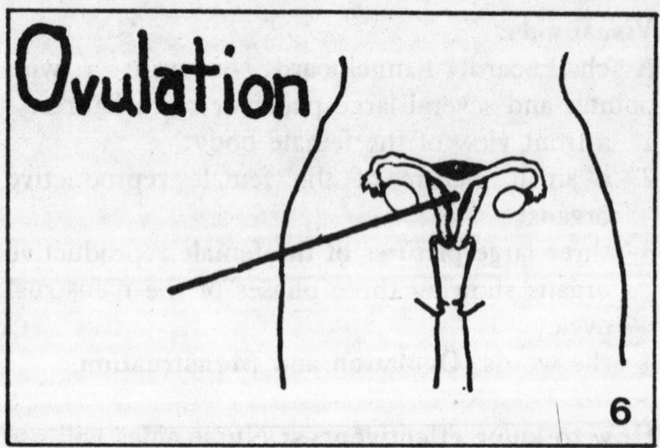

If the egg is not fertilized by a male sperm while in the fallopian tube, it moves through the uterus and outside the body.

How to use:

Move the egg on the wire through the uterus and outside the body.

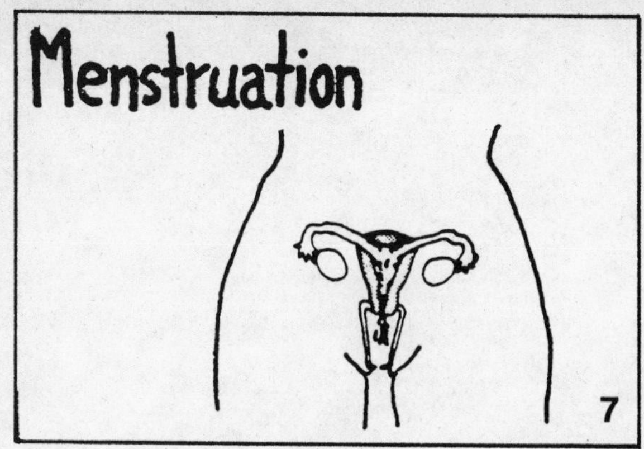

About 14 days after ovulation the uterus begins to shed the thick lining. This is called menstruation.
How to use:
Erase the word **Ovulation**. Write **Menstruation** on the chalkboard. Remove the picture of the thick lining and put up the picture showing menstruation.

Summarize by repeating the same presentation using the visual aids in the same way. Ask one of the nurse aides to explain menstruation using the visual aids.

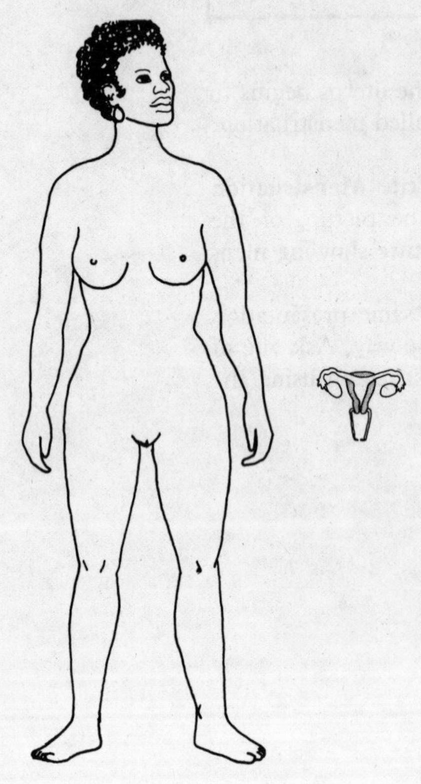

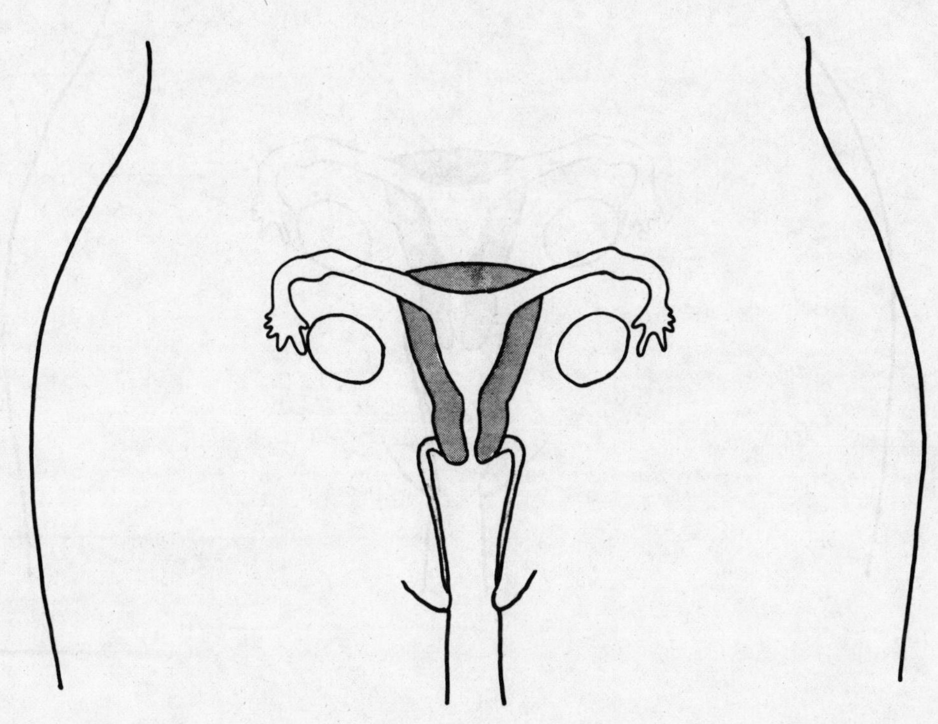

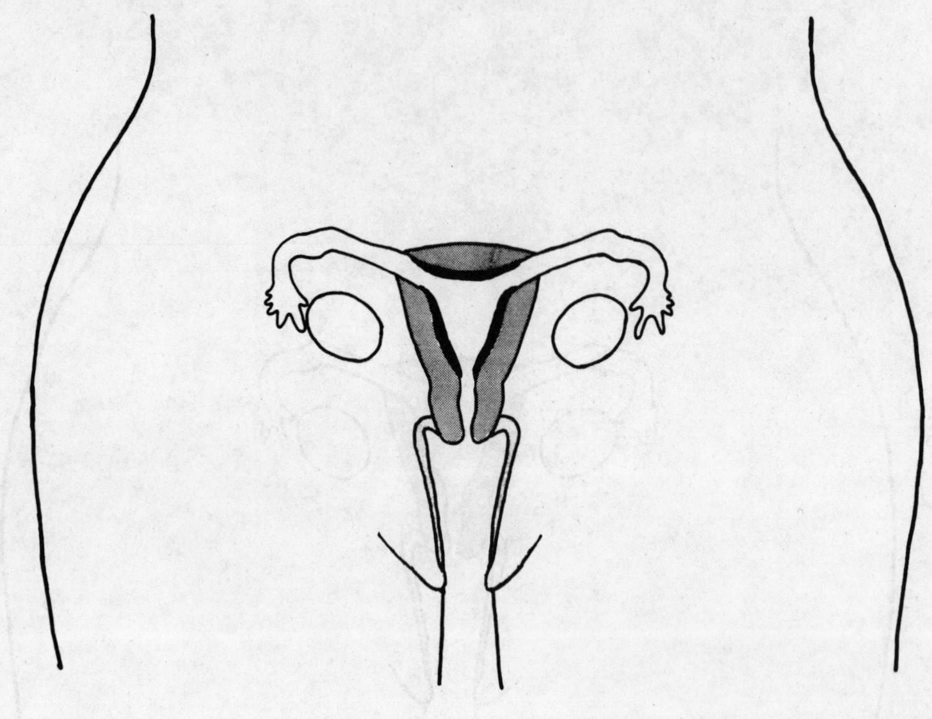

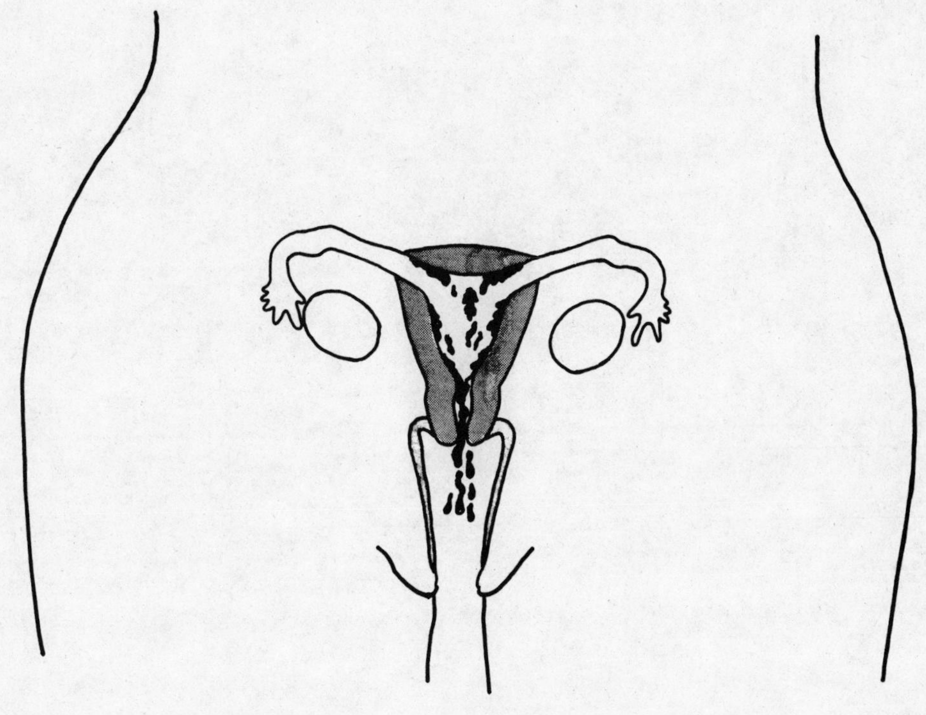

Bibliography

The following list includes all the books, pamphlets, flipbooks, pictures, manuals and other materials that we used to develop the pictures and information in this manual. It is also a useful reference list for anyone who wants to find additional materials on the topics and skills that we have presented here.

American Home Economics Association International Family Planning Project and the East-West Communication Institute. *Handbook of Teaching Strategies and Techniques for Use in Implementing Lessons Relating to Family Planning, Population Education and Quality of Life*. Washington, DC: AHEA International Family Planning Project, 1974.

American Home Economics Association International Family Planning Project and the East-West Communication Institute. *Working With Villagers: Trainers Manual*. Washington, DC: AHEA International Family Planning Project, 1977.

American Home Economics Association International Family Planning Project and the East-West Communication Institute. *Working with Villagers: Media Resource Book*, Field worker Edition. Washington, D.C.: AHEA International Family Planning Project, 1981.

An Introduction to the Arts of Kenya. Washington, DC: Smithsonian Museum of African Art, 1979.

Bale, Kenneth. *Producing Low Cost Visual Media*. London: International Planned Parenthood Federation, 1980.

Barcelona, Delia R., et. al. *Contraception: A Guide to Birth Planning Methods*. Chicago: Community and Family Study Center, University of Chicago, 1981.

British Life Assurance Trust and World Health Organization, *Family Fertility Education: A resource package for teachers of Natural Family Planning Methods*. London: British Life Assurance Trust, Centre for Health and Medical Education, 1982. (Booklets, posters and flash cards).

Bureau d'Etudes et de Recherches pour la Promotion de la Sante. *Je suis fort car je n'ai pas de vers*. Kangu-Mayombe, Zaire: Bureau d'Etudes et de Recherches pour la Promotion de la Sante, n.d. (Picture Series).

Bureau d'Etudes et de Recherches pour la Promotion de la Sante. *Tuberculose Pulmonaire* Kangu-Mayombe, Zaire: Bureau d'Etudes et de Recherches pour la Promotion de la Sante, n.d. (Picture Series).

Centers for Disease Control (CDC), *Family Planning Methods and Practice: Africa*. Atlanta: Centers for Disease Control (CDC), Center for Health Promotion and Education, Division of Reproductive Health, 1983.

Clark, Ann L. and Affonso, Dyanne D. *Childbearing: A Nursing Perspective*. Philadelphia: F.A. Davis Company, 1976.

Collier-Macmillan. *Prenatal Nutrition and Breast Feeding*. New York: Collier-Macmillan, Ltd., 1982. (magnetic board).

Collier-Macmillan. *Why Family Planning?* New York: Collier-Macmillan, 1982.

Courtejoie, J. *La jeunesse et le probleme des naissances desirables*. Kangu-Mayombe, Zaire: Bureau d'Etudes et de Recherches pour la Promotion de la Sante, 1974. (Brochure #11).

Crone, Catherine D. and St. John-Hunter, Carman. *From the Field: Tested Participatory Activities for Trainers*. New York: World Education, 1980.

Emory University School of Medicine. *Producing Low-Cost AV's: A Workbook for Health Professionals and Others Developing Their Own Educational Materials*. Atlanta, Georgia: Regional Training Center for Family Planning, Emory University School of Medicine, n.d.

Hatcher, et. al. *Contraceptive Technology 1982–83*. New York: Irvington, Publishers Inc., 1982.

Hertaing, I. Rotsart and Courtejoie, J. *La tuberculose aujourd'hui: Conceptions recentes de la lutte contre la tuberculose*. Kangu-Mayombe, Zaire: Bureau d'Etudes et de Recherches pour la Promotion de la Sante, n.d.

Hilton, David. *Health Teaching for West Africa: Stories, Drama, Song*. Wheaton, Illinois: MAP International, 1980.

IPPF. *Planning your Family: Strong and Healthy Mothers and Children*. London: Information and Education Department, n.d. (Flipchart).

IFRP. *Maternal Record for Traditional Birth Attendants*. Research Triangle Park, NC: IFRP, draft 1983. (One-page pictorial record keeping form).

Jelliffe, Derrick B. *Child Nutrition in Developing Countries: A Handbook for Fieldworkers*, revised edition. Washington, DC: Office of War on Hunger, Agency for International Development, 1969.

Keehn, Martha (ed.). *Bridging the Gap: A Participatory approach to Health and Nutrition Education*. Westport, Conn.: Save the Children, May, 1982.

Liberia Ministry of Health, Bureau of Preventive Services, Ministry of Health and Social Welfare, *Health Talk on Germs*. New York: Health Education Materials Production Unit, (UNICEF) n.d. (Picture Series).

Liberia Ministry of Health. *The Story of Fatu and Musu*. Monrovia, Liberia: Family Planning International Assistance Program with Preventive Medical Service Project, Family Health and Social Welfare Division, Ministry of Health, n.d. (Flipbook).

Lovedee, I.M., Clarke, W.D., Maglacas, A. Mangay., Shah, K.P. *A TBA Trainer's Kit*, Part 3, *Teaching/ Learning Resources*. London: BLAT Centre for Health and Medical Education, 1982. (Pictorial instructions for making visual aids).

McBean, George; Kaggwa, Norbert and Bugembe, John (eds.). *Illustrations for Development*. Nairobi, Kenya: Afrolit Society, 1980.

Newstrom, John W. and Scannel, Edward. *Games Trainers Play*. New York: McGraw Hill, 1980.

Pett, Dennis. *Audiovisual Communication Handbook*. Indiana: Indiana University, Peace Corps and World Neighbors, n.d.

Ritchie, Jean A.S. *Manual on Child Development, Family Life Nutrition*. Addis Ababa: United Nations Economic Commission for Africa, 1978.

Sierra Leone Home Economics Association and IPPA of Sierra Leone. *The IUD*. Sierra Leone: Sierra Leone Home Economics Association and IPPA, n.d. (Picture booklet).

Sierra Leone Home Economics Association and IPPA of Sierra Leone. *The Pill*. Sierra Leone: Sierra Leone Home Economics Association and IPPA, n.d. (Picture booklet).

Srinivasan, Lyra. *Workshop Ideas for FP Education*. New York: World Education, 1975. (Folder with sample materials).

Stanfield, N.F. *A Handbook of Art Teaching in Tropical Schools*. London: Evans Brothers, 1958.

Werner, David. *Where There is No Doctor: A Village Health Care Handbook*. Palo Alto, Ca.: The Hesperian Foundation, 1977.

Werner, David and Bower, Bill. *Helping Health Workers Learn: A Book of Methods, Aids and Ideas for Instructors at the Village Level*. Palo Alto, Ca.: The Hesperian Foundation, 1982.

Sources for illustrations

Many of the illustrations in this manual have been adapted from pictures developed by others. The list below gives recognition to those sources. Below each source you will find the page numbers from *Teaching and Learning with Visual Aids (TLVA) where borrowed and adapted pictures are located. Following those page numbers are the pages or picture numbers of the pictures borrowed from the source listed above.*

Bale, Kenneth. Producing Low Cost Visual Media. London: International Planned Parenthood Federation, 1980.

Picture at bottom of page 186 (TLVA) copied from picture on page 13.

Pictures on pages 195/6 (TLVA) adapted from pictures on pages 18 and 19.

Barcelona, Delia R., et. al. *Contraception: A Guide to Birth Planning Methods*. Chicago: Community and Family Study Center, University of Chicago, 1981.

Pictures on page 79 and page 199 (TLVA)– adapted from picture on page [126.]

Picture on page 80 (TLVA) adapted from picture on page 21.

British Life Assurance Trust and World Health Organization, *Family Fertility Education: A resource package for teachers of Natural Family Planning Methods*. London: British Life Assurance Trust, Centre for Health and Medical Education, 1982.

Picture on page 276 (TLVA) adapted from picture 2.2.

Pictures on pages 277–9 (TLVA) adapted from picture 4.2.

Bureau d'Etudes et de Recherches pour la Promotion de la Sante. *Je suis fort car je n'ai pas de vers*. Kangu-Mayombe, Zaire: Bureau d'Etudes et de Recherches pour la Promotion de la Sante, n.d. (Picture Series).

Pictures on pages 69–70 (TLVA) traced from pictures no.16, 18 in series.

Picture on page 88 (TLVA) traced from picture 1 in picture series.

Bureau d'Etudes et de Recherches pour la Promotion de la Sante. *Tuberculose Pulmonaire* Kangu-Mayombe, Zaire: Bureau d'Etudes et de Recherches pour la Promotion de la Sante, n.d.

Pictures on pages 148 and 149 (TLVA) traced from picture no.7 in picture series.

Clark, Ann L. and Affonso, Dynanne D. *Childbearing: A Nursing Perspective*. Philadelphia: F.A. Davis Company, 1976.

Pictures on pages 213–4 (TLVA) adapted from page 384 picture 13; page 646 picture A; page 646 picture B lower, page 646 picture D.

Collier-Macmillan. *Prenatal Nutrition and Breast Feeding*. New York: Collier-Macmillan, Ltd., 1982.

Pictures on page 76 and pages 180–82 (TLVA) traced from cover of instructor's notes.

Picture on page 75 bottom (TLVA) traced from picture D23 left.

Collier-Macmillan. *Why Family Planning?* New York: Collier-Macmillan, 1982. Used as models for designing the picture series on pages 56–62 (TLVA).

Crone, Catherine D. and St. John-Hunter, Carman. *From the Field: Tested Participatory Activities for Trainers*. New York: World Education, 1980.

Pictures on pages 74 and 93 (TLVA) copied from pictures on pages 91–92.

Emory University School of Medicine. *Producing Low-Cost AV's: A Workbook for Health Professionals and Others Developing Their Own Educational Materials.* Atlanta, Georgia: Regional Training Center for Family Planning, Emory University School of Medicine, n.d.

Picture on page 199 (TLVA) based on picture on page 33.

Hatcher, et al. *Contraceptive Technology 1982–83.* New York: Irvington Publishers, Inc., 1982.

Picture on page 63 top (TLVA) copied from picture on page 21.

Pictures on pages 77–8 (TLVA) adapted from picture on page 217.

Hertaing, I. Rotsart and Courtejoie, J. *La tuberculose aujourd'hui: Conceptions recentes de la lutte contre la tuberculose.* Kangu-Mayombe, Zaire: Bureau d'Etudes et de Recherches pour la Promotion de la Sante, n.d.

Pictures on page 137 and page 146 (TLVA) traced from picture on cover and page 19.

IPPF. *Planning your Family: Strong and Healthy Mothers and Children.* London: Information and Education Department, n.d.

Picture on page 42 (TLVA) adapted from picture 3.

Pictures on pages 140, bottom 141, 142, 144, and also 171, 175 bottom, 176–9 (TLVA) adapted from picture 1.

IFRP. *Maternal Record for Traditional Birth Attendants.* Research Triangle Park, NC: IFRP, draft 1983. (One-page pictorial record keeping form).

Picture on pages 70–71 bottom (TLVA) adapted from pictorial record-keeping form prepared for IFRP, Zaire.

Jelliffe, Derrick B. *Child Nutrition in Developing Countries: A Handbook for Fieldworkers,* revised edition. Washington, DC: Office of War on Hunger, Agency for International Development, 1969.

Pictures on page 20 and page 183 (TLVA) copied from picture on page 83.

Keehn, Martha (ed.). *Bridging the Gap: A Participatory Approach to Health and Nutrition Education.* Westport, Conn.: Save the Children, May, 1982.

Picture on page 52 bottom (TLVA) based on photograph on page 30.

Liberia Ministry of Health, Bureau of Preventive Services, Ministry of Health and Social Welfare, *Health Talk on Germs.* New York: Health Education Materials Production Unit, (UNICEF) n.d.

Pictures on page 225 and pages 230–31 and 248 (TLVA) adapted from picture 1 in series.

Liberia Ministry of Health. *The Story of Fatu and Musu.* Monrovia, Liberia: Family Planning International Assistance Program with Preventive Medical Service Project, Family Health and Social Welfare Division, Ministry of Health, n.d.

Picture story pages 96–100 (TLVA) copied. Pictures on pages 101, 124, 244 (TLVA) adapted from picture 3. Picture on page 155 (TLVA) copied from picture 7. Pictures on pages 151, 156, 159 (TLVA) copied from picture 1.

Lovedee, I.M., Clarke, W.D., Maglacas, A. Mangay, Shah, K.P. *A TBA Trainer's Kit,* Part 3, *Teaching/Learning Resources.* London: BLAT Centre for Health and Medical Education, 1982. (Pictorial instructions for making visual aids).

Pictures on pages 211–13 (TLVA) adapted from instructions for making ILFRA doll.

McBean, George; Kaggwa, Norbert and Bugembe, John (eds.). *Illustrations for Development.* Nairobi, Kenya: Afrolit Society, 1980.

Pictures on page 75 top (TLVA) copied from pictures on page 44.

Pett, Dennis. *Audiovisual Communication Handbook.* Indiana: Indiana University, Peace Corps and World Neighbors, n.d.

Picture on page 168 (TLVA) adapted from picture on page 54.

Pictures on pages 215, 218 (TLVA) adapted from pictures on pages 16 and 17.

Sierra Leone Home Economics Association and IPPA of Sierra Leone. *The IUD.* Sierra Leone: Sierra Leone Home Economics Association and IPPA, n.d.

Pictures on pages 15 and 23 (TLVA) adapted picture from page 4.

Sierra Leone Home Economics Association and IPPA of Sierra Leone. *The Pill.* Sierra Leone: Sierra Leone Home Economics Association and IPPA, n.d.

Picture on page 80 bottom (TLVA) adapted from picture on cover.

Srinivasan, Lyra. *Workshop Ideas for FP Education.* New York: World Education, 1975.

Picture on page 90 (TLVA) adapted from picture of ambiguous figure.

Werner, David. *Where There is No Doctor: A Village Health Care Handbook.* Palo Alto, Ca.: The Hesperian Foundation, 1977.

Picture on page 49 (TLVA) bottom adapted from picture on page 110.

Werner, David and Bower, Bill. *Helping Health Workers Learn: A Book of Methods, Aids and Ideas for Instructors at the Village Level.* Palo Alto, Ca.: The Hesperian Foundation, 1982.

Pictures on pages 27 and 232 (TLVA) adapted from photograph chapter, page 11–12.

Pictures on page 41 (TLVA) adapted from picture in Chapter 22, page 10.

Picture on page 46 bottom adapted from picture in Chapter 22, page 4.

Pictures on page 47 (TLVA) adapted from pictures Chapter 24, page 18.

Picture on page 71 (TLVA) traced from picture in Chapter 25, page 44.
Picture on page 50 (TLVA) adapted from picture in Chapter 13, page 10.
Picture on page 67 top (TLVA) traced from picture in Chapter 23, page 112.
Picture on page 77 top (TLVA) copied from picture in Chapter 25, page 10.
Picture on page 151 (TLVA) adapted from picture in Chapter 12, page 11.
Picture on page 161 (TLVA) adapted from picture Chapter 9, page 21.)
Picture on page 163 top (TLVA) adapted from picture Chapter 12, page 12.
Picture on page 165 top (TLVA) adapted from picture Chapter 12, page 10.
Pictures on pages 205–7 (TLVA) adapted from pictures in Chapter 24, pages 18–19.
Pictures on pages 209–11 (TLVA) adapted from picture in Chapter 22, pages 8–9.
Picture on page 237 (TLVA) traced from photograph in Chapter 11, page 3.

Index

Evaluation

Teaching and Learning with Visual Aids: A Resource Manual for Family Planning Trainers and Health Workers in Africa and the Middle East

Your profession ________________

Your current position ________________

Your experience in developing visual aids on health or family planning ________________

1 What is your general reaction to this book? ________________

2 Are there parts of this book that are *not* appropriate or realistic for your situation? If so, what parts and why?

3 How have you used this book for teaching? (Mark one or more)

Professional education ________ Talking with community leaders ________

Continuing education ________ Public Health Education ________

In-service education ________ Other ________

4 Are there any important topics relating to visual aids development for family planning that should be added? Yes ______ No ______

If yes, please list ________________

5 Is the book easy or difficult to read and understand?

Easy ______ Difficult ______

If difficult, please explain and give examples from the book.

6 Would you recommend this book to others? Yes ________ No ________

Your Name: (optional) ______________________________

Address ______________________________

Date ______________________________

Please return this form to:

Catherine Murphy
Coordinator
Educational Materials Unit
INTRAH
208 N. Columbia Street
Chapel Hill, NC 27514 USA